Handbook of Behavior Modification with the Mentally Retarded

APPLIED CLINICAL PSYCHOLOGY

Series Editors: Alan S. Bellack and Michel Hersen
University of Pittsburgh, Pittsburgh, Pennsylvania

PARTIAL HOSPITALIZATION: A Current Perspective
Edited by Raymond F. Luber

HANDBOOK OF MARITAL THERAPY: A Positive Approach to Helping Troubled Relationships
Robert P. Liberman, Eugenie G. Wheeler, Louis A.J.M. DeVisser, Julie Kuehnel, and Timothy Kuehnel

PERFECTING SOCIAL SKILLS: A Guide to Interpersonal Behavior Development
Richard M. Eisler and Lee W. Frederiksen

HANDBOOK OF BEHAVIOR MODIFICATION WITH THE MENTALLY RETARDED
Edited by Johnny L. Matson and John R. McCartney

THE UTILIZATION OF CLASSROOM PEERS AS BEHAVIOR CHANGE AGENTS
Edited by Phillip S. Strain

FUTURE PERSPECTIVES IN BEHAVIOR THERAPY
Edited by Larry Michelson, Michel Hersen, and Samuel M. Turner

CLINICAL BEHAVIOR THERAPY WITH CHILDREN
Thomas Ollendick and Jerome A. Cerny

A Continuation Order Plan is available for this series. A continuation order will bring delivery of each new volume immediately upon publication. Volumes are billed only upon actual shipment. For further information please contact the publisher.

Handbook of Behavior Modification with the Mentally Retarded

Edited by

Johnny L. Matson

University of Pittsburgh
Pittsburgh, Pennsylvania

and

John R. McCartney

Partlow State School and Hospital
Tuscaloosa, Alabama

Plenum Press • New York and London

Library of Congress Cataloging in Publication Data

Main entry under title:

Handbook of behavior modification with the mentally retarded.

(Applied clinical psychology)
Includes index.
1. Mentally handicapped—Rehabilitation. 2. Mentally handicapped children—Rehabilitation. 3. Behavior modification. I. Matson, Johnny L. II. McCartney, John R. III. Series. [DNLM: 1. Mental retardation—Rehabilitation. 2. Behavior therapy. WM 308 H236]
RC570.H34 616.85'8806 80-28244

DOI 10.1007/978-1-4615-7130-8

A Division of Plenum Publishing Corporation
233 Spring Street, New York, N.Y. 10013

To our wives and children
Deann and Meggan Matson
Barbara and Andy McCartney

Contributors

ANDREW R. BRULLE, Department of Learning and Development, Northern Illinois University, DeKalb, Illinois

JOSEPH A. BUCKHALT, Department of Counselor Education, Auburn University, Auburn, Alabama

JEFFREY C. HOLDEN, Partlow State School and Hospital, Tuscaloosa, Alabama

ALLEN MARCHETTI, Partlow State School and Hospital, Tuscaloosa, Alabama

JOHNNY L. MATSON, Department of Psychiatry, University of Pittsburgh, School of Medicine, Pittsburgh, Pennsylvania

JOHN R. McCARTNEY, Jemison Center, Partlow State School and Hospital, Tuscaloosa, Alabama

JAMES F. McCOY, Department of Psychology, Auburn University, Auburn, Alabama

JAMES A. MULICK, Rhode Island Hospital and Department of Psychology, Brown University, Providence, Rhode Island

FLOYD O'BRIEN, Department of Psychology, University of the Pacific, Stockton, California

RICHARD A. PACKER, Department of Psychology, University of Alabama, Tuscaloosa, Alabama

ALAN C. REPP, Department of Learning and Development, Northern Illinois University, DeKalb, Illinois

JOHANNES ROJAHN, Phillips-Universitaet Marburg, Marburg, West Germany

FRANK R. RUSCH, Department of Special Education, University of Illinois, Champaign, Illinois

CAROLYN S. SCHROEDER, Department of Psychology, University of North Carolina at Chapel Hill, Chapel Hill, North Carolina

STEPHEN R. SCHROEDER, Department of Psychology, University of North Carolina at Chapel Hill, Chapel Hill, North Carolina

RICHARD P. SCHUTZ, Department of Special Education, University of Illinois, Urbana, Illinois

JOHN W. SCIBAK, Department of Special Education, Unviersity of Indiana, Bloomington, Indiana

RANDY UZZELL, Partlow State School and Hospital, Tuscaloosa, Alabama

LUKE S. WATSON, JR., Partlow State School and Hospital, Tuscaloosa, Alabama

PAUL WEISBERG, Department of Psychology, University of Alabama, Tuscaloosa, Alabama

ROBERTA S. WEISBERG, Department of Special Education, University of Alabama, Tuscaloosa, Alabama

THOMAS L. WHITMAN, Department of Psychology, University of Notre Dame, South Bend, Indiana

Foreword

Mental retardation has probably existed for as long as mankind has inhabited the earth. References to seemingly retarded persons appear in Greek and Roman literature. Examination of Egyptian mummies suggests that some may have suffered from diseases associated with mental retardation. Mohammed advocated feeding and housing those without reason. There is other evidence for favorable attitudes toward the retarded in early history, but attitudes varied from age to age and from country to country.

The concept of remediation did not emerge until the nineteenth century. Earlier, in 1798, Itard published an account of his attempt to train the "wild boy of Aveyron." A rash of efforts to habilitate retarded persons followed. Training schools were developed in Europe and the United States in the 1800s; however, these early schools did not fulfill their promise, and by the end of the nineteenth century large, inhumane warehouses for retarded persons existed. The notion of habilitation through training had largely been abandoned and was not to reappear until after World War II.

Seminal behavioral research beginning in the 1950s ushered in a new age in the care and treatment of the retarded. Laboratory studies of learning and operant conditioning demonstrated a potential for learning even in the most severely mentally retarded. Skinnerian psychology, in particular, offered new approaches to communicating with, and changing the behavior of, nonverbal, "vegetative" human beings. The untrainable could be trained! Even the definition of mental retardation was changed; no longer was it defined as an "incurable" condition. The attitudes of society became more sanguine, the stigma of mental retardation weakened. Much of the hopelessness associated with the condition disappeared.

From modest beginnings in the 1950s, behavioral science efforts in the field increased and gained sophistication and respectability. Academicians became interested in the analysis and remediation of retarded behavior, and graduate students prepared for professional/scientific careers in the field. Research laboratories developed in residential institutions for the retarded. Research reports made their way into respectable journals.

Operant conditioning was an approach that could be applied directly to training problems, and it, therefore, attracted most interest. In the main, the techniques had been developed in research with animals. Verbal instructions were not required; behavior could be changed through seemingly simple principles of reinforcement. New behaviors such as self-help skills could be "shaped" in persons who formerly possessed none. Undesirable behaviors such as self-injury or aggressiveness could be eliminated by the withdrawal of reinforcers or the use of aversive contingencies. The approach was a natural for the residential institution.

The applied aspect of operant conditioning became "behavior modification," and a fairly large literature reports numerous studies in this field. Indeed, a number of new journals have appeared to accommodate the flow of research reports. Since most residential institutions use mainly behavior modification training methods, the bulk of research derives from this source. The present book reviews, analyzes, and interprets this research. It is about training the retarded with behavior modification techniques. In practice, behavior modification is an amalgam of principles from a number of sources including the ingenuity and common sense of the person using the approach. It is a pragmatic approach: "Whatever works is correct!" The behavior modifier does not question whether or not the organism possesses the necessary mental processes to perform a certain skill. Instead, various techniques are tried until one is successful. If none is found, the behavior modifier concludes, safely, that the correct approach has not yet been discovered or that an effective reinforcer has not been found. To be sure, behavior modification, as much of this book will show, can be a very powerful training method. It is most effective in dealing with the person with minimal, or no, verbal skills and in teaching self-help habits. But, contrary to common understanding, it is not an easy method to use. Direct translations of techniques from the pigeon or rat box to human training situations will rarely succeed. Moreover, one must thoroughly understand the training principles in order to use them to advantage. The trainer with a superficial knowledge of the principles cannot expect to succeed with a mechanistic application.

This research, as this volume reveals, has many shortcomings. Some of the reported studies are well conceived and executed. Others provide little useful or reliable information. Most are commendable in that they represent sincere efforts to improve the lot of the retarded. In perspective, we should not be too critical of any of them. Few have had adequate financial support. Most are the products of clinical staff pursuing research interests in their spare time and are conducted in the buzzing confusion of an institutional ward under the most trying of conditions.

Behavior modification efforts are not always successful. Many of the reports cited here yield results that leave much to be desired. But this may not always be the fault of the method or of the investigator. Sometimes, accident, disease, or inheritance reduces behavioral potential to extreme levels. It seems likely that even these powerful methods, under ideal conditions, cannot restore adaptive behaviors to any meaningful extent in some persons.

Hopefully, future research in the field will be more systematic. Adequate funding is a necessity; otherwise, we will continue to see piecemeal, brief, and inconclusive studies. In the past this approach has led to the selection of subjects who exhibited a specific problem, with no attempt to select *representative* samples for study. Consequently, we know little about the training potential of classes or subgroups of retarded persons. For example, we know that some profoundly retarded can be taught certain skills using behavior modification methods, but we cannot generalize from these to the *class* "profoundly retarded." This research has not established the generality of behavior change. Will behavior learned in one setting occur in another? The durability of training has rarely been assessed. The typical study focuses on behavior change over a few weeks; there have been few long-term follow-ups. New research is needed to refine the methods. Vestiges of animal techniques remain that may not be effective with human beings in the complex environments in which the research must be conducted.

These criticisms, fully recognized by the authors in this volume, should not obscure the overall value of this research nor of the significance of applied behavior modification. The present volume brings together the best and a little of the worst of it. These writers are perceptive and they bring out the most useful aspects of this research. They are all scholars, and most are well-known researchers, or shortly will be, in this field. Through efforts such as these interpretive reviews, the foibles of this research will be eliminated, and behavior modification will become an even more effective method in attempts to alleviate the burden of mental retardation. Certainly, as many of the present writers imply, more rigorous research is needed in this field. But the practitioner can learn much from this volume. It is a handy source of information for the clinician confronted with a seemingly intractable behavior problem, and it will have immense heuristic value for researchers as well.

Most retarded persons, even many of the profoundly handicapped, can be improved through training. Our failures with a few should not detract from the overall success of this enterprise. Behavior modification is a training approach that holds promise for the lowest among us.

NORMAN R. ELLIS

University of Alabama

Preface

The emphasis on habilitation of the mentally retarded in the last few years had led to a substantial increase in the amount of research devoted to training adaptive skills and reducing inappropriate behavior in this population. Behavior modification procedures have been the primary basis for these attempts to improve the independence and quality of life of the mentally retarded. These procedures have been successful in achieving behavioral changes when applied appropriately for a broad range of skills, including such diverse behaviors as toilet training and interpersonal behavior.

As in many other areas of scientific endeavor, there has been an information explosion in this field, making it difficult for the practitioner to stay abreast of the literature. The goal of this volume is to provide reviews of the major topics addressed in behavior modification research with the mentally retarded to date. Chapters are based on specific types of behavior that have been treated. They are presented in a roughly developmental sequence to give a more systematic presentation.

Chapter authors have considerable clinical and research experience with the mentally retarded. As a result, they are fully cognizant of the problems facing the practitioner in this area. We feel that the analysis of what treatments work best under different conditions is aptly made by the various authors. Also, and perhaps more important, they have pointed out the limitations of the procedures currently available. Certainly behavior modification is not a panacea for the habilitation of the mentally retarded. However, these methods have proven utility. Thus, it is hoped that this book will be of value to those who are currently involved in research, treatment, and administration at some level of applied work.

No attempt is made to resolve broad general issues regarding the degree of trainability of the severely retarded, the viability of the concept of normalization, or our interpretation of it. These concepts are certainly important and impact strongly on the behavior modification treatments that are used. It is our position that these and related questions are subject to empirical and legal resolutions that fall outside the purview of a discussion of behavior modification technology. Rather, it is our hope that the reader will benefit from the technical information presented in this volume with respect to the current state of behavior modification procedures for treating the mentally retarded.

JOHNNY L. MATSON
JOHN R. MCCARTNEY

Contents

1 Behavior Modification Research with the Mentally Retarded

Treatment and Research Perspectives

Thomas L. Whitman and John W. Scibak

Introduction

Within modern times, there has been considerable variation in society's attitudes toward mentally retarded individuals, particularly with reference to their educability and curability. At one extreme mentally retarded persons have been viewed as having an incurable condition, and at the other extreme they have been seen as possessing a normal learning potential capable of realization in a proper educational environment. In general, those emphasizing an organic condition have been more pessimistic concerning its remediation, and those who have maintained that mental retardation is caused by environmental factors have been proponents of active habilitation programs.

Historically, these contrasting positions were documented by Jena Itard in his extensive case history, *The Wild Boy of Aveyron*. According to Itard, the wild boy, about 11 or 12 years old, had for a number of years been seen wandering about in the countryside in France. At the time of his capture in 1799, his behavior was more animal-like than human. He neither spoke nor responded to verbal inquiry or instruction, showed no ability to function in a social environment, was alternately shy and aggressive in his behavior, and was seen as "indifferent to everything and attentive to nothing" (p.4). After his capture the boy was seen by Philippe Pinel, often referred to as the father of modern psychiatry, who declared him to be incurably affected with

Thomas L. Whitman • Department of Psychology, University of Notre Dame, South Bend, Indiana 46556. John W. Scibak • Department of Special Education, University of Indiana, Bloomington, Indiana 47401.

"idiocy," and "not capable of social-ability or instruction" (p. 6). In contrast, Itard viewed the boy's condition as a consequence of the social and educational deprivation which had occurred during his early childhood. Based on this speculation, Itard felt that the child could be fully educated, and consequently proceeded with an elaborate program of instruction. Although he succeeded in teaching the boy numerous adaptive responses, he failed to normalize his behavior. Whether this failure was a function of the educational program delivered or was due to the nature of the boy's condition is a matter for conjecture. Whatever the reason, Itard became less optimistic about what environmental-intervention programs could accomplish, even though he showed that the child's idiocy was at least in part "curable."

Since the nineteenth century, there has been considerable refinement in our knowledge of and conceptualization concerning the nature of mental retardation and its treatment. However, the basic issue, concerning the extent to which this condition, particularly in its more severe form, is modifiable, remains largely unresolved. Mental retardation is now typically viewed as consisting of a heterogeneous grouping of individuals, who vary both in the causes of their deficiency and in their potential for acquiring adaptive behavior (Robinson & Robinson, 1976). Specifically, the mildly, and to a lesser extent the moderately, retarded are seen as being educable and capable of reaching some degree of independence in the community. The severely retarded are usually characterized as being capable of learning only the most basic of the self-help behaviors and the most rudimentary academic, social and vocational skills. Finally, the profoundly retarded are often regarded as being unable to acquire sufficient skills to care for their basic needs (Chinn, Drew, & Logan, 1975). As the severity of retardation increases, organic rather than social-environmental factors are usually seen as more instrumental in producing the behavioral deficiencies, and there is a corresponding increase in skepticism concerning the possibilities of effectiveness of habilitation programs.

It is important to note, that this skepticism regarding remediation is not reflected in the recent definition of mental retardation published by the American Association on Mental Deficiency (AAMD) (Grossman, 1973). According to this definition, mental retardation is described as involving "significantly sub-average general intellectual functioning existing concurrently with deficits in adaptive behavior, and manifested during the developmental period" (p. 11). This definition is completely descriptive in nature, and makes no assertions concerning etiology, and no prognostic statements stipulating levels of potential achievement for individuals so labeled. Prognosis is related more to "associated conditions, motivation, treatment and training opportunities than to mental retardation itself" (p. 12). This AAMD definition is in distinct contrast to earlier definitions of mental retardation, such as that given by Doll (1941), who asserts that this disorder is of constitutional origin and is essentially incurable.

Even though the recent definition makes no absolute statements about the nature and treatability of mental retardation, it is obvious that society, and more particularly the parents, professionals, and paraprofessionals who interact on a daily basis with this population, are generally more pessimistic concerning the potential for achievement of the retarded in contrast to normal individuals. Moreover, it is clear that society's expectancies also differ, depending on the extent of the retarded individual's behavioral and intellectual deficiency. Gottlieb (1977) notes that adults are significantly more receptive to the idea of mainstreaming mildly rather than severely retarded pupils, because they feel that the former group would be less likely to present behavioral problems. This negative attitude concerning the educability of the severely/profoundly retarded appears to be based also on several other assumptions. First, it is assumed that persons with lower IQs, as measured by an intelligence test, have less potential for achievement. Second, it is asserted that there is a direct relationship between the degree of present behavioral deficiency manifested by an individual and his potential for future behavioral development. Specifically, it is believed that persons who are more behaviorally deficient have less potential for behavioral development. Third, it is believed that persons who learn when placed in educational programs have a greater potential than those who learn only a little or do not learn at all. A corollary to this assumption is that an individual who shows minimal or no progress after being in an education program for a "reasonable" amount of time, is probably not capable of learning. Although numerous logical counterarguments can be brought to bear concerning the validity of these assumptions, they nevertheless often influence decisions concerning the type and extent of educational services offered to the retarded.

Recently, these types of assumptions have been seriously challenged by investigators working in the area of behavior modification, who have been developing and evaluating new programs for educating severely and profoundly retarded individuals. Specifically, as a result of their endeavors, doubt has been cast on the belief that low-IQ individuals, who are quite behaviorally deficient and who have had a history of not progressing in institutional programs, cannot learn.[1] These behavior modification programs and questions concerning their general efficacy will be discussed in the next section.

Behavior Modification Programs with the Severely and Profoundly Retarded

When behavior modifiers first entered institutions for the mentally retarded in the 1960s, they were confronted with a major challenge. At that time, institutional programming was directed primarily toward providing residents with basic physical care and general types of stimulation programs. Systematic training programs were generally nonexistent, because of the prevailing attitudes about the uneducability of this clinical population, because of inadequate numbers of staff, and, most important, because of ignorance concerning the specific nature of such programs. However, through the efforts of behavior modifiers, a technology has been developed within the past two decades which has greatly influenced programming provided for mentally retarded individuals. In fact, the introduction of behavior modification technology into residential institutions has been one of the major reasons why programs have changed from a custodial to a habilitative orientation.

The goals of most behavior modification programs have been similar, focusing on increasing adaptive behavior in the self-help (e.g., self-feeding, toileting, grooming, and oral hygiene), social, language, preacademic, and prevocational areas, and on decreasing inappropriate behaviors, including self-stimulating self-injurious, aggressive, and tantrum responses (Whitman & Scibak, 1979). At present, educators concentrating on these behavioral objectives with the severely and profoundly retarded have a choice of numerous behavioral treatment techniques. In retrospect, it can be stated that an extensive behavior modification technology has developed as a result of research with the mentally retarded in the last 15 years, and that this technology has greatly influenced the types of educational programs offered to them. Perhaps the ultimate significance of the behavior modification movement lies in

[1] Throne (1970), drawing on earlier statements by Ogden Linsley, has stated that retardation merely reflects the fact that an individual does not learn under ordinary conditions, not that he could not learn under other conditions. In this regard, it has also been frequently asserted that the failure on the part of the severely and profoundly retarded individuals to learn is more a function of inadequate and ineffective educational programs than of the condition of retardation itself.

the fact that it has questioned traditional beliefs and created a more positive attitude concerning the educability and "curability" of the more severely retarded person.

Despite the many published reports which suggest that behavior modification programs can be successfully employed in teaching retarded persons, there is disagreement about whether this technology can really be generally employed in educating those individuals who are most deficient in adaptive skills, that is, the severely and profoundly retarded. In a recent court case (Wyatt v. Hardin, 1979a,b), it has been argued in the defendant's response (1979b) to an Amici Associations' post-trial brief that substantial numbers of mentally retarded individuals in institutions may be unable to learn basic self-help skills, even though exposed to the best training methods currently available (p. 106, Volume 1). It was stressed in this brief by the defendants: (1) that the behavioral technology now available is not sufficient to overcome the obvious disabilities that many retarded persons exhibit, (2) that the potential of severely and profoundly retarded individuals to benefit from such programs is limited, and (3) that the residents who fail to improve after extensive attempts at educating them have occurred should not be subjected to further training or education, but rather should be provided with a full program of enriching recreational and leisure-time activities. By way of example, they pointed out that "if a person is twenty-one years old and can't walk and is not toilet trained and efforts to learn these skills have not succeeded, there is little reason to believe they will succeed in the future." Additionally, they note that when no improvement is shown after every attempt is made to train a retarded person, then "it is wrong to simply continue training indefinitely" (pp. 114, 117).

The plaintiffs, in an Amici Associations' post-trial brief (1979a), argued that the negative conclusions reached by the defense regarding the learning potential of severely and profoundly retarded persons are not supported by the findings reported and testimony given. They suggested that the assertion that residents cannot make significant gains is based on the erroneous assumption that residents who do not learn have been provided adequate training. Testimony by expert witnesses for the plaintiff stressed that "every severely and profoundly retarded person has the ability to learn, "and that when these individuals fail to learn in educational programs, training procedures must be changed and improved, rather than terminated (p. 34). Furthermore, it was stated that "flexibility is crucial," and that when first and second attempts to educate fail, other attempts must be made, and that one can always find an approach that works (p. 34). It was further argued that placing residents in general enrichment programs, as suggested by the defense, would be counter-productive, and developmental gains achieved by residents prior to their placement in such a program might be lost.

The issues raised and argued in the Wyatt v. Hardin case are interesting from an historical perspective. A ruling in favor of the defense might be seen as reaffirming earlier views concerning the incurability of retardation, such as those espoused by Pinel and Doll. In contrast, a ruling in favor of the plaintiff would seem to reinforce the more recent optimistic attitude that severe and profound retardation is a treatable condition. In either case, the decision by the court may well determine the nature and extent of treatment given to retarded residents in institutions in the future.[2]

If one could choose an ideal forum to address issues concerning the educability and treatability of the severely and profoundly retarded, it probably would not be within the adversary system of the courtroom. The very nature of this system forces issues to be examined basically in a dichotomous fashion. Through the judicial system, people are judged as guilty or not guilty, insane or sane, treatable or not treatable. Expert witnesses typically must give evidence on one side of the issue or the other. Even the judge who weighs the evidence presented by the opposing sides is compelled ultimately by the system to rule on one side or another. The case of Wyatt v. Hardin is no exception. However, one should be careful not to make too harsh a judgment of the judicial system, because historically professionals in medical, social science, and educational areas have taken similar categorical positions concerning the nature of mental retardation and its treatability.

Any forum examining questions concerning treatability and curability of mental retardation should recognize from the outset that they cannot be answered in a dichotomous fashion, and that answers to these questions today should not be viewed as irrevocable proclamations concerning the nature of a given condition. In addition, this forum should carefully consider the available empirical evidence bearing on these questions. Presently, there exist

[2] Shortly after this chapter was written, the final ruling in this case was handed down. The Court found that the defendants were in "substantial and serious noncompliance" with orders to provide adequate habilitation programming. This ruling was based on evidence which indicated that several residents were not receiving habilitation programming suited to their needs. In making this ruling, the judge pointed out that "formal ritualistic training regimens which are not modified when unsuccessful do not constitute adequate habilitation programming." He concluded that the evidence *did not* justify modifying minimum constitutional standards "to allow defendants to cease providing habilitation programming and to provide instead an enriched environment."

within professional journals a large number of research reports evaluating techniques for modifying the behavior of individuals. Although this research literature certainly was considered by a number of expert witnesses in the Wyatt v. Hardin case, the post-trial briefs suggest that it was never really given the careful consideration it deserved, and that impressionistic information was more important than were empirical data.

In order to show how such research might be employed in assisting society in planning appropriate programs for the mentally retarded, the remainder of the chapter will be devoted to a general examination of behavior modification research which has been conducted with the severely and profoundly retarded. This analysis has been limited to studies with this subpopulation to restrict its scope, given the large amount of research which has been done with retarded individuals generally, and because it is with these individuals that the most serious questions concerning educability have arisen. During this overview, the scientific acceptability of this research, as it relates to the adequacy of the measurement procedures and experimental designs employed, and the effectiveness and efficiency of the techniques utilized in these studies, will be discussed. Finally, the implication of this research as it bears on the question of whether the severely or profoundly retarded are educable will be addressed.

Behavior Modification Research with the Severely and Profoundly Retarded

Methodological Considerations

The major rationale for the use of behavior modification techniques in clinical/educational situations should be that there is scientific evidence that these techniques are effective. However, it is important to recognize that the task of evaluating any technology is a very complex one and is never really completed. Techniques are evaluated not only to establish their effectiveness, but also to assist in their refinement and in the development of new and better techniques. Although a single study can provide valuable information about the usefulness of a technique, the effectiveness of a technology can only be established through repeated examination of its effects as it is employed by different therapists, with different clients and in various situations. For such studies to be scientifically valid, it is critical that reliable measurement systems and appropriate experimental designs be used which allow lawful relationships between a technique and behavior changes to be assessed. Moreover, it is important to evaluate whether a technique has produced short-term effects as well as generalized changes in behavior over time and situations. These standards, and the extent to which existing behavior modification research with the severely and profoundly retarded conforms to them, will be briefly considered in this section.

Measurement Considerations

Basic to the scientific evaluation of any technology is the notion of measurement. In order to assess whether change has really occurred, a reliable measurement system must be employed. Measurements of behavioral data are reliable to the degree that they accurately represent the behavior of the person being observed, rather than some transient characteristic of the instrument employed in rating that behavior (Kazdin, 1978). In most behavior modification research with the severely and profoundly retarded, single-case experimental designs are employed, and overt client behaviors are assessed in a repeated fashion, often daily, during baseline and intervention conditions. Although automated or semiautomated recording procedures are occasionally employed in such assessments, human observers are typically used to rate client behaviors. Whichever measurement procedure is employed, it is imperative that its reliability be established. Kazdin (1978) points out that when measurement error is present it contributes to the variability of the behavior being observed, and when variability owing to this type of error is sufficiently large evaluation of an intervention may be impossible.

Internal Validity

The goal of science is to discover and describe lawful relationships among events. Although the reliability of a measurement system reflects the accuracy of an observation of a behavior, it has only an indirect bearing on the decision concerning whether that behavior has changed as a result of an intervention. In order to examine this relationship, research is conducted in which one variable, the independent variable, is manipulated, and its effects on a second variable, the dependent variable, are observed. In behavior-modification research, the focus is on examining for possible functional relationships between the application of a treatment technique (i.e., independent variable) and changes in socially important behaviors (i.e., dependent variable). Internal validity is concerned with the conditions under which it can be stated with some certainty that such a functional relationship exists or, in other words, that it was the systematic introduction of a treatment which produced an observed change in behavior, and not some other uncontrolled and unspecified variable (Campbell & Stanley, 1963).

Whether the results generated by a particular research project are internally valid depends on the experimental design employed and its ability to control for confounding variables which can produce changes in the target behavior (i.e., the dependent variable). Through the experimental design, a scientist arranges the conditions of the experiment so that the effect of a treatment intervention can be specifically evaluated. Kazdin (1978) points out that traditional group as well as single-case research designs are similar, in that they both involve a comparison of performance under different conditions, and that it is only in the manner that the comparison is made that the two approaches differ. Although traditional group studies focus on differences *between* subjects who have or have not been exposed to the treatment intervention, single-case research is primarily concerned with comparisons *within* subjects over time.

In research with the retarded, single-case designs typically have been employed. Although a variety of single-case designs have been used in these studies, the reversal (ABAB) and the multiple-baseline strategies are the most frequently employed of the designs generally considered to possess good internal validity (cf. Hersen & Barlow, 1976). In most behavior modification research, it is assumed that if the client's behavior changes and a legitimate design is employed, the intervention procedure was responsible for the change. However, even if these requirements are met, the internal validity of an experiment may be further increased if data are gathered showing that the intervention was applied as stipulated (Kazdin, 1978). Where this information is lacking, it is possible that the behavior changes observed were not a function of the treatment *per se*, but some other therapist- or treatment-related variable. This issue will be addressed in greater detail later in this chapter.

Response Change Assessment

The answer to the question whether a treatment procedure is effective is not a simple one. The reason is that the effects of training can be evaluated across a number of dimensions. In order for a technique to have any clinical value, it must at a minimum effect direct changes in the target behavior. Ideally, a treatment should produce positive generalized changes in a client's behavior over time, over situations, and in other behaviors. That is, a technique should produce not only immediate, but also longterm changes in behavior; it should change the client's behavior both in the treatment situation and in the natural environment; and it should effect positive changes in client behaviors which are not specifically the focus of the treatment intervention, such as increasing other appropriate behaviors, or decreasing other maladaptive responses in the client's repertoire. To the extent that these types of generalized changes do not occur, time-consuming extensions of the treatment program become necessary.

From a design perspective, assessments of these generalized changes have several implications for the investigator. In order to evaluate whether response effects are maintained over time, a follow-up must be conducted. Such follow-ups may be conducted over a period of days, weeks, or months. Obviously, the longer the time period over which the follow-up is conducted, the more information one has concerning the power of the technique. In addition to these temporal characteristics, follow-ups also differ in terms of what happens therapeutically while they are in effect. The treatment procedure may be sustained with its form unaltered, it may be continued but the manner of application changed (usually abbreviated and simplified in some fashion—cf. O'Brien & Azrin, 1972), or it may be discontinued altogether (cf. Christian, Hollomon, & Lanier, 1973). From a pragmatic standpoint, a technique which can produce long-term effects even though it is not applied during the follow-up period or is applied in an abbreviated format is more valuable than a technique which must be continued in its original form to control behavior.

In most programs, a treatment technique is usually applied by one or two individuals in a limited number of situations. It is hoped that during treatment the client will show a change in response not only in the treatment situation with the treatment agent, but also in other social situations in the presence of other individuals. In order for situational generalization effects to be evaluated, it is necessary to observe the subject's target response in the treatment situation and also in other settings before, during, and, ideally, after treatment. To assess empirically whether there is a functional relationship between a treatment intervention and a response change in untreated situations, an appropriate experimental design must be employed. One design sometimes used for this type of assessment is the multiple baseline across subjects and situations. With this design, each subject's behavior is measured and, if necessary, treated successively across situations. When situational generalization occurs, replication of this effect across subjects is essential in order to ascertain whether the correlated change in behavior across situations is fortuitous. A hybrid design in which a reversal procedure is used in combination with a multiple-baseline strategy can also be employed for this purpose (cf. Hersen & Barlow, 1976). Although time consuming, these types of extended observations are necessary if the generalized effects of a technique across situations are to be properly evaluated.

Response generalization is hypothesized when a change in an untreated behavior occurs concurrently with a change in the treated behavior. These side effects may be desirable, undesirable, or mixed in their social value. For obvious clinical reasons, it is important to know whether such effects are occurring. As with situational generalization, response generalization can only be assessed if the multiple responses are observed before and during treatment. The experimental designs used to evaluate response generalization effects are also similar to those employed in assessing situational generalization effects, and include the multiple baseline across responses and subjects, and a hybrid of the multiple-baseline and reversal procedures.

External Validity

In contrast to internal validity, which deals with the direct implications of an experiment, external validity is concerned with the more ultimate meaning of an experiment, or what Campbell and Stanley (1963) refer to as the question of generalizability. In behavior modification research, this concern is reflected when questions are asked about whether the relationship observed between a treatment technique and a target behavior holds across populations, settings, and therapists. To the extent that a particular study can answer these various questions, it has external validity. At a minimum, the results of a specific study suggest that, if the experiment were replicated with similar subjects, therapists, and environmental circumstances, the outcome would be similar. However, if in a particular study a large, heterogeneous sample of subjects and therapists is employed, and if the experimental hypothesis is examined across a number of diverse situations, more general kinds of conclusions can be drawn.

In general, single-case designs, such as the reversal and multiple-baseline, do not have considerable external validity. One of the major reasons is that, typically, only one or a few subjects are used when these designs are employed, thus restricting the types of inferences which can be made. For example, it is difficult to conclude that severely retarded children, in general, will respond in a certain fashion to a specific treatment technique, just because one or two severely retarded children responded in this way in a particular experiment. In contrast, if 10 severely retarded children respond in a unitary fashion to a treatment, then a stronger inference can be made about the effects of the treatment with this population of individuals. Hersen and Barlow (1976) emphasize this point. They state that isolating the active therapeutic variable for a given client through a rigorous single subject experimental design provides little basis for inferring that this therapeutic procedure would be equally effective when applied to clients with similar behavior disorders (client generality), when applied by different therapists (therapist generality), or when applied in different settings (setting generality). Because of these problems associated with generalizing from a specific case, group designs are suggested and preferred by many investigators.

Unfortunately, practical logistical problems, such as subject unavailability, monetary constraints, or time limitations, often render group research investigations impossible. These problems are among the major reasons why single-subject designs have become increasingly popular with clinical researchers. Hersen and Barlow (1976) point out that the external validity of an experiment with one client can be increased if the results of an original experiment are *directly* replicated three or four times with similar clients. In a direct replication series, the same therapist applies the procedure being evaluated in the same setting to clients with nearly identical target behaviors. Thus, the issue of general efficacy of a procedure across clients is addressed. Hersen and Barlow also indicate that, through a *systematic* replication strategy, questions concerning the general effectiveness of a treatment procedure can be more extensively examined. In systematic replication studies, an attempt is made to replicate findings from a direct replication series while varying the setting, behavior change agent, type of client, or some combination of these parameters.

Although direct and systematic replication strategies can be employed to increase the external validity of findings associated with single-subject designs, they require a considerable expenditure of time and energy. Although it is not unusual to see a direct replication series in which the effectiveness of a particular procedure is examined across three or four subject with a particular behavioral problem or deficiency, systematic replication series evaluating a procedure across behavior change agents occur with considerably less frequency.

Critique and Evaluation[3]

In order to examine the scientific status of behavior modification studies conducted with the severely and profoundly retarded and the types of conclusions which can be drawn about the techniques employed, a systematic review of the research literature in this area was conducted, using the parameters just discussed. The data assessed was generated by a survey of research which appeared in the following journals: *AAESPH Review*, *American Journal on Mental Deficiency*, *Behavior Modification*, *Behavior Research and Therapy*, *Journal of Behavior Therapy and Experimental Psychiatry*, *Mental Retardation*, *Journal of Applied Behavior Analysis* and *Journal of Experimental Child Psychology*. In addition, reference lists from several other reviews, including Berkson and Landesman-Dwyer (1977) and Birnbrauer (1976), were examined, and relevant articles critiqued from a number of other journals. The following items of information were recorded from each study for analysis purposes: authors, journal name, year, number of severely retarded, profoundly retarded, and other retarded subjects, target behaviors addressed, training procedures employed, who applied the procedures, the situation in which the procedures were applied, whether the reliability of the measurement procedure was appropriately assessed, whether a valid experimental design was employed and technique application was monitored, whether generalization of effects over time, situations, and responses were evaluated, and, finally, whether the social validity of the results were assessed. Except for the first three items of information response codes were developed and the reliability of the rating procedures assessed. In all instances, the reliability coefficients exceeded 80.

Since 1962, 280 studies evaluating the effects of behavior modification techniques with the severely and profoundly retarded were found in the professional journals just cited. Table I shows the number of studies appearing annually in each of these journals from 1962 through 1979. As depicted in this table, there has been a gradual increase over the years in the number of studies published. Not surprisingly, journals which are exclusively concerned with mental retardation are publishing a greater amount of research in this area. In the last four years, over a third of the research published has appeared in the *AAESPH Review* and *Mental Retardation*. However, the *Journal of Applied Behavior Analysis*, which has no constrictions regarding subject population addressed, has published 51 studies since 1968. Perhaps

[3] The data reported in this section represent only a small percentage of that collected and analyzed. A more complete presentation of the data will appear in a forthcoming article.

TABLE I
Behavior Modification Research with the Severely and Profoundly Retarded Published in Various Journals from 1962 to 1979

Year	AAESPH	AJMD	BM	BRAT	BT	BTEP	MR	JABA	JECP	Other	Total
1962	—[a]	1	—	—	—	—	—	—	—	0	1
1963	—	2	—	0	—	—	0	—	—	1	3
1964	—	0	—	0	—	—	3	—	—	0	3
1965	—	3	—	0	—	—	2	—	—	0	5
1966	—	3	—	0	—	—	0	—	—	0	3
1967	—	7	—	1	—	—	3	—	—	0	11
1968	—	1	—	0	—	—	0	3	1	2	7
1969	—	6	—	0	—	—	0	7	1	0	14
1970	—	5	—	0	0	0	2	5	0	1	13
1971	—	6	—	0	2	0	3	9	0	1	21
1972	—	5	—	1	1	0	4	4	0	2	17
1973	—	5	—	2	1	1	8	6	0	1	24
1974	—	7	—	0	4	1	10	4	0	1	27
1975	—	5	—	5	4	2	5	2	0	4	27
1976	3	3	—	1	0	4	4	3	0	0	18
1977	5	3	5	1	3	5	5	5	0	1	33
1978	10	6	4	2	1	3	10	3	1	1	41
1979[b]	4	1	0	1	1	1	4	0	0	0	12
Total	22	69	9	14	17	17	63	51	3	15	280

Note. The journals reviewed are the following: *AAESPH Review*, *American Journal on Mental Deficiency (AJMD)*, *Behavior Modification (BM)*, *Behavior Research and Therapy (BRAT)*, *Behavior Therapy (BT)*, *Behavior Therapy and Experimental Psychiatry (BTEP)*, *Mental Retardation (MR)*, *Journal of Applied Behavior Analysis (JABA)*, *Journal of Experimental Child Psychology (JECP)*, and other miscellaneous journals.

[a] Indicates journal not in existence that year.

[b] Research published in journals during the first three to six months of 1979.

because of the current availability of other outlets, the number of studies published annually in JABA is on the decline.

Closer examination of the studies reviewed shows that 26% of them employed profoundly retarded subjects exclusively; 33%, severely retarded individuals; 15%, subjects from both these populations; 18%, a combination of mildly, moderately, and severely retarded subjects; and 8% of the investigations reported using retarded individuals, but did not report the level of retardation. From the behavioral description given of the subjects in this last group of studies, it appears that most, if not all, were in the severe and profound range of retardation.

In the greater part of the research reviewed, the subjects chosen for inclusion in the studies did not appear to have been randomly selected. In most instances, it is not clear whether behavioral criteria were employed other than the presence of the particular target behavior or target deficiency which provided the focus for the treatment program. If these subjects were selected because in some sense they were the elite of the severely or profoundly retarded residents in an institution, data concerning technique effectiveness from these subjects cannot legitimately be used to make inferences about how the technique would affect the larger population of the severely or profoundly retarded. For example, the fact that a behavior-shaping program works with a cooperative, physically nonhandicapped, higher functioning, profoundly retarded individual does not mean that it would work with a profoundly retarded individual with less positive behavior characteristics. If general conclusions about the efficacy of behavioral techniques with the severely and profoundly retarded are to be reached, it is imperative that random subject selection procedures be employed.

Further analysis of the data from this survey shows that 63% of the studies were directed to increasing appropriate behavior, and 37% focused on decreasing inappropriate responses. Table II presents a further breakdown of the target behaviors addressed by these studies. As can be seen in this table, the majority of the studies were directed to modifying self-help, language, self-stimulation, or self-injurious behaviors. Within the self-help area, studies were most frequently focused on developing toileting ($N = 25$), self-feeding ($N = 13$), or a combination of self-help skills ($N = 12$). In contrast, little attention has been given to the evaluation of techniques for developing dressing ($N = 5$), grooming ($N = 2$), and oral-hygiene ($N = 1$)

TABLE II
General Target Behaviors Addressed in Behavior Modification Research with the Severely and Profoundly Retarded

Target behaviors	Number of studies	Relative percentage
Self-help	58	20.7
Social behavior	21	7.5
Language	46	16.4
Other appropriate	52	18.6
Self-stimulation	33	11.8
Self-injurious	29	10.4
Aggression & tantrum	11	3.9
Other inappropriate	30	10.7
Total	280	100.0

behaviors. In the language area, only eight of the studies were concerned with the development of receptive language skills, most of the remaining being concerned with increasing expressive language. Other appropriate behavior frequently addressed included the development of prevocational, imitative, and attentional skills. Besides those inappropriate behaviors tabulated, the only other maladaptive response to receive considerable attention was rumination behavior ($N = 10$). Although a number of other responses, such as ambulation, coin usage, pica, coprophagy, stealing, and stripping, have provided the focus for treatment, the number of studies concerned with each has been small.

Procedurally, a wide array of techniques for changing behavior has been evaluated across studies. Techniques employed in 5% or more of the studies include positive reinforcement, verbal instruction, modeling, differential reinforcement of other behaviors (DRO), and a wide variety of punishment procedures, including time-out and overcorrection. In the majority of the studies, about 75%, various combinations of two or more techniques were used. Although many of the techniques employed across studies can be conceptually categorized together, these techniques at a procedural level vary considerably from study to study. For example, the nature of the stimuli involved in punishment programs have been quite diverse, and have included aversive agents such as shock, slaps, lemon juice, and aromatic ammonia.

Table III shows the agents who administered these procedures and the setting in which the training programs have been conducted. As indicated in this table, most programs have been delivered by experimenters, research assistants, institutional staff members, or teachers in experimental rooms, ward-or dayrooms, classrooms, or workshops. Several points concerning the information provided by this table are worthy of mention. The clinical validity of any behavior modification program is best established when the techniques are administered by the agents who daily interact with the retarded clients, such as teacher or ward personnel, and when these techniques are delivered in the client's natural setting. When this does not occur, questions concerning whether programs can be transferred to these agents and across settings arise. In this regard, it should be noted that, though 42% of the programs were administered by natural treatment agents and 57% did occur in the client's daily environment, a large percentage were administered by an experimenter or research assistant (39%), and in an experimental room (30%). Table III also shows that a high percentage of studies did not clearly specify who applied the technique (21%) or where training took place (11%).

TABLE III
Therapists Applying Procedures and Settings in which Behavior Modification Research with the Severely and Profoundly Retarded Has Been Conducted

Therapists	Number of studies	Relative percentage
Experiment research assistant	109	38.9
Institutional staff	69	24.6
Teacher	27	9.6
Parent	5	1.8
Volunteer-foster grandparent	7	2.5
Mechanical delivery	1	.4
Other	3	1.1
Not specified (unclear)	59	21.1
Total	280	100.0
Settings	**Number of studies**	**Relative percentage**
Experimental room	85	30.4
Classroom	37	13.2
Home	6	2.1
Hospital ward-dayroom	96	34.3
Workshop	21	7.5
Other	4	1.4
Not specified (unclear)	31	11.1
Total	280	100.0

Because this information is lacking, it is impossible to make inferences concerning the clinical validity of the programs, specifically, who might be able to apply such programs and where they can be effectively implemented.

Since the inception of behavior research programs with the severely and profoundly retarded, the measurement procedures employed have been more frequently and extensively evaluated. From 1962 through 1967, reliability data were reported in only a few investigations. More recently, there has been a marked increase in the number of studies in which measurement instruments have been examined. However, in over 50% of the research published in the last five years, investigators still either have not made this assessment, or have used measurement systems which have failed to meet suggested standards. Studies in the latter category have either not evaluated the reliability of their rating instruments during each experimental condition, or have reported reliability coefficients of less than .80. It should also be pointed out that, although in over 90% of the studies reviewed, observers were employed in the collection of data, attempts to eliminate potential sources of rater bias which can influence reliability estimates (Kazdin, 1977) have been infrequent.

From a design perspective, there has also been an improvement in the quality of research conducted in the last few years. Whereas from 1962 through 1967 less than 50% of the studies conducted used appropriate research designs, over 75% of the designs employed in the last five years have enabled scientifically valid statements to be made concerning the relationship between treatment procedures and target behaviors. However, in only one of the studies reviewed was an attempt made to monitor directly the treatment procedure itself, and determine whether it was implemented as stated by the investigators. It should be noted that this methodological deficiency has been present in most of the published research in the behavior modification area and is not restricted to studies conducted with the severely and profoundly retarded. Moreover, though the failure to monitor technique implementation somewhat reduces the confidence which may be placed in statements about the functional relationship between a treatment intervention and behavior change (Kazdin, 1978), this shortcoming does not completely invalidate the conclusions that may be reached about such relationships.

Although the methodological quality of the behavior modification research conducted with the severely and profoundly retarded has been improving, the focus of almost all early research and most recent investigation has been primarily on evaluating the short-term effects of the treatment intervention. Although an increasing number of studies are examining the effects of treatment programs over time, the absolute number of such studies is still small, and the length of the follow-up and maintenance periods are relatively short. Thus, more definitive statements concerning the effects of maintenance procedures, and whether initial behavior changes are sustained over time, cannot be made (see Table IV and Figure 1). Even greater ignorance exists concerning our knowledge about the generalized effects of training procedures on target behavior in nontreatment situations and the side effects of these procedures on behaviors not directly treated (see Table IV and Figure 1).

The aforementioned statements are descriptive of the overall picture of behavior modification research with the severely and profoundly retarded. A closer analysis of research with this population reveals that, though numerous techniques have been evaluated and their effectiveness established across subjects within a study, there have been few attempts across studies to examine systematically the general effectiveness of a technique when it is administered by other therapists in other settings. Moreover, systematic

TABLE IV
Number and Percentage of Studies from 1962–1979 Which Have Included Maintenance and Generalization Assessments

	Number of Studies	Percentage[a]
Maintenance[b]	59	21.1
Follow-up[b]	29	10.4
Situation generalization	56	20.0
Response generalization	41	14.6

[a] The percentages were derived by dividing the actual number of studies which made the assessments by 280, the number of studies reviewed.
[b] The term "maintenance" was applied to all studies which continued to examine the effects of the training procedure after it was modified in some way. For example, during the maintenance period, the therapeutic procedure may have been abbreviated, or responsibility for its application may have been taken over by a teacher, ward attendant, or parent. In contrast, "follow-up" was used to describe studies where the training procedure was not changed and its effects over time were evaluated.

attempts to test the general utility of such techniques when they are employed with numerous subjects who reflect the total range of deficiencies which characterize severe and profound retardation are nonexistent.

In summary, many studies have been conducted which evaluate the efficacy of behavioral techniques with the severely and profoundly retarded. In general, the methodological quality of these studies has been improving. As we have pointed out elsewhere (Whitman & Scibak, 1979), an extensive technology for teaching mentally retarded children a variety of adaptive behaviors and suppressing numerous deviant responses has been developed. However, based on our present analysis of the research literature, it is obvious that a great deal more research must be conducted before it can be stated with certainty that effective techniques for modifying the behavior of the severely and profoundly retarded exist. Specifically, there is considerable variation in the number of studies conducted in different behavioral areas. For example, little work has been done in the areas of self-grooming, oral hygiene, and self-dressing. Even in those behavioral areas where considerable research has been completed, few attempts to examine systematically the effectiveness of particular behavior change procedures in different situations have been made. Moreover, although research indicates that this technology has often produced dramatic short-term positive changes in behavior in the treatment situation, evaluations of the long-term and generalized effects of these procedures have seldom taken place. Although there might be a temptation to criticize investigators in this area for not incorporating follow-up and generalization assessments in their studies more frequently, it seems strategically appropriate that the initial emphasis in the evaluation of a technology be placed on examining the direct and immediate effects of treatment techniques. Presently, however, it is imperative that maintenance and generalization questions be examined and that systematic examination of the effects of techniques across diverse clinical situations be conducted.

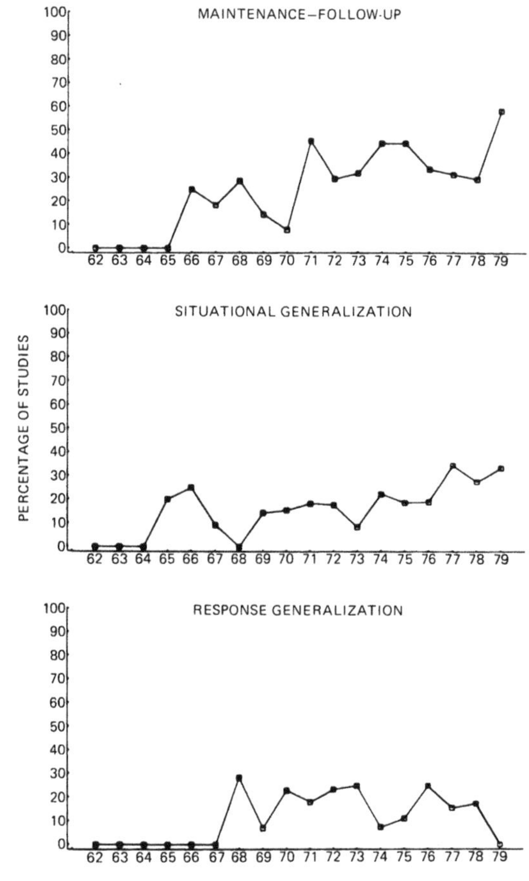

FIGURE 1. Percentage of studies annually from 1962–1979 which include maintenance–follow-up and situational and response generalization assessments.

Future Directions

Social Validity

In particular, it is important that the social validity of the results be evaluated, that the treatment techniques be completely specified and monitored and their efficiency evaluated, and that the response of the public to these techniques be assessed. Behavior therapists generally agree that it is not sufficient for an intervention to produce only reliable change in the behaviors of concern, but also that these changes should be therapeutically important and meaningful. In order for a treatment to be considered effective, it must not only increase adaptive behavior or decrease maladaptive behavior *per se*, but it must change behavior to an extent that the client is viewed more positively by significant others. That is, it is critical that social agents, such as teachers and parents, perceive and evaluate positively the behavioral changes produced by the treatment programs.

Two methods, social comparison and subjective evaluation, have been used by researchers in making decisions concerning the therapeutic significance of a behavioral change (Kazdin, 1978). In the social comparison method, criterion reference subjects, along with experimental subjects, are monitored during a study. In contrast to traditional control subjects, criterion reference subjects are not only omitted from treatment, but they are behaviorally different from the experimental subjects. Whereas the treatment subjects are selected because they are deficient or deviant in their behavior, the criterion reference subjects are chosen because they are viewed by significant social agents as behaviorally competent and are objectively rated as displaying a higher frequency of socially desirable behaviors. At the termination of a treatment procedure, a program is considered successful to the extent that the treatment subjects approximate the criterion reference subjects in their behavior.

In contrast to the social comparison method, the subjective evaluation approach to assessing therapeutic significance is less objective. Typically, clients are evaluated on some type of rating scale by significant others who interact with them on a routine basis. The rating scales are used to assess whether, from a more global, impressionistic perspective, the client is different after treatment. Although self-report measures are more likely to be biased by a variety of external factors, their use as a convenient and economical supplementary evaluation procedure has been strongly recommended (O'Leary & Turkewitz, 1978). With the exception of a handful of studies (cf. Azrin & Armstrong, 1973; Reid & Hurlbut, 1977) behavior modification research with the mentally retarded has not included either of these two procedures for assessing therapeutic significance.

Technique Specification and Monitoring

In examining the results of any research, it is necessary to have complete information concerning the independent variable. In particular, it is important that the treatment technique is completely specified, its application monitored, its efficiency evaluated, and the response of the public to the technique assessed. As O'Leary and Turkewitz (1978) point out, the failure to specify therapeutic procedures in detail constitutes one of the most common and serious problems in psychotherapy research. In order for a treatment technique to be subjected to continued empirical evaluation and/or to be employed in a standardized fashion in clinical situations, the technique must be clearly and sufficiently articulated. The major vehicle for conveying this information to the scientific and clinical community has been research appearing in professional journals. Unfortunately, treatment procedures have been typically only briefly described in published research with the mentally retarded.

Although the benefits that might accrue from publishing more extensive descriptions of treatment procedures seem obvious, journals typically have not allowed space for such information. Recently some journal editors have been encouraging authors to submit a treatment manual, which is reviewed and, although not published, is made available on request from the author or a central information source. O'Leary and Turkewitz suggest that such treatment manuals should include a description of the treatment procedure, information on how the therapist was trained, and data concerning the amount and extent of therapist and therapy supervision required. To the extent that such essential information about a treatment technique is not developed and made available, the scientific base for the evaluation of behavior modification techniques is undermined, and standardization of the technology becomes impossible.

At some point in the evaluation of a technique, a decision must be made concerning its effectiveness. Usually, this decision is made after examining for changes in the target behavior across conditions of an experiment. For example, if an appropriate target behavior (dependent variable) shows a reliable increase in frequency during a treatment condition when contrasted with its baseline level, and this effect is replicated within an appropriate experimental design, the assumption is usually made that the treatment produced the changes in the target behavior (independent variable). However, even if the experimental results are replicated and design requirements met, confidence in the conclusions concerning the functional relationship between a treatment and target behavior can be increased by gathering supplementary data showing that the intervention was conducted as specified (cf. Kazdin, 1978; Koegel, Russo, & Rincover, 1977). As mentioned earlier, this type of evaluation has seldom been conducted in research with the mentally retarded. Without monitoring the intervention and knowing empirically that it was implemented as stipulated, it is more difficult to conclude that changes in a target behavior during a treatment condition were a function of that treatment, and not some other therapist- or treatment-related variable. For example, it is possible that a response change may occur during treatment even though administration was not appropriate, suggesting that the misapplied treatment was nevertheless an effective therapeutic package. Conversely, when change is minimal or nonexistent during treatment, several alternative explanations are also plausible. It could be that the technique is ineffective, *or* that it was not administered in an appropriate fashion.

In summary, if it can be determined that a given technique is actually administered as prescribed, a stronger statement can be made about its effectiveness or lack of effectiveness. In order to monitor a treatment, the technique and its mode of application must be fully specified in advance. It is also important that the reliability of the monitoring procedure be established. In discussing these issues, O'Leary and Turkewitz (1978) suggest that, by having a more detailed assessment of the independent variable, investigators will be automatically prompted to provide more adequate treatment descriptions.

Technique Efficiency

At the inception of the behavior modification movement, emphasis was almost exclusively placed on developing techniques that worked, that is, procedures that resulted in behavioral change. However, as a variety of effective techniques has evolved for dealing with particular behavioral deficiencies and problems, other indices for evaluating this technology have become increasingly relevant. One of these indices has to do with the efficiency of the procedure being employed. In this context, efficiency refers to the amount of time it takes for a procedure to effect behavior changes (O'Dell, 1974). Given that all other factors are equal, a technique which works faster must be judged superior. When the technologies used in educational programs with the mentally retarded are examined, a considerable variation in their efficiency is seen. For example, some early behavior modification programs directed at developing self-help behaviors, such as toileting skills, have taken months and sometimes years to produce desired effects (Baumeister & Klosowski, 1965). In contrast, more recent self-help programs, such as the toileting program developed by Azrin and Foxx and their colleagues (1971, 1973), have reported considerable success in training retarded individuals in a matter of days. Unfortunately, from both a clinical and a developmental perspective, technique efficiency data seldom are reported, even in more recently published studies. Such information ideally should include the number of days and hours per day a program was in effect, the number of staff involved in the administration of the program, the time spent to train the staff, and the amount of time each staff member had to devote to the program. Because such detailed information is not usually reported, it is impossible for staff in clinical settings to judge whether it would be practical or possible to incorporate the technique into their educational programs.

Although information about the efficiency of a particular technique should be helpful in therapeutic planning, caution must be exercised when making inferences concerning the relative efficiency of two techniques or, more specifically, when making judgments about their potential value in another setting. Although a procedure employed in one study may seem more efficient than in another, differences may be related to therapist, population, or setting variables, rather than to the technique *per se*. From a scientific perspective, in order to compare systematically the efficiency of two different techniques, a group study should be conducted, where confounding factors, such as those just mentioned, are controlled through either matching or randomization procedures.

Social Perception of Behavioral Techniques

During the early history of the behavior modification movement, a great deal of notoriety was associated with behavior therapists, and negative public reaction was voiced regarding behavior techniques. In part, this reaction was probably due to the vigor with which those in the behavioral movement rejected medical and psychoanalytic models for treating "psychological" problems and asserted their own approach. Perhaps even more important was the fact that behavioral techniques were seen as controlling and dehumanizing, and as not being applicable to man. Whatever the reason, behavior modification, like many other scientific disciplines, has had to contend with public skepticism and rejection, even when a technique's effectiveness has been established.

Ultimately, if behavior modifiers are to enhance the face validity of their technology, they will, to some extent, have to change their own behavior. One solution involves developing techniques which are more acceptable to the public. From a methodological perspective, if this is to be done, it is imperative that behavior modification researchers assess the perceptions of those trained to utilize behavioral techniques, those toward whom the techniques are directed, and those who view these techniques being employed. This type of assessment, which would require the administration of some type of rating form or attitudinal scale, can be readily incorporated into any study. Such an assessment would not only provide information concerning how a technique is viewed, but would also provide cues to the investigator for changing the technique so as to make it more socially appealing. Again, unfortunately, this type of evaluation has been conducted in only a few studies (Webster & Azrin, 1973). A second solution requires changing the way the technology is presented to the public. In this regard, it is striking how many behavior modifiers have recently begun to describe their procedures in less technical terms and have started using "everyday" language in discussing their approach to the study of human behavior. A third solution for gaining public acceptance of behavior modification technologies is to educate the public regarding behavior modification and how it lies "on a continuum" with therapeutic efforts of the past. The negative attitudes of the public toward behavior modification have often occurred as a result of misconceptions on their part concerning its true nature. If this strategy for changing public reaction to behavior modification is to work, active dialogue and interchange must occur between its advocates and its potential consumers.

As behavior modification technology with the mentally retarded evolves within various therapeutic domains, there is little doubt that there will be increasing emphasis on refining and strengthening existing techniques. In addition to the methodological and procedural modifications just discussed, it is imperative that future studies focus on assessing: (1) the relative effectiveness of different treatments, (2) the gains to be made by combining already established techniques, and (3) the importance of specific subcomponents of complex treatment packages. Such evaluations will require that group designs be employed. In evaluating the results of these types of studies, there will be an increased focus on isolating small but reliable differences between techniques which, in and of themselves, have already been shown to be educationally valuable.

Treatment Implications of Behavior Modification Research

In the first part of this chapter, questions concerning the behavioral potential and the educability of the severely and profoundly retarded were raised. It was pointed out that historically there has been extensive debate on these questions and that, presently, this debate continues as evidenced by the issues brought forth in the Wyatt-Hardin court case. It was further noted that there is considerable empirical evidence bearing on these questions, and that these data must be considered if more definitive answers are to be found. In the second section, behavior modification research conducted with the severely and profoundly retarded was evaluated and its scientific acceptability along with the scope and extent of its inquiry examined. On the basis of this evaluation, it can be concluded that many of the deficiencies presented by the severely and profoundly retarded can be at least temporarily remediated and that individuals so handicapped are capable of learning a multitude of new behaviors. Virtually all the studies reviewed show that short-term changes in behavior occur. Furthermore, the majority of these studies, particularly those which are more recent, are methodologically sound. However, it was also noted that randomized subject selection procedures were often not employed, and that most of these studies did not examine whether behavioral changes were sustained over time or generalized over situations. Although the need for further research in some behavioral areas (e.g., social behaviors) is particularly great, it is also obvious that more work generally must be conducted across all areas before more definite conclusions concerning the educability of this population can be reached. Despite the limitations of past research, there are little data at present to suggest that educational programming and evaluation of these programs should not be vigorously pursued and that guarded optimism concerning their ultimate success is warranted. However, future studies need to be conducted to broaden the scope of their evaluation and assess more directly the social significance of their results, as well as to monitor technique applications and information about the efficiency of the intervention and the public's perception of these techniques.

It should be recognized that the basic question concerning whether retarded persons are educable cannot be categorically answered, and that any answer must take into account the fact that both the issue of educability and the phenomenon of retardation are concepts on a continuum. In one sense, it can be stated with a high degree of certitude that, although mentally retarded persons differ in their learning potential, all are educable, in that each is capable of learning at least some new behaviors, however simple. Thus, the basic question centers around the extent to which various mentally retarded persons are educable. Most scientists and practitioners now recognize that the answer to this question, for any specific individual, cannot be arrived at on an *a priori* basis, but must be based on careful evaluation of the individual's response to the educational programming that he or she receives. In this regard, it should be recognized that even when a person fails to learn under a particular teaching regimen, it cannot be concluded that he or she is not capable of learning in other situations when other approaches are employed.

Ultimately, the issue concerning the educability of the mentally retarded is really a practical rather than a theoretical one. That is, the emphasis on educating this population and more to society's value system concerning the importance of such educational programs and how much time and resources it is willing to devote to the development of these programs. Whereas in the first half of this century there was considerable emphasis on custodial care and eugenics programs for the mentally retarded, there currently is a commitment to recognizing the rights of these persons and providing them with the best treatment and education possible. The extent to which society continues this commitment in the future will be at least in part a function of the success of current programs. It is hoped that both future program development and society's evaluation of these programs will be based on the findings of scientifically acceptable research.

REFERENCES

AZRIN, N.H., & ARMSTRONG, P.M. The "mini-meal"—A method for teaching eating skills to the profoundly retarded. *Mental Retardation*, 1973, *11*, 9–13.

AZRIN, N., & FOXX, R. A rapid method of toilet training the institutionalized retarded. *Journal of Applied Behavior Analysis*, 1971, *4*, 89–99.

AZRIN, N., SNEED, T., & FOXX, R. Dry bed: A rapid method of eliminating bedwetting (enuresis) of the retarded. *Behavior Research and Therapy*, 1973, *11*, 427–434.

BAUMEISTER, A.A., & KLOSOWSKI, R. An attempt to group toilet train severely retarded patients. *Mental Retardation*, 1965, *3*, 24–26.

BERKSON, G., & LANDESMAN-DWYER, S. Behavioral research on severe and profound mental retardation (1955–1974). *American Journal of Mental Deficiency*, 1977, *81* (5), 428–454.

BIRNBRAUER, J. Mental Retardation. In H. Leitenberg (Ed.), *Handbook of behavior modification and behavior therapy*. Englewood Cliffs, N.J.: Prentice-Hall, 1976.

CAMPBELL, D., & STANLEY, J. *Experimental and quasi-experimental designs for research*. Chicago: Rand-McNally, 1963.

CHINN, P., DREW, C., & LOGAN, D. *Mental retardation: A life cycle approach*. St. Louis: Mosby, 1975.

CHRISTIAN, W., HOLLOMON, S., & LANIER, C. An attendant operated feeding program for severely and profoundly retarded females. *Mental Retardation*, 1973, *11*, 35–37.

DOLL, E.A. The essentials of an inclusive concept of mental deficiency. *American Journal of Mental Deficiency*, 1941, *46*, 214–219.

GOTTLIEB, J. Attitudes toward mainstreaming retarded children and some possible effects on educational practices. In P. Mittler (Ed.), *Research to practice in mental retardation* (Vol. 1). Baltimore: University Park Press, 1977.

GROSSMAN, H. (ED.). *Manual on terminology and classification in mental retardation* (rev. ed.). Washington, D.C.: American Association on Mental Deficiency, 1973.

HERSEN, M., & BARLOW, D. *Single case experimental designs: Strategies for studying behavior*. New York: Pergamon, 1976.

ITARD, J. *The wild boy of Aveyron*. New York: Appleton-Century-Crofts, 1962.

KAZDIN, A. Artifact, bias and complexity of assessment: The ABCs of reliability. *Journal of Applied Behavior Analysis*, 1977, *10*. 141–150.

KOEGEL, R., RUSSO, D., & RINCOVER, A. Assessing and training teachers in the generalized use of behavior modification with autistic children. *Journal of Applied Behavior Analysis*, 1977, *10*, 197–205.

O'BRIEN, F., & AZRIN, N.H. Developing proper mealtime behaviors of the institutionalized retarded. *Journal of Applied Behavior Analysis*, 1972, *5*, 389–399.

O'DELL, S. Training parents in behavior modifications: A review. *Psychological Bulletin*, 1974, *81*, 418–433.

O'LEARY, K.D., & TURKEWITZ, H. Methodological errors in marital and child treatment research. *Journal of Consulting and Clinical Psychology*, 1978, *46*, 747–758.

REID, D., & HURLBUT, B. Teaching nonvocal communication to multihandicapped retarded adults. *Journal of Applied Behavior Analysis*, 1977, *10*, 591–603.

ROBINSON, N., & ROBINSON, H. *The mentally retarded child: A psychological approach*, New York: McGraw-Hill, 1976.

THRONE, M., A radical behaviorist approach to diagnosis in mental retardation. *Mental Retardation*, 1970, *8*, 2–5.

WEBSTER, D., & AZRIN, N. Required relaxation: A method of inhibiting agitative-disruptive behavior of retardates. *Behavior Research and Therapy*, 1973, *11*, 67–78.

WHITMAN, T., & SCIBAK, J. Behavior modification research with the severely and profoundly retarded. In N.R. Ellis (Ed.), *Handbook of mental deficiency: Psychological theory and research* (2nd ed.). Hillsdale, N.J.: Erlbaum, 1979.

WYATT v. HARDIN. Amici associations' post-trial brief. Filed in United States district court for middle-district of Alabama, northern division. Civil Action No. 3195–N, 1979.

WYATT v. HARDIN. Defendant's post-trial brief. Filed in United States district court for middle-district of Alabama, northern division. Civil Action No. 3195–N, 1979.

2 Toilet Training for the Mentally Retarded

JOHN R. MCCARTNEY AND JEFFREY C. HOLDEN

INTRODUCTION

The systematic application of learning principles to modify the behavior of humans has perhaps one of its most basic and important functions in the training of toileting skills in mentally retarded persons. Many of these persons have no language and lack the ability to dress, feed, and groom themselves. However, in many instances the most degrading aspect of their behavior, both to the client and to his or her parents or caretakers, is the absence of toileting skills (Baumeister & Klosowski, 1965; Bettison, Davison, Taylor, & Fox, 1976; Ellis, 1963; Osarchuk, 1973).

The absence of toileting skills presents a significant problem for habilitation efforts. Inability to remain clean and dry is not acceptable behavior in the community, except for young children. As a result, the older child, teenager, or adult who exhibits this behavior is severely restricted in his or her interactions with the environment. Indeed, admission to an institution is often the result. Even within the institution, the lack of independent toileting skills leads to further restrictions on habilitative opportunities by limiting educational and leisure time experiences (Bettison *et al.*, 1976; Rentfrow & Rentfrow, 1969). Toileting skills are prerequisite for training more advanced skills (Baumeister & Klosowski, 1965; Rentfrow & Rentfrow, 1969).

Another important consideration related to the absence of toileting skills is the effect on the attitude and morale of parents and/or institutional staff (Bettison *et al.*, 1976; Ellis, 1963). Cleaning up accidents and escorting clients to the toilet are unpleasant jobs that consume large amounts of time and energy. A feeling of hopelessness and lowered expectations results, attitudes which may further interfere with habilitation attempts.

The economic costs involved in caring for non-toilet-trained patients,

---

JOHN R. MCCARTNEY AND JEFFREY C. HOLDEN • Partlow State School and Hospital, Tuscaloosa, Alabama 35401.

though certainly not as important as the humanistic concerns mentioned previously, are significant (Baumeister & Klosowski, 1965; Ellis, 1963; Osarchuk, 1973; Rentfrow & Rentfrow, 1969; Smith, Britton, Johnson, & Thomas, 1975). Soiled linens and clothes are a major burden for institutional laundries. Also, staff time used in helping residents to void appropriately and in cleaning up after accidents is enormous. Certainly it would be desirable to spend this money in more productive ways.

Finally, health problems are exaggerated in environments where non-toilet-trained individuals reside. The incidence of dysentery and intestinal infection is increased in such settings (Rentfrow & Rentfrow, 1969).

Although the absence of toileting skills is a significant problem, little attempt was made to increase toileting skills in severely and profoundly retarded persons until the 1960s. Before that time, the "caring" or custodial approach was used with this population (Smith *et al.*, 1975). It was assumed that these persons could not learn toileting skills, or any other skills for that matter, and they were sheltered in crowded wards with high resident–staff ratios (Rentfrow & Rentfrow, 1969). However, with the emergence of interest in using formal learning principles to solve applied human problems during the last two decades, the training of toileting and other self-help skills has been approached with increased fervor.

This more energetic approach to the problem of incontinence was fueled by a theoretical analysis presented by Ellis (1963) of the S–R principles that might be used to train the severely retarded resident to eliminate in the toilet. He postulated that, prior to toilet training, the patient eliminates in response to rectal tension or bladder distension alone. However, after training, by the principles of contiguity and drive reduction, the elimination response occurs only after approaching the toilet and in the presence of cues associated with the toilet. Ellis proceeded to propose a detailed procedure for training appropriate elimination responses using these principles.

Ellis' article suggested a methodology for the training of toileting skills; however, its primary effect was to reverse the old assumption that severely retarded persons could not be toilet trained. Although he postulated damage to the central nervous system as one possible cause of the problem, he stated that the major causes are a lack of training and decreased learning ability in these persons. He strongly suggested that effective use of learning principles might overcome these latter problems.

Since 1963 there have been a number of attempts to train toileting in mentally retarded persons. At least 40 articles can be related directly to this problem. As in most research areas, the early experiments were relatively unsophisticated and had limited objectives; but in recent years more extensive procedures have been used, and successful attempts to train full toileting independence have been reported (e.g., Azrin & Foxx, 1971; Smith *et al.*, 1975; Van Wagenen, Meyerson, Kerr, & Mahoney, 1969).

The object of this chapter is to provide a critical review of the literature on toilet training of mentally retarded persons. A brief theoretical analysis of the training techniques described in this literature will be presented, as well as a detailed coverage of the training methods, so that more practical factors can be considered. Weaknesses in experimental design will be discussed, as well as administrative issues. An attempt is made to provide the applied researcher with a more thorough understanding of what is currently known about toilet training, as well as to provide the clinician with needed information for treating the problem in the clients that he or she serves.

Toilet Training Procedures

Procedures for training toileting skills in the mentally retarded can be divided into two basic categories, including procedures for decreasing inappropriate toileting behaviors (e.g., toilet accidents) and procedures for increasing appropriate toileting behavior (e.g., dressing skills associated with toileting). The primary techniques used, as well as some theoretical rationale, will be presented in the following sections.

Decreasing Inappropriate Toileting Behavior

The basic theoretical rationale for techniques used in reducing toileting accidents is that these behaviors are operant responses controlled by their consequences. Since sphincter muscles can be controlled voluntarily if they have matured sufficiently and there is no central nervous system damage, this assumption seems appropriate.

Punishment, the application of a contingent aversive event for the purpose of reducing the frequency of a behavior, is a commonly used procedure. Mild corporal punishment (i.e., spanking) was used by Ando (1977) and Azrin, Bugle, and O'Brien (1971), whereas Baumeister and Klosowski (1965), Smith (1979), and Waye and Melnyr (1973) allowed their subjects to wear soiled clothes for a period of time after each accident. The former procedure in particular must be used with care, and only if approved by appropriate guardians, human rights groups, etc.

Azrin and Foxx (1971) and Smith *et al.* (1975) used a verbal reprimand such as "Stop!" or "No, you're wet!" at the onset of an accident, with the aid of an electronic signaling device. Such reprimands may act as punishers, but they also inhibit the voiding response in some cases. After consistently pairing these reprimands with bladder distension, classical conditioning may occur causing bladder distension to become a conditioned stimulus for the inhibition of voiding, thus reducing toileting accidents. The principle here is the same as that often used in dealing with the nocturnal enuresis of normal children (Doleys, 1977).

Response cost is also an aversive contingency that has been applied to toilettng. In this procedure, certain specific privileges or rewards that a client possesses are withdrawn contingent upon an accident. For example, Luiselli (1977) withdrew special outings or evening TV watching if an accident occurred.

Time-out from positive reinforcement is very common in the toilet training literature (Ando, 1977; Azrin & Foxx, 1971; Azrin, Bugle, & O'Brien, 1971; Smith, 1979; Smith *et al.*, 1975). After an accident, the subject may be ignored for 10 minutes to an hour, hopefully removing any opportunity for reinforcement which may unintentionally strengthen the inappropriate toileting response.

Another technique used to reduce toileting accidents is restitution overcorrection (Ando, 1977; Azrin & Foxx, 1971; Bettison *et al.*, 1976; Doleys & Arnold, 1975; Smith *et al.*, 1975; Trott, 1977). This method requires the client to clean the residue produced by the toileting accident. For instance, he or she may be required to undress, take a shower, wash the soiled clothes, and mop up any traces of soil on the chair or floor where the accident occurred (Azrin & Foxx, 1971). The restitution overcorrection technique includes many components. First, the social consequences of having an accident are stressed by this procedure, which is the primary intention (Azrin & Foxx, 1971). Second, the technique is probably an aversive event to most persons, which suggests that punishment may be operating to suppress accidents. Finally, the technique entails time-out from positive reinforcement, since edibles, praise, and other reinforcers are withheld during this procedure. Thus, the technique is actually a combination of many learning principles.

Increasing Appropriate Toileting Skills

Skills necessary for fully independent toileting are: (1) approaching the toilet, (2) dressing skills associated with toileting, and (3) eliminating in the toilet. A truly continent individual must be able to approach the toilet area on his own, lower his pants and underwear, eliminate in the toilet, use tissue appropriately, and pull his clothes back on. However, researchers differ on the method they use to attain such results. These three categories will be discussed separately; however, in a number of studies an attempt is made to train all three.

The majority of the studies reported on toilet training involve systematically reinforcing appropriate elimination. The client is given praise, edible reinforcement, or both, immediately after appropriate eliminations. Although this approach appears simplistic, it is complicated by the fact that the occurrence of a voiding response may not always be readily discernable. For this reason, signaling devices have been used by several researchers. An electronic device is located in the toilet bowl, and a signal is elicited when the slightest elimination occurs. Once appropriate elimination has been increased by the use of positive reinforcement, it is necessary to fade out the continuous-reinforcement schedule by gradually introducing partial-reinforcement schedules, which are thinned until extrinsic positive reinforcement can be eliminated totally.

Although nearly all attempts to toilet train the mentally retarded focus on increasing appropriate elimination behavior, not all researchers have addressed the issue of ensuring that the individual can arrange his or her clothes properly before and after elimination. In most of these studies, dressing was not targeted, because the subjects chosen for the study were capable of pulling their pants and underpants up and down. However, in attempting to generalize training effects to more severely retarded residents, one must recognize the importance of the client's possessing at least minimal dressing skills before he can be considered toilet trained.

Those toilet training studies which have been designed to target dressing skills have typically utilized manual guidance and fading (e.g., Azrin & Foxx, 1971; Smith *et al.*, 1975; Van Wagenen *et al.*, 1969). In using these procedures, the individual is given the minimum physical guidance necessary to insure appropriate lowering of his pants and underwear. As the client begins lowering his or her garments independently, the guidance provided by the trainer is reduced. The crucial factor is that the trainer allows the mentally retarded individual to function as independently as possible. Some researchers differ in their method for fading out manual guidance. Several researchers (e.g., Azrin & Foxx, 1971) have suggested that, once the mentally retarded individual has demonstrated completely the ability to pull down his pants and underwear, the trainer should no longer be allowed to reintroduce manual guidance. Other researchers (e.g., Van Wagenen *et al.*, 1969) continue to give as much guidance as necessary. Attempts to increase appropriate dressing skills for toileting are never taught in isolation, but rather as one component of a chain of toileting behaviors. In these cases, reinforcement is not given to the trainee until he or she completes the final toileting response (i.e., elimination).

As with dressing skills, acceptable approaching skills are generally taught as a component of a chain of behaviors. Approaching behaviors include any response that brings the person to a position where appropriate elimination can occur. This factor is crucial, since many mentally retarded persons, particularly the severely and profoundly mentally retarded, often have no difficulty in eliminating appropriately when they are taken to the bathroom. However, these same individuals have numerous accidents when this procedure is not followed. Apparently, they are failing to approach the toilet in response to physiological cues (e.g., a full bladder).

The two procedures used to teach approaching behaviors are backward and forward chaining. The backward chaining of approach skills involves initially breaking down approaching behavior into components (e.g., approaching toilet from 1 ft., 5 ft., 15 ft., etc.). Training then commences, beginning with the final step of the chain (i.e., elimination). This technique enables the trainer to reinforce the terminal response on every trial while still requiring the client to perform the designated response on his own. As soon as the individual performs the final response reliably, he is required to perform the next step in the chain in addition to the final step before reinforcement is delivered. Gradually, the individual is required to perform a complete chain of behaviors which is longer and more difficult. In teaching approaching behaviors using this method, the end of the program occurs when the trainee is able to chain all components together and approach the toilet from any location, with no prompt from the trainer.

Forward chaining has also been used to train approaching skills to the mentally retarded (Van Wagenen *et al.*, 1969). With this procedure, the individual is required to complete all components of the approaching response in the appropriate sequence. If the individual will not perform the entire chain, the trainer manually guides him through the sequence until the terminal response is performed. This guidance is faded out as the person exhibits more of the chain independently. With this procedure, reinforcement is given initially for an increasing number of completed steps or only for the terminal step.

Literature Review

The following review is not exhaustive, in that a number of studies that trained toileting skills as one component of a large general self-help skill training program are not presented, primarily because of a lack of detail about specific training procedures. Also, technical articles concerned only with an apparatus used in toilet training are not presented, although it is recognized that this equipment may facilitate the implementation of certain techniques. In addition, the reader will note that the object of training, bowel or bladder control, is not specified in many cases. Few studies have focused on bowel training, so the reader should assume that bladder control is the object of training, unless otherwise specified. Finally, the organization of this review is quite rudimentary, because of the unsystematic nature of the research. Therefore, our approach is to present this literature as a continuum, initially reviewing studies using relatively simple techniques with limited objectives and progressing to those studies using more complex training packages with fully independent toileting as the goal.

Several studies, especially some of those published early on, emphasized treating accidental defecations and/or urinations, with little expressed concern for training fully independent toileting (Baumeister & Klosowski, 1965; Levine & Elliott, 1970; Olofson & Karan, 1976; Waye & Melnyr, 1973). In one of the first studies, Baumeister and Klosowski (1965) attempted to apply some of the procedures outlined by Ellis (1963) to 11 profoundly mentally retarded males living in a cottage housing the lowest functioning residents in an institution. Mean chronological age (CA) was approximately 18 years, and mean IQ was 13. Criteria for inclusion as a subject were good mobility, deficient toileting habits, and toileting accidents that were predictable, based on a 30-day sample of behavior. Training was conducted in a dormitory with an adjacent toilet. Stimulus conditions were held constant by isolating the subjects in this area during treatment. Trainers were cottage attendants who received inservice in reinforcement principles. They were instructed to reinforce all adaptive responses associated with using the toilet with edibles or whatever proved to be reinforcing, based on prior experience with each subject. After accidents, subjects were left in wet clothing for at least 45 minutes. Results were not particularly encouraging. The percentage of times the subjects defecated or urinated in the toilet apparently increased, but the degree of improvement was not specified. Only one subject became fully independent in his toileting.

A number of problems exist with this study. The subject sample was a select group, being some of the lowest functioning individuals in the institution, thus limiting generalization to other populations. Baseline data were not presented, making the degree of improvement impossible to determine. In addition, little detail was given about the training methods. The authors also found that a slight change in stimulus conditions (i.e., addition of a daily recreation period) produced a significant decrease in appropriate responses. As a result, they suggest that greater attention to maintaining constant stimulus conditions is warranted. However, such a finding may suggest just the opposite. If training is expected to generalize to other settings, perhaps it should occur in a more normal environment, so that abrupt changes will be less likely to disrupt performance after training is completed.

A toileting program initiated spontaneously by a charge attendant in a residential institution for the mentally retarded is described by Dayan (1964). Twenty-five males ranging from 6 to 12 years of age and with IQs of 30 or below were placed on the toilet every two hours, and rewarded for elimination. The dependent measure, the number of pounds of laundry used per resident each week, showed a decline from 26 pounds at the beginning of the program to approximately 19 pounds after nine months of training.

Using a measure as indirect as the number of pounds of laundry soiled does not allow for a clear evaluation of treatment effects. Frequency counts of the number of accidents and/or appropriate eliminations would have provided a more precise evaluation. In addition, the two-hour "potting" procedure was apparently never terminated, so that any increase in ability to inhibit inappropriate voidings was impossible to determine.

A comparison of conventional training, operant reinforcement principles, and a no-treatment control condition was performed by Hundziak, Maurer, and Watson (1965). Twenty-six severely mentally retarded boys ranging in age from 7 to 14 and with Vineland Social Maturity Scale social quotients between 8 and 33 served as subjects. Each subject had toileting accidents according to staff reports, and random assignments were made to the training groups. The conventional training group was taken to the bathroom several times a day and scolded for having accidents. The operant conditioning group received the same training, with the addition of edible reinforcement, a light, and a tone provided by a special mechanical device attached to the toilet after an appropriate voiding response. The no-treatment group received no training. In addition to the training methods, the two experimental groups spent their days in a special training unit.

With the number of defecations and urinations in the toilet as the dependent measures, performance prior to training and after training was compared, and a posttraining test at the home living unit was performed for the two training groups. A significant increase in appropriate urinations and defecations for the operant conditioning group, a significant increase in appropriate urinations for the no-treatment group, and no significant changes for the conventional training group were found.

Although the authors were able to show the superiority of operant conditioning techniques in increasing the number of voidings in the toilet, one must question the social significance of these findings. The number of toilet accidents was not decreased, and only one subject became better at communicating the need to void, and/or perhaps trainers became more proficient in detecting his needs. One noteworthy point was that the behaviors learned on the special training unit were maintained at the same level when the subjects returned to their home unit, an encouraging finding, given the lack of generalization found by Baumeister and Klosowski (1965); however, no attempt at long-term follow-up was made.

The use of basic operant techniques in the previous studies was extended to the training of a blind, profoundly mentally retarded boy by Waye and Melnyr (1973). The subject was 15 years old, nonverbal except for one or two words, and had been institutionalized since the age of 7. During the week prior to the initiation of training, the frequency and time of all eliminations were charted. During training, the basic procedure was to place the subject on the commode at the times when the subject normally voided, as indicated by the charting record. He remained on the commode until voiding occurred and was then awarded with a pat or a hug by the staff. After accidents, the subject was left in his soiled clothes for one-half hour.

When the amount of time spent on the commode before voiding and the number of accidental defecations were plotted as a function of time in training, a significant improvement was found. By the 10th week of training, the subject voided immediately on being placed on the commode. The mean frequency of accidental eliminations had decreased to less than one per day by the 13th week. The authors also report positive effects of training after one year, although no empirical data are presented to substantiate this claim.

Connally and McGoldrick (1976) attempted to train nine severely mentally retarded children with a mean age of 8.8 years who were participating in a day program. During a one-week baseline period, inappropriate wetting and soiling as well as appropriate eliminations were recorded. During the first two weeks of training the subjects were taken to the toilet at 30-minute intervals, and during the last two weeks, at 45-minute intervals. Subjects were verbally praised when dry and/or when they eliminated appropriately. When wetting or soiling had occurred, or when appropriate elimination was not forthcoming, the subject was ignored.

After training, the baseline conditions were reinstated, and a 14% decrease in wetting accidents, as well as a 75% decrease in soiling accidents, was found. At a six-week follow-up, the improvement in inappropriate urinations had been maintained, but inappropriate defecations had increased to just under the original baseline rate. The authors report that two subjects became fully toilet trained as a result of the training. It is not made clear what "fully toilet trained" means to these authors, but, considering the relatively simple procedures used, it is apparent that these two subjects no longer had accidents; however, there is no evidence that self-initiated toileting occurred.

Olofson and Karan (1976) were successful in eliminating the accidental urinations of a 24-year-old severely mentally retarded woman working in a sheltered workshop. Training proceeded in five phases. A bell-and-pad apparatus was used to signal the occurrence of inappropriate urinations. In Phase I, when the bell sounded indicating an accidental urination, the subject was sent to the bathroom to finish eliminating and to change her clothing. In Phase II the procedure was the same except for the addition of increased fluid intake. In Phase III, the bell was replaced by a light visible only to staff members, purportedly to reduce the external cues used by the subject and to force reliance on internal cues. In Phase IV, fluid intake was reduced to a normal level, and in Phase V the bell-and-pad apparatus was removed. Staff praise was used to reinforce being dry, and the frequency of this praise was decreased as the training continued. Toileting accidents were reduced from an average of 2.87 to zero per day within 11 weeks.

A study reported by Luiselli (1977) focused on training an institutionalized 15-year-old mentally retarded male who apparently had toileting skills but failed to demonstrate them. He had recently developed a "phobia" toward the toilet, as indicated by his avoidance of the commode and the fearful behaviors he exhibited when forced to sit on it, resulting in numerous wetting accidents. Techniques used were reinforcement for voiding in the toilet and time-out and loss of privileges for having accidents. Reinforcers were special outings, edibles, TV watching, etc., which were delivered when a given number of stars or pencil marks were earned for appropriate voiding. Reinforcing events were faded out as appropriate behavior increased. Accidents were followed by 40 minutes of being ignored by the ward staff.

A three-week baseline period resulted in a mean of 15.6 wetting accidents per week. After 28 weeks of training, this rate dropped to zero accidents weekly. Follow-ups of 4, 6, and 12 months were obtained. The subject had one accident during the 4-month follow-up, but no accidents after 6 and 12 months.

Profoundly mentally retarded children with behaviors characteristic of autism were the target of a toilet training program developed by Ando (1977). Five institutionalized males ranging from 5 to 9 years in age were the subjects. They had no expressive language, and few self-care skills. Only two of the five children responded to verbal commands. The children in this subject sample had the lowest level of toileting skills in the entire institution.

A baseline period of one to two months was implemented with time of occurrence and frequency of urinations (1) in places other than the toilet, (2) in the toilet after being prompted, and (3) in the toilet without prompting, serving as the dependent variables. This baseline, as well as subsequent training, was carried out seven days a week, 24 hours a day. For treatment, the children were taken to the toilet every 2 hours, or when they expressed a need to urinate. During the initial stages of training, reinforcers (e.g., social praise, candy, hugs, etc.) were always delivered after the child eliminated in the toilet; however, as training progressed, reinforcers were given only after self-initiated toiletings. Following toileting accidents, aversive consequences such as spankings and scoldings were administered, as well as a 10-minute time-out period.

Although the author reported that his methods were effective compared with other procedures that had been tried with these children, the results reported are not encouraging. Two of the five subjects appeared to self-initiate on 60% of the occasions that they urinated, while the remaining subjects showed little or no improvement in self-initiated toileting. Even after 12 months of training, two of the subjects exhibited no significant improvement.

Perhaps the operant techniques used in the present study are not so effective with children exhibiting autistic behavior as with other mentally retarded children. However, the failure to present enough detail about training techniques precludes any judgment about how effectively these procedures were applied. For example, if prompts to go to the toilet were not faded appropriately, continued dependence on such cues may have resulted. Until these questions are answered, the utility of current toilet-training approaches with "autisticlike" mentally retarded children is questionable.

A number of authors have increasingly focused not only on decreasing toileting accidents, but also on increasing appropriate toileting behaviors with the mentally retarded. These behaviors include approaching the toilet at the appropriate time, removing and replacing clothing, etc., the learning of which leads to fully independent toileting.

Levine and Elliott (1970) attempted to toilet train 103 profoundly retarded residents of a large institution. Unlike previous studies, there was some attempt to train self-initiated toileting by rewarding approach to the toilet and removal of clothing, as well as elimination in the commode. Staff received a minimum of nine hours of training in the practical application of operant conditioning techniques, although no information was given on the exact procedures used. Staff-to-resident ratios never exceeded 1:10.

Unfortunately, only the number of accidental defecations and the amount of laundry used were reported as dependent measures. Accidents were reduced by 59% after 10 weeks of training, compared to baseline, and the amount of soiled clothing was decreased by approximately 42%. If self-initiated toileting was a serious objective of this training, data on the number of independent uses of the toilet would have been valuable, but they were not reported. The authors correctly suggested that improvement may not have been due totally to the operant techniques used, but also to factors such as increased staff awareness and a regular training schedule. In addition, follow-up data needed to evaluate the long-term effects of training were not reported.

Litrownik (1974) trained a 7-year-old profoundly mentally retarded male in the home. Although no IQ or other standardized test data were reported to verify the degree of mental retardation, the subject was nonverbal and unresponsive to simple commands, as well as being incontinent. Training was carried out between the hours of 3:30 and 9:00 P.M., after a one-week baseline period indicated that the subject had four to six accidents per day during this interval. During the first nine weeks of training, the parents used traditional toilet training methods. The subject was prompted to go to the bathroom, lower his pants, and sit on the toilet three times a day. During this period, the subject learned to sit quietly on the commode, which he had never done before; however, despite all attempts to get him to eliminate, he did so only twice during the nine weeks. As a result, a pants alarm apparatus that signaled the occurrence of an accident was employed. As training began, the parents said "potty" and took the subject to the bathroom immediately when the alarm sounded, followed by food and praise. After two days, the same procedure was followed, but in addition the subject had to remove his clothes and sit on the toilet before receiving reinforcement. After eliminations began to occur, reinforcement was given only after eliminating in the commode. As training progressed, the subject emitted anticipatory responses (e.g., pulling at his pants) prior to eliminating, allowing the parents to say "potty" and send him to the bathroom without the aid of the auditory signal. After 35 days, the subject was consistently indicating his need to go to the toilet. To establish more independent behavior, the parents began walking him by the toilet at appropriate times to prompt him to approach the toilet on his own. By the 50th day of training, independent toileting was occurring on a consistent basis.

The results of this study are encouraging. Training was done at home by parents, certainly a desirable state of affairs. The author also reported generalization to other settings, such as school and a relative's home during a two-week visit; however, no data to verify the degree of generalization in these settings were presented. In addition, a five-month follow-up phone call to the parents indicated continued continence on the part of the subject. Again, clear data to substantiate long-term effects were not reported.

A recently institutionalized 4½-year-old severely mentally retarded male was trained by Singh (1976). He was epileptic, obeyed simple commands, and could say "mama" and "papa." Training was carried out 5 days a week during a 5-hour school session. A baseline period was conducted during which the frequency of accidents over a 5-day period preceding the training was assessed. The mean frequency of accidents was five per day. In addition, the child's ability to approach the commode, lower his pants and underwear, sit on the toilet, wipe himself, pull up underwear and pants, and wash and dry his hands was assessed. Unfortunately, no data were presented to indicate the subject's pretraining level on these latter skills.

During training, the teacher employed verbal prompting, manual guidance, and edible and social reinforcement to achieve correct responding. At times when the child was most likely to eliminate, based on behavioral observations and baseline data, the subject was reminded to go to the toilet. Then, using as little prompting and manual guidance as possible, the child was encouraged to walk to the toilet, perform the steps mentioned above, and return to his playroom. If a voiding response was not forthcoming, he remained on the toilet 5 to 10 minutes and then continued with the sequence of appropriate toileting behaviors. After each behavioral component was successfully completed, edibles and/or social praise were given.

During the next stage of training, after the child could toilet himself without manual guidance, he was required to indicate his need to void by pulling the teacher toward the bathroom. When this was done consistently, the child was simply instructed to go to the bathroom at 30 minute intervals. Finally, all instructions and manual guidance were omitted. Rewards were faded out as each component behavior was performed successfully without instructions. Training lasted 14 days, at the end of which no accidents were occurring.

A posttraining, or maintenance, phase was instituted after training. The child was checked before meals and snacks, and praised for being dry. If an accident had occurred, the subject changed his clothes and practiced the full toileting sequence. This maintenance phase lasted for 10 weeks, with only one accident occurring.

Singh's results demonstrated rapid success, which might be expected in a recently institutionalized, young child who may not actually have been severely retarded, as suggested by the behavioral observations reported. If the data on the child's initial ability to perform the approach, dressing, and hand-washing behaviors had been reported, doubts about his initial level of independent toileting would have been resolved. A long-term follow-up assessing the subjects continued ability to toilet himself after all training had ceased is also needed.

Giles and Wolf (1966) attempted to train five profoundly mentally retarded residents of an institution to toilet themselves indpendently. Subjects ranged in age from 6.8 to 18.5 years, and in social age on the Vineland Social Maturity Scale from 1.55 to 2.56 years. The subject with the highest level of adaptive skills could play cooperatively and follow simple commands, but none of the subjects had speech. Some minimal feeding and dressing skills were present in three of the five subjects.

A baseline record of toileting accidents was taken over a 4-week period, followed by a 60-day training period. Training occurred between the hours of 5:30 A.M. and 8:00 P.M., and was carried out in the cottage where the subjects lived. Three basic procedures were used: positive reinforcement for appropriate toileting behavior, aversive consequences for toilet accidents, and shaping. Behaviors such as approaching the toilet, removing underwear, and eliminating in the toilet were rewarded with praise, sweets, physical contact, etc. If positive procedures alone were unsuccessful, accidents were followed by varying aversive events, such as ignoring the subject, tying him to a toilet, and terminating meals, procedures which would be severely restricted at the present time. Closer approximations to self-initiated toileting were required as training continued. In the beginning, rewards were given simply for approaching the toilet; however, sitting on the toilet in addition to approach was required at a later point. Finally, approach, removing clothes, sitting, and eliminating were required for reinforcement in the latter stages of training. Manual guidance was used when necessary to achieve the desired behavior.

In addition to the above procedures, various agents to increase the frequency of bowel movements, such as suppositories and milk of magnesia, were used to increase the number of training experiences and rewardable behaviors. Finally, appropriate bowel movements were trained initially, with appropriate urinations being trained after subjects were consistently defecating in the toilet.

Giles and Wolf (1966) had marked success in training subjects to use the toilet when prompted to do so, but independent toileting was achieved only on an intermittent basis, with one exception. All subjects had some self-initiated toiletings, but training was terminated before a convincing criterion could be reached in all cases. Only one subject self-initiated on every occasion in which elimination occurred in the last nine or more days of training. However, accidents were reduced from approximately 33 during the first 10 days of baseline to approximately 11 during the last 10 days of training.

Giles and Wolf (1966) demonstrated that operant principles are helpful in improving the toileting behavior of mentally retarded persons. In spite of the low functioning level of their subjects, the number of toileting accidents was significantly reduced, and self-initiated and prompted voidings were increased. If their training had continued, no doubt more of the subjects would have become fully independent, as they all appeared to be improving at the end of training. A deficiency in the study was the lack of follow-up data on the degree to which trained behaviors were maintained after training was concluded. Additionally, many of the procedures used might be considered as violations of basic human rights today.

A positive aspect of the Giles and Wolf (1966) study was their reporting of training effects on nighttime toileting accidents. Although exact reports on the frequency of nighttime accidents prior to training were not given, the authors did report that nighttime soiling dropped to zero, even in those cases in which the subject was regularly restrained to the bed at night.

One significant development in training toileting skills was made by Van Wagenen, Meyerson, Kerr, and Mahoney (1969). Instead of beginning with placing a subject on the commode at frequent intervals and rewarding voidings, and then gradually adding dressing, approaching, etc., to the chain of behaviors, their training procedure emphasized training the child to perform the final criterion behavior (i.e., inhibiting voiding, approaching the commode, removing clothes, voiding, replacing clothes) from the very beginning of training. In addition, training was carried out when a voiding response naturally occurred. To do this, subjects wore a pants alarm in their normal living environment. At the onset of voiding, the pants alarm sounded and the following events occurred in sequence: The trainer approached the child and yelled "No!" (which was incorporated as a method to startle the child and inhibit voiding); the trainer escorted the child to the bathroom; the child was prompted with manual guidance to remove clothes; the child was encouraged to continue voiding; the child was prompted to replace clothes. This sequence was followed in a rapid, forward-moving manner, and the child was reinforced at the end of the complete chain of behavior.

In the Van Wagenen *et al.* (1969) study, eight profoundly mentally retarded subjects were trained to be fully independent in urinating. They ranged in age from four to nine years and had limited speech. However, several could lower and pull up their pants and respond to basic commands, and all were ambulatory. A baseline period of 5 days was used to determine the initial toileting skills of the subjects. During training, each child was fitted with a pants alarm. Three children were trained simultaneously for a 3-to 4-hour period, during which time each child was encouraged to drink large quantities of liquids. In addition, training was carried out in a small playroom that adjoined a bathroom, utilizing the procedure discussed above.

It was found that each subject reached criterion performance (i.e., independently walked to the toilet, removed clothes, urinated in commode, replaced clothes). The number of training sessions required to reach this level ranged from 5 to 22. Follow-ups on individual subjects ranged from 3 weeks to 7 months (eight of nine subjects). Little regression was noted, although follow-up data were based on subjective reports, thus decreasing their validity. The experimenters did note that any periods of incontinence were related to a parent's prompting the child to go to the bathroom, leading the child to depend on this prompting. When the prompting ceased, the accidents stopped.

Mahoney, Van Wagenen, and Meyerson (1971) used a procedure similar to that of Van Wagenen *et al.* (1969), with one major modification. Prior to actually having the subject urinate in the commode, he or she was trained to approach the commode and remove his or her clothing in response to an auditory signal, which was later generated by the pants alarm. This modification was justified by the authors because of the fact that voiding responses are low in frequency, resulting in a waste of training time if treatment occurs only at the onset of a reflex voiding.

Subjects were three normal and five mentally retarded children (data are reported only for the mentally retarded children). Four of the mentally retarded subjects were four years old, and the fifth was nine. Their IQ scores ranged from 10 to 45, and only one child had expressive language. All subjects were found to have toileting accidents consistently during baseline.

Training time ranged from 17 to 48 hours, with independent toileting being achieved in four of the five subjects. Follow-up was performed for only one of the mentally retarded subjects. Six months after training, the child averaged four accidents per week. Experimenter observation indicated that the parent was prompting the child excessively, creating a dependence on these cues.

Any improvement over the basic forward-moving training of Van Wagenen *et al.* (1969) produced by the Mahoney *et al.* (1971) modifications was not apparent. Except for minor discrepancies, training appeared to proceed no more rapidly than with the former technique. Certainly, more research comparing the two techniques is needed. Also, the limited amount of follow-up data provided was unfortunate, since generalizations about treatment effects based on one subject are difficult to make.

To date, the most extensive toilet training package for the mentally retarded has been proposed by Azrin and Foxx (1971). The package involves an intense application of several behavioral procedures. First, the procedure involved positive reinforcement for appropriate voiding and related behaviors. Second, electronic urine-sensitive devices which serve to signal the occurrence of voiding to the trainer and/or the trainee were used. Third, an increase in the operant level of the eliminations was effected by giving the mentally retarded individual large amounts of fluid. Fourth, trainees were taught dressing and undressing skills. Fifth, toilet approaching behaviors were taught. Finally, the package included an overcorrection procedure which involved punishment for the toileting accidents. The rationale for this broad and complex procedure is stated succinctly by Foxx and Azrin (1973): "[N]ormal toileting is not simply a matter of learning to respond to bladder and bowel pressures by relaxing, but rather is a complex operant and social learning process that has been hindered by a reduced learning capacity and by institutionalization" (p. 89).

In an early attempt to toilet train the mentally retarded using Full Cleanliness Training, Azrin and Foxx (1971) trained nine incontinent institutionalized mentally retarded individuals ranging in age from 20 to 62 years. These persons had been institutionalized from 6 to 45 years, and their IQs ranged from 7 to 45. A baseline measure of incontinence was obtained over a three-day period, after which the subjects were randomly assigned to either a control or an experimental group. The subjects were matched on the number of accidents during baseline. To ensure that all eliminations would be immediately detected by the trainer, a pants alarm and a toilet seat alarm were used. When the subjects urinated or defecated, either in their pants or in the toilet, detec.ion was immediate. (For a more detailed description of this apparatus, see Azrin, Bugle, and O'Brien, 1971.) All subjects were required to stay in the toilet area for the entire 8-hour daily session. To increase the frequency of urinating, which is a low-frequency response, each half hour the subjects were given as much liquid as they could consume. Initially, the subject stayed in a chair in front of the toilet, and every half-hour was required to sit on the toilet for 20 minutes, or until an elimination occurred, whichever came first.

To increase the number of appropriate eliminations, subjects were given both edible and social reinforcers every five minutes while their pants remained dry and immediately following voiding in the toilet. To decrease toileting accidents, when an inappropriate elimination occurred Full Cleanliness Training was used. The subject was verbally reprimanded, shaken, and required to take a shower, change clothes, wash out the dirty clothes, and hang them up. When the subject returned to the toilet area, he was required to clean the soiled area with a mop. This procedure was followed by a one hour time-out period during which the subject received no edible or social praise, or fluids. To ensure that the subjects could independently toilet themselves, Azrin and Foxx (1971) taught pulling up and pulling down pants and underwear for those who lacked these skills. Manual guidance and fading were the primary techniques used to achieve this goal.

Following the successful completion of this training phase, a post-training maintenance phase was implemented. The subjects were returned to their normal daily routine, but they were checked six times daily for toileting accidents. If the subject was dry, social praise was delivered in addition to scheduled snacks or meals. If the resident had an accident, he or she was reprimanded and given Full Cleanliness Training. In addition, the scheduled snack was omitted or the meal was delayed. Gradually the daily dry checks were faded to the point that the subjects were never checked; however, detection of an accident continued to result in Full Cleanliness Training.

The number of accidents was reduced from two per day to one every fourth day for each subject. Accidents were reduced by 90% for the nine subjects. This low frequency of daytime toileting accidents continued for at least four months following the termination of training, with the number of training sessions ranging from 1 to 14 days, with a mean of 4 days.

The identification of a method for toilet training profoundly and severely mentally retarded individuals in only several days is indeed an important breakthrough. Before widespread use of these procedures can be recommended, however, they require more analysis. First, the authors discuss the importance of toilet training the profoundly retarded. However, their study used individuals whose IQs ranged into the moderate range of mental retardation. The level of mental retardation is crucial in predicting the success of training procedures. Another concern with this study is the immediate effects of training. By the end of the first day, accidents had been reduced approximately 75%. Because of such an immediate change, one must question whether we are dealing with learning or performance. Certainly there is a significant difference between teaching toileting skills and motivating the individual to exhibit skills previously acquired, but not currently being performed.

Subsequent to this study, Foxx and Azrin (1973) wrote a book which more thoroughly described the procedure used in their 1971 study. Furthermore, they proposed an additional component to be used following an accident: positive practice. This latter procedure follows Full Cleanliness Training and consists of having the subject repeatedly approach and sit on the toilet, thereby giving the individual experience performing the desired behavior sequence.

Trott (1977) used the basic Foxx and Azrin (1973) procedure in attempting to toilet train an 11-year-old mentally retarded boy, whose level of mental retardation was unspecified. Prior to the onset of training, the child was wet every hour except one during pants checks for a five-day baseline taken during the day at school. By the third day of training, the child was returned to the regular classroom following completion of the intensive toileting procedure proposed by Azrin and Foxx (1971). After reentering the classroom, the child had "occasional accidents" (Trott, 1977, p. 338).

It is difficult to evaluate Trott's results because of the limited information furnished. Although the child was reported to be mentally retarded, no mention of his level of retardation was made. The anecdotal description of the frequency of toileting accidents also limits the ability to analyze the results of the study. Following the completion of training, the child was placed in the classroom, where he began having accidents, with each accident being followed by positive practice or overcorrection. No explanation was offered on the effects of training for reducing the number of accidents. This problem raises the question of whether the effects of the toileting program actually generalized to the classroom. The author stated further that the effects of toileting had generalized to the home, however, no data were presented, and there was no mention of the long-term effects of training. Although no one would question the applied utility of this case study for the individual involved, its importance for the further understanding of toilet training of the mentally retarded is questionable.

Sadler and Merkert (1977) compared the Foxx and Azrin method with a no-training group and a scheduling group which was taken to the toilet four times a day. They used 14 profoundly mentally retarded children who had never been involved in a toilet-training program. These children were randomly assigned to one of the three conditions. Following a one-week baseline, Phase I of training involved exposing subjects to one of the three aforementioned conditions which lasted four months, with assessments made at three and four months. Phase II involved taking half the no-training group and all the scheduling group and training them using the Foxx and Azrin method. All the other children continued in their original groups. This phase lasted two months and was then followed by a return to baseline for one week.

The results of the study were impressive. During Phase I, children in the Foxx and Azrin group reduced the number of toileting accidents by nearly 90%, the scheduling groups reduced toileting accidents by 40%, and the no-training group failed to change. During Phase II, those children who continued in the Foxx and Azrin group had a continued reduction in toileting accidents. Those children who had shifted from the scheduling groups to the Foxx and Azrin groups exhibited better than an 80% decrease in the number of accidents. Finally, those children who had previously been in the no-treatment group and then shifted to the Foxx and Azrin group showed a 75% decrease in toileting accidents. Although these results appear to offer more evidence for increase the in effectiveness of the Foxx and Azrin (1973) approach, one must question the adequacy of the dependent measure. Successful toilet training was defined in terms of a reduction in the number of times the child was found to have wet pants. This measure is not a sensitive index of continence if independent toileting is the goal. No data were presented indicating the number of residents who achieved fully independent toileting. Furthermore, no data were presented on the maintenance of the attained skills. In addition to assessing the effects of different types of toilet training, Sadler and Merkert (1977) also addressed the issue of training costs. They found that, though the Foxx and Azrin approach was more effective than scheduling, it involved significantly more staff time. The mean number of hours required to train a child using the Foxx and Azrin method was 35.

In an attempt to cross-validate the Foxx and Azrin (1973) approach, a British research group (Smith *et al.*, 1975) conducted a study with five profoundly mentally retarded adults who were ambulatory but nonverbal. The authors used the basic procedure described earlier in the Azrin and Foxx (1971) study. The results of this study were impressive, in that the frequency of wetting accidents was decreased by 84%. However, more crucial was the increase in the number of self-initiations from zero during baseline to a high of nearly 100% during training. During the maintenance phase, self-initiations fell to approximately 50%, before leveling off. At the final follow-up (30 weeks), four subjects continued to improve, and the fifth individual exhibited a slight relapse.

As Smith *et al.* (1975) point out, certain modifications in the original Foxx and Azrin method (Azrin & Foxx, 1971; Foxx & Azrin, 1973) were necessary. First, time-out periods following accidents were shorter than the 60-minute time-out used by Azrin and Foxx (1971). Second, Smith *et al.* (1975) stated that they failed to follow strictly the prescribed Full Cleanliness Training procedure. Unfortunately, the authors did not detail how they modified the procedure, and this limits the utility of the promising results.

Bettison *et al.* (1976) also attempted a cross-validation of the Foxx and Azrin approach, in this case with an Australian population. Subjects were eight moderately to profoundly mentally retarded individuals who ranged in age from 12 to 50 years and had been institutionalized from 3 to 45 years. Training was conducted by two to four trainers, including the senior author, in addition to ward personnel. They employed the Foxx and Azrin (1973) procedure.

Five subjects reached the training criterion (9 out of 10 successive self-initiated eliminations) and advanced to the maintenance phase, which took place in the normal ward setting. Maintenance lasted until the subject went 14 days without an accident, or for six months, whichever occurred first. One of the five subjects failed to remain continent during the maintenance phase. Eight to 11 months following the withdrawal of the training, a three-day follow-up was conducted. The four residents who graduated from maintenance were observed every hour for dry pants. Only two residents continued to self-initiate while having no accidents.

Smith (1979) conducted a study in which he compared three toilet training procedures: (1) a modified Foxx and Azrin (1971) procedure, (2) group toileting procedure, and (3) an individual timing procedure. The first program was similar to the procedure used by Foxx and Azrin (1971), with the exception that Full Cleanliness Training (i.e., overcorrection) was not used; instead, a forceful reprimand followed by a 10-minute time-out period was applied.

The second training condition in the Smith (1979) study involved a group approach similar to those informally used in many institutions. Every 45 minutes the subjects were guided to the bathroom. If the resident urinated in the toilet, reinforcement was delivered immediately. When an accident occurred on the war, the resident was ignored for five minutes before the wet pants were changed. Prompts to use the toilet were faded when possible.

The third condition involved a procedure somewhat similar to that used by Mahoney *et al.* (1971) and Van Wagenen *et al.* (1969). During training, the subject was seated near the toilet and reinforced every five minutes for dry pants. Every half hour the subject was prompted to the toilet, using physical, verbal, gestural, and radio-controlled alarm prompts. These prompts were then faded out as the subject began exhibiting self-initiated responses. Gradually, the residents were moved farther and farther away from the toilet. When accidents occurred, the individual was reprimanded and prompted to use the toilet. When further urination occurred, reinforcement was immediate. Each of the programs was conducted from 8:00 A.M. to 5:00 P.M., seven days a week.

Each training condition involved five institutionalized children ranging in age from 5 to 18 years and in social age from .94 to 2.2 years. During the 12 weeks of training, the two individual approaches produced significantly better results than the group-training method. By the end of the 12th week, the modified Foxx and Azrin (1971) approach yielded the greatest reduction in incontinence, 95%. The individual approach using the radio-controlled prompting device showed a more modest decrease in urinary accidents, approximately 80%. Finally, the group approach resulted in a 40%–50% reduction in accidents. It should be noted that, although the group approach was less effective than the individual methods, it required approximately one-half the staff time.

It is unfortunate that Smith (1979) attributed so little importance to the long-term effects of the three training procedures. He stated that it was sufficient to know how many children were continent at the termination of training. A study purporting to evaluate the relative efficiency of different training procedures should acknowledge the crucial role of long-term training effectiveness.

Smith and Smith (1977) conducted a study to assess the relationships of chronological age and social age in the success of a modified Azrin and Foxx (1971) training procedure. Procedures were identical to Azrin and Foxx (1971) with the exception of Full Cleanliness Training. Following a toileting accident, the trainees were reprimanded and given time-out from reinforcement. Thirteen subjects were used, ranging in age from 6 to 52 years, with social ages ranging from 1.24 to 2.59 years. Based upon these ages, subjects were assigned to one of three categories: (1) Old-Low social age, (2) Young-Low social age, or (3) Young-High social age. The older (25–56 years) subjects were significantly less successful than the younger subjects (6–17 years) in acquiring toileting skills. Whereas Young-Low social-age subjects demonstrated a 100% reduction in wetting accidents by the 17th week, four of five Old-Low social-age subjects had not attained this level by the same time. It was further demonstrated that social age was positively correlated with the speed of attaining urinary continence. Subjects in the Young-High social-age group attained total continence by the 9th week, whereas subjects in the Young-Low social-age group did not reach this level until the 17th week of training.

Follow-up data were also collected. For the Old-Low social-age subjects, the results indicated they had regressed somewhat, but were still significantly more continent than prior to training. For the Young-Low social-age subjects, three had maintained full continence, and two had regressed minimally, having one accident per week. Finally, for the Young-High social-age group, all subjects maintained their toileting skills.

The authors strongly suggest that retarded individuals who are young have a greater probability of successfully responding to toilet-training procedures, and may have a greater chance of maintaining acquired skills. Also, those individuals with lower social ages, like older individuals, have more difficulty in acquiring and maintaining toileting skills. These conclusions must, however, be viewed with skepticism, due to the fact that follow-up measures were taken from 6 to 18 months after training, with no indication of when the different groups were evaluated. Therefore, it is difficult to compare the results for the three groups. Had the groups been assessed at the same time, the results would be far more conclusive.

Luiselli, Reisman, Helfen, and Pemberton (1979) toilet trained two retarded children in a classroom setting using a modified Azrin and Foxx

(1971) approach. One subject was 7 years old with a social age of 1.7 years, and the other was 9 years old with a social age of 1.8 years.

For three hours a day, four days a week, the subject sat on the toilet once every 30 minutes for a period of 20 minutes, or until urination occurred. Subjects were reinforced for appropriate eliminations and for having dry pants between placements on the toilet. Accidents were followed by Full Cleanliness Training. However, due to limited afternoon staff, the intensive one-to-one training was confined to the morning hours. In the afternoon, a maintenance procedure was used whereby the children were returned to the classroom. They were checked every 15 minutes for dry pants. The children were reinforced if dry, and given Full Cleanliness Training if wet.

Following a 24- to 26-day baseline, intensive training was begun, being terminated when the subject eliminated appropriately 70% of the time (when taken to the toilet) during the 3-hour session. This level of continence was attained in 14 days for the first subject and 13 days for the second, and was then followed by maintenance. At this point, both subjects were exposed to the same contingencies during the morning and the afternoon sessions. Both children stayed in the classroom all day and were taken to the bathroom five times during this period, with appropriate voidings being reinforced as usual. Also, each subject was checked for dry pants at 15-minute intervals. Dry pants resulted in reinforcement, and wet pants resulted in Full Cleanliness Training. This training phase lasted 20 days for the first subject and 22 days for the second.

At termination of this phase, the schedule for taking the subjects to the toilet was four times daily (same as during baseline). Accidents were followed by Full Cleanliness Training, and appropriate urinations were followed by reinforcement. This phase lasted 13 days for the first subject and 28 days for the second.

The goal of increasing appropriate eliminations and decreasing accidents was attained. By the end of training, the first subject was eliminating 60% of the time when placed on the toilet, and the second subject 30% of the time. Accidents, meanwhile, were reduced from greater than one per day to less than one per six days for both subjects. A one-year follow-up suggested that these results were maintained. Although the goals of this study were achieved, one must question the practical implications of training. Following more than a month of fairly intensive training, toileting accidents had been brought under control, but only when the subjects were taken to the bathroom and seated on the commode. It would have been beneficial if in fact an assessment of the change in self-initiated toiletings had been conducted, even though self-initiation had not been trained directly.

Song, Song, and Grant (1976) demonstrated the importance of generalization and long term follow-up of toilet training using a modified Azrin and Foxx (1971) procedure. The authors report training a 16-year old, profoundly retarded blind boy to self-initiate appropriate urination in the toilet. Initially, a two-week baseline was conducted, followed by 23 days of training at a school within a residential facility for the mentally retarded. Training was essentially the same procedure described by Azrin and Foxx (1971), with minor modifications which were dictated by the blindness of the client. Unlike the Azrin and Foxx (1971) procedure, that of Song *et al.* broke training down into four phases, with each phase requiring fewer physical and verbal prompts. Curiously, the training phase was terminated while the client was continuing to exhibit an average of one accident per day. The authors made no attempt to explain the basis for their decision to terminate the training phase, which was immediately followed by a maintenance phase lasting 25 weeks. During maintenance, the client was given normal classroom contingencies in addition to food and social reinforcement following self-initiation of appropriate voiding. During the first six weeks of maintenance, the client averaged approximately one accident per week, at which time accidents ceased totally for the remainder of the maintenance phase.

Concurrent with the classroom training, data were being collected on accidents in the living cottage, where each resident was taken to the toilet on a regular basis, but with no attempt at training. The results obtained in the cottage were most revealing. By the end of training in the classroom, accidents in the cottage had been reduced to zero, but had increased to one to nine per week immediately upon initiation of the maintenance phase in the classroom. After about 10 weeks, a maintenance procedure was introduced in the cottage setting. Within two weeks, daytime toileting accidents had been reduced to zero.

It is impossible to draw definitive conclusions regarding the effects of training on cottage behavior, since no baseline data were obtained. It appears that, although some success was achieved, the intensity and duration of the training procedure forces one to question the cost effectiveness. Another concern is that, although the authors claimed to have effected complete toilet training, edible and social reinforcement was never faded out. Fully independent toileting can occur only when artificial contingencies have been replaced by naturally occurring ones.

Doleys and Arnold (1975) applied Azrin and Foxx's (1971) Full Cleanliness Training in an attempt to alleviate encopresis (i.e., soiling). The study was conducted with an 8-year-old trainable mentally retarded child. The child reportedly had urinary continence, and soiled himself only in certain settings. Furthermore, clear indications existed that the child had developed a phobia of sitting on the toilet. Before attempting to eliminate the occurrences of soiling, the authors focused on the phobia.

During one day of training, the child's behavior was shaped to approach and sit on the toilet. They used another child as a model, with the retarded child being reinforced for imitating successive approximations to the toilet. By the end of the day, (i.e., 7 hours), the child would sit on the toilet at the request of the mother. The following week, training was extended to the school setting, where within a three hour period the child was sitting on the toilet at the teacher's request. Elimination of soiling immediately followed the treatment of the phobia. The parents checked the child's pants every 15 to 20 minutes and reinforced him if they were clean. Second, they had the child sit on the toilet every hour for 10 minutes, reinforcing him for attempts to defecate. Third, every time the child went to the toilet, he was asked if he had to defecate. This questioning was done to increase the child's awareness of internal stimuli. Located in the bathroom was a selected toy which could be played with following defecation. Also, a data chart was located in the bathroom, and following each defecation a square was colored in. After attaining the first toy, the child could earn a second toy by coloring 20 squares. Following a fecal accident, Full Cleanliness Training was used. The parents would reprimand the child and then require him to clean his clothes for at least 15 minutes, following which he had to bathe himself.

In addition to a significant decrease in soiling accidents, an increase in bowel movements in the toilet was found by the end of the 16th week of treatment, at which time accidents had been virtually eliminated, as compared with the baseline mean of three per week. At a 10-week follow-up, fecal continence was maintained. However, 24 weeks following treatment, accidents had increased to one a week. The authors attribute this finding to the failure of the mother to carry out Full Cleanliness Training following accidents. Also, the teacher had lost control in getting the child to sit on the toilet at school.

In analyzing this study, many questions arise. First, the child is described as trainable mentally retarded; unfortunately, no other information is given regarding his functioning level. The second question concerns the effect of treatment for the phobia. From the author's accounts, the phobia appeared to be the major factor in the encopresis. However, no attempt was made to analyze the effects of treating the phobia independently of the encopresis training. The authors state, "Because the toilet phobia training occurred at the same time as the introduction of Full Cleanliness Training it is difficult to determine the relative effects of each" (Doleys & Arnold, 1975, p. 16). This confounding is even more disturbing, given that on initiation of the two training programs, an immediate increase in the number of bowel movements in the toilet and a decrease in accidents was seen. Consequently, it is impossible to draw any definitive conclusions regarding the effects of either the phobia training or the encopresis training as separate treatment techniques. This confounding may not be crucial, considering the applied nature of the problem, but in terms of furthering our understanding of incontinence in the mentally retarded, it is unfortunate.

Critical Issues

Methodological problems were frequently mentioned in the research reviewed, and the practitioner about to embark on a training program should be sensitive to these problems before choosing treatment procedures. A serious problem evident in the toilet-training literature is the failure to provide enough information about the subject sample, such as specific adaptive behaviors present before training. This information can be used to substantiate the level of retardation indicated, as well as to provide the reader with information useful in predicting generalization in the population in which he or she is interested. Trainer characteristics, particularly the amount of training in behavioral techniques, should also be reported, as well as significant detail about the training methods employed, so that replication is possible.

Inappropriate dependent variables were often used to measure the effects of training in the articles presented. If self-initiated toileting is the goal of training, the number of accidents alone is an inadequate measure, since the number of accidents could decrease owing to increased vigilance on the part of the trainer, rather than the subject's increased sensitivity to bowel and bladder cues. We suggest that, if self-initiated toileting is the goal of a training program, both accidents and the frequency of self-initiated toiletings should be recorded.

A final major methodological criticism is the failure to provide appropriate control procedures to establish that any change in the dependent variable results from the manipulation of the independent variable rather than any extraneous factors. We would suggest that many of the more sophisticated behavioral analysis procedures developed in recent years (e.g., the multiple baseline procedure), if sometimes difficult to carry out in applied settings, are worth the extra effort required, because of the additional confidence they produce in the reliability of the findings.

A number of practical issues important to the clinician and applied researcher seem evident, based on this survey of the toilet training literature. A primary issue is determining the objectives of a toilet training program. With the simple application of environmental contingencies, the clinician is virtually assured of a decrease in accidents, even with the lowest functioning individual; however, increased effort on the part of the trainer may produce closer approximations of fully independent toileting. With the reported success of program packages such as those described by Azrin and Foxx (1971) and Van Wagenen *et al.* (1969), perhaps fully independent toileting should be the goal of training. Certainly this goal should not be quickly abandoned, considering the evidence.

The actual costs in terms of staff or parental time and training is also a crucial issue in choosing training procedures. Complex training programs (e.g., Azrin & Foxx, 1971) require large numbers of staff and long hours. Because of this, it is important for applied researchers to try to isolate the effective components of training programs. Constituent analysis may indicate that some aspects of a program are not active in producing behavior change, and elimination of the excesses may reduce costs.

As in any applied research, the persistence of toileting skills when conditions that existed during training are changed (e.g., trainer, location, etc.) is crucial. Little value can be given to a procedure which improves toileting skills during training but which results in deterioration in these skills on movement to a different setting. Fortunately, most training procedures reported addressed this problem, with the individual being taught in the environment where he or she normally lives. Although several studies conducted early training in an isolated area with special trainers, they later moved training to the regular ward with the usual staff.

The issue of the long-term effects of training has not been as adequately addressed as has generalization of training to other settings. Many studies presented no data following training (Baumeister & Klosowski, 1965; Giles & Wolf, 1966; Levine & Elliott, 1970). Other researchers state that they collected follow-up data, but the data are anecdotal (Litrownik, 1974; Van Wagenen *et al.*, 1969). However, several studies have more adequately assessed the long-term effects of training. For example, Azrin and Foxx (1971) had excellent success in suppressing toilet accidents up to five months following training. However, this finding is somewhat misleading, since the subjects were continually reinforced for having dry pants and punished for accidents throughout the five-month period. Therefore, one could argue that training was still in effect. No training contingencies should be used if long-term efforts are being studied—or it should be specified that maintenance procedures are necessary to maintain trained skills at acceptable levels.

The ethical issues raised by certain training procedures must also be considered. In the Azrin and Foxx (1971) procedure, for example, the number of punishing events used is of particular concern. Following a toileting accident, the individual is reprimanded, bodily shaken, forced to shower, wash soiled clothes, and mop the floor. Furthermore, some studies using this approach require the individual to go through positive practice,wherein he is required to practice going to the toilet for as long as an hour (Foxx & Azrin, 1973). Anyone who has witnessed an individual during this procedure can attest to its apparent aversiveness. Certainly this method is no more questionable than some others (Ando, 1977; Giles & Wolf, 1966); however, more research is needed to substantiate the effectiveness of such training procedures before they can be justified as the least aversive method of attaining a clinically relevant goal.

The training package developed by Van Wagenen *et al.* (1969) offers a viable alternative to the Azrin and Foxx procedure, particularly when limited resources and punishment considerations are taken into account. The results attained were impressive. All five profoundly retarded subjects were totally toilet trained; independently walking to the commode, removing clothes, voiding, and replacing clothing after several days of training. Also, rather than involving eight hours a day of training, each daily session lasted only three hours. This compares favorably with the Azrin and Foxx (1971) study which effected a 90% reduction in toileting errors at the end of 12 days. However, that study possessed two residents who were not toilet trained by that time. The crucial point to be made is that success in toilet training the retarded has been found using a procedure which involves staff time (i.e., three vs. eight hours) and no significantly less staff time punishment techniques—which are, at best, questionable. Before we accept a procedure as complex and serious as the Azrin and Foxx approach, we should be certain other procedures are not as effective.

CONCLUSIONS

Much has been learned regarding training toileting skills in mentally retarded persons since Ellis' 1963 article. Researchers have demonstrated that a reduction of toileting accidents can be achieved. Furthermore, several studies have demonstrated that fully independent toileting skills can also be taught, using more complex training packages. However, the sophisticated research needed to establish, with confidence, the most efficient method of toilet training retarded persons has yet to be conducted.

A definite need currently exists for constituent analysis of the more complex training packages represented in the literature (e.g., Azrin & Foxx, 1971; Van Wagen *et al.*, 1969). It may be that through such an analysis those components of the package which could be omitted and consequently reduce cost and time consumption could be identified. Direct comparisons of different training procedures are also needed. Results of published procedures are difficult to compare, since they typically differ in subject populations, trainer experience, length of training, location of training, dependent measures, etc. Only through a well-controlled comparative study can one draw definitive conclusions concerning the relative effectiveness of different procedures.

The practitioner who is interested in training toileting skills in the mentally retarded should consider several factors when attempting to choose an appropriate training package. First, one's goals should be considered. If a reduction in accidents is sufficient, then a complex procedure which focuses on several behaviors may not be necessary. However, if the goal is to develop fully independent toileting skills, then one must be prepared to use a procedure which is complex and targets several behaviors, and which demands a significant expenditure of time and effort.

If one chooses to teach fully independent toileting skills, certain practical issues should be addressed. First, staff issues must be considered. Whether a parent, aide, or professional person conducts the training, the individual must have extensive supervision and be highly motivated. Second, the resident–staff ratio needs to be as low as possible. Third, the trainer should consider the client's characteristics, especially adaptive behaviors. For example, the probability of success in teaching independent toileting skills if the client cannot follow simple commands is low. Finally, consideration must be given to the application of aversive contingencies. In many settings, the use of any type of punishment is prohibited or greatly limited. In such situations one may be forced to use a training package that does not use punishment or to modify a procedure that does.

The choice of a toilet training program cannot be based solely on the results of experimental studies. Rather, the choice should be made after weighing a multitude of methodological and practical variables in addition to the reported success of any given procedure. This will enable the practitioner to develop and implement a procedure which is suited to his or her specific needs and limitations.

REFERENCES

ANDO, H. Training autistic children to urinate in the toilet through operant conditioning techniques. *Journal of Autism and Childhood Schizophrenia*, 1977, *7*(2), 151–163.

AZRIN, N., & FOXX, R. A rapid method of toilet training the institutionalized retarded. *Journal of Applied Behavioral Analysis*, 1971, *4*, 89–99.

AZRIN, N., BUGLE, C., & O'BRIEN, F. Behavioral engineering: Two apparatuses for toilet training retarded children. *Journal of Applied Behavioral Analysis*, 1971, *4*(3), 249–253.

BAUMEISTER, A., & KLOSOWSKI, R. An attempt to group toilet train severely retarded patients. *Mental Retardation*, 1965, *3*(6), 24–26.

BETTISON, S., DAVISON, D., TAYLOR, P., & FOX, B. The long-term effects of a toilet training programme for the retarded: A pilot study. *Australian Journal of Mental Retardation*, 1976, *4*(4), 18–35.

CONNALLY, J., & MCGOLDRICK, M. Behavior modification toilet training procedure in a special care unit. *Child Care, Health and Development*, 1976, *2*, 267–272.

DAYAN, M. Toilet training retarded children in a state residential institution. *Mental Retardation*, 1964, *2*, 116–117.

DOLEYS, D. M. Behavioral treatments for nocturnal enuresis in children: A review of the recent literature. *Psychological Bulletin*, 1977, *84*(6), 30–34.

DOLEYS, D., & ARNOLD, S. Treatment of childhood encopresis: Full Cleanliness Training. *Mental Retardation*, 1975, *13*(6), 14–16.

ELLIS, N. R. Toilet training the severely defective patient: An S–R reinforcement analysis. *American Journal of Mental Deficiency*, 1963, *68*, 99–103.

FOXX, R. M., & AZRIN, N. H. *Toilet training the retarded: A rapid program for day and night time independent toileting*. Champaign, Ill.: Research Press, 1973.

GILES, D., & WOLF, M. Toilet training institutionalized, severe retardates: An application of behavior modification techniques. *American Journal of Mental Deficiency*, 1966, *70*, 766–780.

HUNDZIAK, M., MAURER, R., & WATSON, L. Operant conditioning in toilet training of severely retarded boys. *American Journal of Mental Deficiency*, 1965, *70*, 120–124.

LEVINE, M., & ELLIOTT, C. Toilet training for profoundly retarded with a limited staff. *Mental Retardation*, 1970, 766–780.

LITROWNIK, A. A method for home training an incontinent child. *Journal of Behavior Therapy and Experimental Psychiatry*, 1974, *5*, 77–80.

LUISELLI, J. Case Report: An attendant administered contingency management programme for the treatment of a toilet phobia. *Journal of Mental Deficiency Research*, 1977, *21*(4), 283–288.

LUISELLI, J. L., REISMAN, J., HELFEN, C. S., & PEMBERTON, B. W. Toilet training in the classroom: An adaptation of Azrin and Foxx's rapid toilet training procedure. *Behavioral Engineering*, 1979, *5*, 89–93.

MAHONEY, K., VAN WAGENEN, R., & MEYERSON, L. Toilet training of normal and retarded children. *Journal of Applied Behavioral Analysis*, 1971, *4*, 173–181.
OLOFSON, G., & KARAN, O. Toilet-training in the sheltered workshop. Why not? *Rehabilitation Counseling Bulletin*, 1976, *20*(1), 69–72.
OSARCHUK, M. Operant methods of toilet-behavior training of the severely and profoundly retarded: A review. *Journal of Special Education*, 1973, *7*, 423–437.
RENTFROW, R., & RENTFROW, D. Studies related to toilet training of the mentally retarded. *American Journal of Occupational Therapy*, 1969, *23*(5), 425–430.
SADLER, W., & MERKERT, F. Evaluating the Foxx and Azrin toilet training procedure for retarded children in a day training center. *Behavior Therapy*, 1977, *8*(3), 499–500.
SINGH, N. Toilet training a severely retarded non-verbal child. *Australian Journal of Mental Retardation*, 1976, *4*(1), 15–18.
SMITH, P. A comparison of different methods of toilet training the mentally handicapped. *Behavior Research and Therapy*, 1979, *17*(1), 33–43.
SMITH, P., & SMITH, R. Chronological age and social age as factors in intensive daytime toilet training of institutionalized mentally retarded individuals. *Journal of Behavior Therapy and Experimental Psychiatry*, 1977, *8*(3), 269–273.
SMITH, R. S., BRITTON, P. G., JOHNSON, M., & THOMAS, D. Problems involved in toilet training of institutionalized mentally retarded individuals. *Behavior Research and Therapy*, 1975, *3*, 301–302.
SONG, A. Y., SONG, R. H., & GRANT, P. A. Toilet training in school and its transfer in the living unit. *Journal of Behavior Therapy and Experimental Psychiatry*, 1976, *7*, 281–284.
TROTT, M. Application of Foxx and Azrin's toilet training method for the retarded in a school programme. *Education and Training of the Mentally Retarded*, 1977, *12*, 336–338.
VAN WAGENEN, R., MEYERSON, L., KERR, N., & MAHONEY, K. Field trials of a new procedure for toilet training. *Journal of Experimental Child Psychology*, 1969, *8*, 147–159.
WAYE, M., & MELNYR, W. Toilet training of a blind retarded boy by operant conditioning. *Journal of Behavior Therapy and Experimental Psychiatry*, 1973, *4*, 267–268.

3 Self-Injurious Behavior

An Analysis of Behavior Management Techniques

STEPHEN R. SCHROEDER, CAROLYN S. SCHROEDER, JOHANNES ROJAHN, AND JAMES A. MULICK

INTRODUCTION

Defining self-injurious behavior (SIB) presents some difficulties. It has been broadly described as behavior that produces injury to the individual's own body (Tate & Baroff, 1966a), and thus could be seen as including suicide, self-neglect, substance abuse, malingering, and so on—all terms that infer some intent on the part of the client. The research literature on modification of SIB, however, has settled on a narrower definition: overt acts directed toward oneself that have restricted spatial and temporal topographies, whose rate of occurrence is reliably observable, and whose consequences are actual or threatened physical damage. Even this definition is not satisfactory, though. Schroeder, Mulick, and Rojahn (1980) have pointed out that it suffers from three flaws: (1) the consequences specified by the term do not pertain functionally to the reinforcing stimuli responsible for maintaining the behaviors; (2) researchers disagree about the membership of various topographies in the response class of SIB; and (3) no single intervention strategy is indicated for the particular "class" of SIB as opposed to other behaviors.

Because of these problems with the definition of SIB, perhaps the best

This research was supported by USPHS Grant #HD-03110, MCH Project 916, NICHD Grant #HD-10570, and NIEHS Grant #ES-01104. We especially acknowledge DDSA H.I.P. Grant #51P2052 entitled "Modifying Retardates' Self-Injurious Behavior," to Murdoch Center from 1974–1977, Stephen R. Shcroeder, Project Director.

STEPHEN R. SCHROEDER AND CAROLYN S. SCHRODER • Department of Psychology, University of North Carolina at Chapel Hill, Chapel Hill, North Carolina 27514. JOHANNES ROJAHN • Phillips-Universitaet Marburg, Marburg, West Germany. JAMES A. MULICK • Rhode Island Hospital and Department of Psychology, Brown University, Providence, Rhode Island 02912.

way to begin a discussion of it is by an example. Tate's (1972) description of Suzie presents a typical client and the behaviors chosen for treatment:

> Suzie developed slowly. She walked at 20 months but still crawled up stairs at age 5 years. Self-injury began at age 4 but did not become frequent until immediately after all her deciduous teeth were extracted when she was 7-years-old. Suzie was admitted to a state institution for the mentally retarded when she was 11-years-old. Nurses on duty the day of her admission stated that she was battered and bruised. The injuries were presumably self-inflicted. Within hours after her admission she was restrained in bed to prevent further damage to herself from headbanging. During the following 5 years she remained in restraints and received drug therapy, physical therapy, and much tender loving care from the hospital staff. None of these treatment appeared to be appreciably beneficial. When Suzie was 16 an unsuccessful attempt was made to stop the self-injury by using response contingent electric shock. In retrospect, the procedure probably failed because the shock was too weak. (p. 73)

To gain a better understanding of SIB and to insure an effective, long-term treatment program for Suzie, one would have to ask several critical questions about her environment, her caretakers, and the topographies of her particular SIB. For instance, did Suzie's headbanging consist of only one response topography, such as hand-to-head, head-to-knee, head-to-object? Did these different responses form one response class? Was there any other type of SIB involved, such as hair-pulling or gouging? How were Suzie's headbanging responses related to the rest of her behavioral repertoire? How did people in her environment react to her headbanging?

Finding ways to answer these questions is important not only for Suzie's case, but for any SIB case. In this chapter we shall attempt to analyze critically the research literature on SIB in pursuit of answers to these questions. A brief review of the various etiological models of SIB will be followed by a discussion of antecedent conditions and the ecology of SIB, response-contingent management techniques, evaluation of treatment effects, and, finally, programmatic considerations with SIB.

Etiological Models of SIB

There are several excellent recent reviews of etiological models of SIB (Bachman, 1972; Baumeister, 1978; Baumeister & Rollings, 1976; Carr, 1977; Frankel & Simmons, 1976). Only a summary of this work will be given here.

Studies of the etiology and pathogenesis of SIB suggest that it is not a unitary phenomenon. It is exhibited in a wide variety of behavioral topographies and environmental settings. At present only two organic syndromes are known to have SIB as symptoms: Lesch–Nyhan and Cornelia de Lange's syndromes. There exist several motivational conditions conducive to the development of SIB: arrested development, avoidance conditioning, stimulus discrimination for positive reward, and stereotyped behavior arising from disruption of homeostasis.

Medical Etiology

Lesch–Nyhan Syndrome

Physicans have developed increased interest in the physiological components of self-injurious behavior since the description of the Lesch–Nyhan syndrome in 1964 (Lesch & Nyhan, 1964; Nyhan, 1967, 1968a, b.). The Lesch–Nyhan syndrome is a sex-linked disorder of purine metabolism in which the child demonstrates spasticity, choreoathetosis, possible mental retardation, elevated urine uric acid (the serum uric acid may also be elevated), self-mutilation, and aggressive behaviors. Mutilation, especially biting of the oral structures and fingers, is most common; this mutilation does cause pain, and the child may welcome restraints to prevent further injury. Patients can cause such severe self-mutilation that the mouth orifice is totally deformed or the fingers lost.

The self-mutilation appears to be, at least in part, under voluntary control, and may be partly related to attention-getting behaviors. However, in most cases the patient's self-mutilation seems to be rather compulsive and uncontrollable. In addition patients develop other forms of self-destruction, such as sticking their fingers in the spokes of their wheelchairs or throwing themselves off furniture, and may also show aggressive behaviors toward others. These other self-destructive and aggressive behaviors seem to be less compulsive and more geared toward attention-getting.

It should be noted that the self-mutilation occurs in patients who are of near-normal intelligence and verbally communicative as well as in those with more severe intellectual and communication handicaps (Nyhan, 1976).

The Lesch–Nyhan syndrome represents the first condition with a demonstrated biochemical defect in which very specific abnormal behaviors are described. However, the exact connection between the defect and the self-mutilation is unknown. Although the serum uric acid level may be elevated, reduction of the uric acid level with Allopurinol does not alter the neurological or behavioral phenomena. In addition, a survey of serum uric acid levels in an institutionalized mentally retarded population (Brandon Training School in Vermont) resulted in no definite correlation between serum uric acid levels and self-injurious responses. Thus, the uric acid level does not seem to be the determinant of the abnormal behavior. It is frustrating to know the specific biochemical defect in a condition, and yet not be able to determine its relationship to behavior. Hopefully, though, this defect is a clue toward more complete understanding of self-injurious behaviors.

Cornelia de Lange's Syndrome

Self-mutilation may also be a common accompaniment in Cornelia de Lange's syndrome (Bryson, Sakati, Nyhan, & Fish, 1971; Marie, Royer, & Rappaport, 1967). This syndrome is characterized by low birth weight, retarded growth, hirsutism, a distinctive facies, and digital abnormalities. No specific genetic etiology has been demonstrated, no consistent chromosomal abnormalities have been found, and no biochemical defect has been identified. As a result there is little apparent similarity between this and the Lesch–Nyhan syndrome, except for the tendency to self-mutilation. In the Cornelia de Lange's syndrome, the self-abusive behaviors include self-inflicted blunt trauma (hitting the face, extremities, trunk) as well as self-biting. Each patient appears to have his own stereotyped forms of self-abuse, and not all the case reports have noted the very destructive biting which is always involved in the Lesch–Nyhan syndrome. The compulsive quality of the self-injury, so striking in the Lesch–Nyhan syndrome, is also absent. Operant programs have been noted as being effective in the management of both disorders (Duker, 1975b).

There are no other known physiological conditions with such a high incidence of self-injurious behavior. Patients with peripheral neuropathies or insensitivity to pain also will demonstrate self-mutilation, but here the origin is more accidental and is related to the lack of awareness of the damage being inflicted.

Psychodynamic Interpretations

Psychodynamic interpretations (e.g., Crabtree, 1967; Fitzherbert, 1950; Frederick & Resnick, 1971; Freud, 1954; Greenacre, 1954; Slawson & Davidson, 1964; Stinnett & Hollander, 1970) have viewed SIB as symbolic behavior related to infantile or fetal drives, or displacement upon oneself or one's anger and aggression toward others, or symbolic suicidal or masochistic tendencies, or self-stimulation related to parental rejection (see Lester, 1972, and Sandler, 1964, for a review). What little research is available on these theories does not support such interpretations, and most psychotherapeutic methods have been ineffective in treating SIB. It is difficult to see how such interpretations apply to the severely retarded, where SIB is most prevalent, since these people to a large extent appear to have impaired symbolic thought processes insofar as we know. In addition to these problems, they often lack expressive language to relate such thoughts, assuming that they occur.

Behavioral Motivational Interpretations

Behavioral motivational interpretations of SIB assume that it is behavior that is functionally related to consequences of reward in the subject's environment. There are at least four behavioral analyses, which are not mutually exclusive, of how SIB might come to be learned.

The Avoidance Hypothesis

The basic notion involved here is one first proposed by Skinner (1953) and demonstrated very reliably with animals (Byrd, 1969; Kelleher, Riddle, & Cook, 1963; Sidman, Herrnstein, & Conrad, 1957; Stretch, Orloff, & Dalrymple, 1968; Waller & Waller, 1963). It states that individuals may expose themselves to aversive stimulation—like SIB—in order to avoid even more aversive consequences. This, of course, is a commonplace of everyday life and is known experimentally as avoidance learning. In avoidance learning, the behavior is associated with a strong emotional response and is very resistant to extinction, even long after the avoidance stimulus has been withdrawn. Both these characteristics are frequently observed with SIB.

This explanation of SIB requires a history of aversive stimulation and avoidance conditioning. Reported clinical studies of SIB that have developed from conditioned avoidance of present or prior aversive stimulation are very few. Green (1968) reported a relationship between parental physical abuse and SIB among schizophrenic children. Thus, in some cases SIB may develop to avoid more severe attacks. There is also some clinical justification for suggesting that SIB is related to avoidance of social contact. For instance, autistic children often display "tactile defensiveness," that is, they tend to avoid physical contact. The retarded often perform high rates of SIB on release from restraint (Corte, Wolf, & Locke, 1971; Peterson & Peterson, 1968). Sometimes they even attempt to tie themselves down again (Tate, 1972). Social contact or particular ward attendants may serve as aversive rather than positively rewarding stimuli. Nevertheless, there are many instances where SIB in the retarded has developed in environments in which no primarily aversive social consequences could be identified. Although the avoidance hypothesis alone is inadequate to account for the pathogenesis of SIB, it does point out that the history of rewards and punishments is critical to the strategy for treatment.

Stereotyped Response

In this view, SIB is considered an extreme case of the stereotypy frequently observed among retarded persons, especially those who are institutionalized (Baumeister & Forehand, 1973). It is seen as an instrumental response developed from more benign types of stereotyped acts. For example, headbanging may have had as its antecedants such things as bodyrocking, bodytwirling, and handwaving, which were then shaped into headbanging.

This explanation again is only a partial one. Stereotyped acts are repetitious, topographically invariant motor behaviors or action sequences in which reward is unspecified or noncontingent and the performance of which is considered pathological (Schroeder, 1970). SIB fits this definition in certain forms, such as headbanging. However, many types of SIB, such as gouging and digging, are nonrepetitious, and are often unpredictable and highly variable in their occurrence.

In addition, when approaching SIB in terms of stereotyped behavior, one must deal with the uncertainties about the pathogenesis of stereotyped behavior (Baumeister, 1978; Berkson, 1967). The most widely accepted explanation of stereotyped behavior, however, is that it is a symptom of imbalance of internal homeostasis, perhaps CNS arousal, which is precipitated by such things as sensory deprivation, sensory overload, and frustration (Berkson & Mason, 1964a,b; Green, 1967). When applied to SIB, this would mean that environmental contingencies, such as parental neglect in infancy or lack of stimulation on a ward, could be the setting for homeostatic imbalance, and SIB a mechanism for raising or lowering arousal to restore balance. But this idea is difficult to document experimentally. Recently Kohlenberg, Levin, and Belcher (1973) recorded skin conductance as a psychophysiological measure of arousal before, during, and after treatment of a severe case of SIB. They found that SIB resulted in increased levels of arousal after the client was removed from physical restraints, but before removal of restraints, there was no relationship between rates of SIB and amount of increase in skin conductance level.

Furthermore, reduction in SIB after punishment produced effects on arousal different from those owning to SIB itself. A simple homeostatic relationship of SIB to arousal levels did not occur, which argues against the homeostatic and therefore the stereotyped-behavior explanation of SIB.

Another argument against the general arousal hypothesis is that, as the subsequent literature review shows, SIB most often occurs in a specific context under specific environmental conditions. In addition, treatment of SIB does not generalize to other situations easily. This result would be unexpected if nothing but internal homeostasis were involved. Although stimulus deprivation or stereotypy may be variables related to the pathogenesis of SIB, they cannot be considered an adequate explanation of it.

The Developmental Hypothesis

The developmental hypothesis is based on the assumption that SIB is a vestige of earlier motor behaviors which were adaptive (Lourie, 1949) for motor and personality development, but have never been outgrown (e.g., headbanging in the crib). Perhaps headbanging is maintained by coincidental reinforcement, or persists after a disruption in child–caretaker relationships. There is some support for this view from animal studies of developmental insult related to maternal deprivation (Davenport & Berkson, 1963; Erwin, Mitchell, & Maple, 1973; Gluck & Sackett, 1974) and the significance of vestibular stimulation in infancy for later development (Clark, Kreutzberg, & Chee, 1977; Gregg, Haffner, & Korner, 1976; Sallustro & Atwell, 1978). The latter has been the stimulus for occupational-therapy-oriented sensory integration programs designed to decrease SIB (Bittick, Fleeman, & Bright, 1978; Lemke & Mitchell, 1972). However, there is not enough research on the sensory integration hypothesis of SIB to evaluate it as yet. It is not known whether the need for vestibular stimulation can account for the occurrence of SIB, although this speculation is interesting.

The Discriminative Stimulus-Conditioned Reinforcer Hypothesis

This explanation of SIB, also posited by Skinner (1953), is based on the assumption that an aversive stimulus (SIB) might be paired with a positive reward that maintains it. This result has also been reliably demonstrated in animals and humans (Ayllon & Azin, 1966; Brown, Martin, & Morrow, 1964; Holz & Azrin, 1961, 1962; Murray & Nevin, 1967; Stubbs & Silverman, 1972). Thus aversive stimulation during SIB under appropriate conditions could act as a signal informing the subject of impending positive rewards like attention, affection, and contact.

The discrimination hypothesis can account for a great deal of SIB that develops among the retarded. SIB is most prevalent among the severely retarded who also lack communication skills. For this type of individual, performing SIB, a response that cannot be ignored, could be tantamount to establishing communication and command of one's environment.

A number of studies involving treatment of SIB have noted that it occurred only under specific conditions of presentation or withdrawal of discriminative social stimuli (Corte, Wolf, & Locke, 1971; Lane & Domrath, 1970; Lovaas, Schaeffer, & Simmons, 1965; Lovaas & Simmons, 1969; Peterson & Peterson, 1968) and was maintained by its (SIB) consequences. Although this explanation is suggestive, the necessary research differentiating it from competing hypotheses remains to be done. Many of the studies were conducted under conditions that did not permit adequate experimental control. That SIB is more than just a communication disorder seems almost certain. If it were not, teaching language alone should suffice to eliminate SIB. Teaching discrimination and communication skills may be important, but it is usually not a sufficient condition for elimination of SIB. The discrimination hypothesis does, however, point out the need to replace SIB with more appropriate alternative behaviors if it is to be successfully eliminated.

Summary

The above explanations are not mutually exclusive, and none alone accounts satisfactorily for the development of SIB. All are analogically inferred from observation of current repertoires. It is likely that some or all of these conditions could be present in a single case of SIB. Research must be done that determines how each of these antecedents contributes to the development of SIB before an adequate and preferable treatment mode can be recommended. The ecobehavioral approach to be discussed in the next section focuses on methods that look more closely at antecedent stimulus conditions.

Antecedent Conditions and the Ecology of Self-Injurious Behavior

Viewing self-injurious behavior as an operant response has had tremendous heuristic as well as practical value. It offers testable hypotheses, variables that are generally readily accessible, and a history of treatment procedures that permits optimism. Although in using this approach one cannot completely isolate antecedent stimuli from a response (or its parameters) or from the contingencies of reinforcement affecting the response, each of these interdependent aspects should be considered. In the next three sections we shall discuss each of these as they occur in SIB, particularly as they are relevant to treatment.

This section, which is concerned with antecedent stimulus conditions and their importance for understanding the development and management of SIB, will present a compilation of some empirical data from the current literature from the points of view of (1) environmental conditions as setting occasions for SIB, (2) differential stimulus control of SIB, (3) interaction of environmental conditions with effectiveness of intervention, and (4) environmental conditions and response selection. Suggestions will also be offered on how these data relate to research and future directions. Before beginning, however, it will be helpful to mention some concepts that will be relevant to our discussion.

Ecology is a term shared by scientists in many fields. Its meaning, which varies greatly across disciplines, is still evolving with the purpose and perspective of the users (Rogers-Warren & Warren, 1977). At least two different, though interdependent, dimensions of ecology can be identified when it is applied to behavioral assessment of persons in small groups. The first refers to the system of *intrapersonal behavior,* where the person is viewed as demonstrating a complex of interdependent behaviors. In this context, it is assumed that by changing one behavior, other behaviors of the same person will be affected. The second refers to a person within his or her *physical* and *social* context. Here, the arrangement of settings is seen as influencing a person's behavior, and this person in return is seen as affecting his or her environment (Rogers-Warren & Warren, 1977).

Ecological types of research with the mentally retarded have been pursued mainly by experimental animal psychologists who have been influenced by ethology and have carried out studies about complex nonverbal social behavior such as territoriality, dominance, foodsharing, social behavior with peers, and communication, derived from theories of animal behavior (Berkson & Landesman-Dwyer, 1977). Researchers engaged in ecological psychology have not given much attention to research with the developmentally disabled (Schoggen, 1978), but the basic assumptions of this approach have been recognized. Because of the increasing concern with stimulus conditions in natural environments, and the need for a new rationale and technology, behavior analysts have begun to adapt technologies that attempt to describe carefully persons, environments, and their interactions. These methods show promise of revealing complex constellations of stimulus–response interrelationships involved in long-term behavior change.

This approach has been labeled ecobehavioral analysis by Warren (1977). It can be understood as the second step of the experimental behavior analysis beyond the operant animal laboratory. Applied behavior analysis has attempted to transfer the close control over stimulus–response functions from the controlled environment of the laboratory to the natural environment of humans, and the application of operant principles "to the problems of social importance" (Baer, Wolf, & Risley, 1968). The ecobehavioral approach holds the promise of providing a better understanding of how the environment and the behavior of its inhabitants impact on one another with respect to their long-term relationships. It has already yielded important results with the emotionally disturbed (Wahler, House, & Stambaugh, 1976), with autistic children (Lichtstein & Wahler, 1976), and with SIB in the mentally retarded (Mulick, Hoyt, Rojahn, & Schroeder, 1978; Rojahn, Mulick, McCoy, & Schroeder, 1978; Schroeder, Rojahn, & Mulick, 1978a). The following review of how environmental antecedent conditions affect the occurrence of SIB will indicate the impact that the ecobehavioral approach can have on the treatment of SIB.

Environmental Conditions as Setting Occasions for SIB

The growing interest in the ecology of the developmentally retarded is reflected in the increased recognition of environmental variables in such areas as observational research, the development of functional architecture, and the building of barrier-free living environments. A few naturalistic observational studies of ward environments have yielded interesting results. For example, strong territorial behavior and aggression were found in a series of studies on groups of physically healthy moderately to severely retarded boys (Paluck & Esser, 1971a); protecting one's territory was unaffected on reentering an experimental dayroom even after 20 months (Paluck & Esser,

1971b). Territoriality, which refers to the staking out of specific individual areas in a space common to a group (Paluck & Esser, 1971a), was also investigated in a group of profoundly retarded male adults (Hereford, Cleland, & Fellner, 1973). It was demonstrated that increasing individual territories in the dormitory markedly decreased nocturnal enuresis and encopresis. Visual boundaries between individual areas further decreased these behaviors. Enuresis and encopresis were interpreted, after ethological theories, as scent-marking, and thus a means of territorial defense. Rago, Parker, and Cleland (1978), stressing the residents' need of space, showed that increased space per person reduced aggressive acts. Rago (1977) related individuals' ranking in the dominance hierarchy to amount of aggression, stereotypy, and receptiveness to programming.

Other research on ecological features found that hearing impairment (Talkington & Hall, 1969), the level of communication skills (Talkington, Hall, & Altman, 1971), and institutional diet control procedures (Talkington & Riley, 1970) all were related to aggressive behavior, stereotypy, and SIB. An interesting, but not yet fully interpretable, result was achieved by Frankel, Freeman, Ritvo, Chikami, and Carr (1976) in an investigation of ambient noise level and stereotyped behavior. These researchers found that stereotypic behavior increased with rising noise in low-IQ (mean of 34.7) autistic children, contrasting with a decrease in a matched group of higher-IQ (mean 73.3) autistic children.

These naturalistic studies clearly demonstrate the importance of environmental variables to the occurrence of maladaptive behaviors in institutional ward-type settings. The behaviors are likely to occur in many social settings for the severely and profoundly retarded. Many other ecological phenomena and their relationship to the occurrence of problem behaviors have also been studied (see Berkson and Landesman-Dwyer, 1977, for a review).

Differential Stimulus Control of SIB

In the following section, experimental studies on stimulus conditions and how they differentially affect the occurrence of SIB will be discussed. These studies are presented as illustrations in the context of larger topics that seem particularly to call for ecobehavioral research. The analysis of specific stimulus conditions can not only bring about important conclusions for the treatment of topographically similar cases of SIB, but can also add to the understanding of basic etiological paradigms (e.g., SIB as an escape response) that could provide guidelines for the prevention of new problem behaviors.

Situational Demands

Carr, Newsom, and Binkoff (1976) attempted to isolate situational demands that had controlled the SIB of a mildly retarded child. The subject was exposed to several demand and nondemand situations. Then the situations were changed so that demands occurred only in the context of positive social interaction between the child and the experimenter. The levels of SIB were high in demand situations, and were decreased in nondemand and conversational situations. In further support of the idea of the escape response function of self-hitting, the child abruptly stopped hitting himself when he was presented with the stimulus that normally signaled termination of a demand period. Other stimuli that were never related to the termination did not decrease SIB. In addition, SIB during demand sessions showed a scalloped pattern, the type of responding generally encountered on fixed-interval schedules of escape in lower organisms (cf. Carr, 1977). As noted previously, several other authors have indicated that self-injury may function as an escape response from a variety of aversive situations (e.g., Carr, 1977; Myers & Diebert, 1971; Wolf, Risley, Johnson, Harris & Allen, 1967) or as conditioned avoidance of social contacts (Corte *et al.*, 1971; Peterson & Peterson, 1968).

Physical Restraints

In a study by Favell, McGimsey, and Jones (1978), the positively reinforcing function of physical restraint (rigid arm splints) was demonstrated. Rapid and complete reduction of SIB was achieved when the subjects were physically restrained contingent on increasing periods without self-injury and on providing toys and attention during intervals between the wearing of restraints. When physical restraint was applied contingent on toy play, this response increased. Several interpretations were offered to explain the results. It was argued that (1) stimulus-change components of restraint may constitute positive reinforcement in nonstimulating environment; or that (2) restraint may be paired with a reduction in aversive stimuli, such as staff-imposed demands, and that self-injury in some individuals may function as an escape *into* restraint conditions; or (3) restraint also could be paired with adult attention, and may therefore provide relative physical comfort. The points raised for the explanation of these somewhat paradoxical properties of restraints are well taken.

Using an ecobehavioral approach, Rojahn, Mulick, and Schroeder (1979) investigated the effects of restraints (a camisole and a fencing mask) on three mentally retarded persons with pica. Twenty-two client behaviors and six staff behaviors were simultaneously observed in a descriptive observational study. The study attempted an analysis of social dynamics in a special unit for profoundly mentally retarded clients with SIB (for the data-collection system see Schroeder, Rojahn, & Mulick, 1978a). Although this was not an attempt to replicate the study by Favell *et al.* (1978), the results lend support for their second explanation: the self-protective devices tended to decrease social interactions between the restrained subjects and their caretakers. Staff behaviors, such as non-programmatic positive attention, instructions, and reinforcement in the form of verbal praise for specific tasks, decreased for all three subjects during the time they were wearing restraints, relative to restraint-free periods; this pattern of responsiveness by the staff could reflect an increased demand situation for these clients when they were released from restraints. However, there was no indication with these three clients that the restraints had any reinforcing properties by themselves, or provided an escape function of SIB (by performing pica). How much self-protective devices and their situational consequences lawfully contribute to the development and maintenance of problem behaviors such as SIB beyond their preventive function is an important question for ecobehavioral research.

Daily Routine Activities

Schroeder and Humphrey (1977) carried out a comprehensive analysis of the effect of daily routine activities during an intervention program with a severe case of SIB. The client had been totally blind from birth and deaf for 2 years. SIB consisted of several headbanging topographies, self-kicking, self-pinching, and hairpulling. It appeared that the client was using her multiple SIB very systematically to shape staff behaviors in order to meet her needs. The type and pattern of SIB seemed to vary according to the scheduled activity and the time of day. Data were collected on 13 behaviors (among them five SIB topographies) during 40 consecutive everyday activities, 13 hours per day, 7 days per week, for 4 months; and then for an hour and a half per day for a year during follow-up. The analysis revealed a variety of environmental-context effects. For example, SIB was much higher in training sessions immediately following her weight check, a very stressful activity, than after a quiet period of sitting in her chair later in the afternoon (see Figure 1). Fine

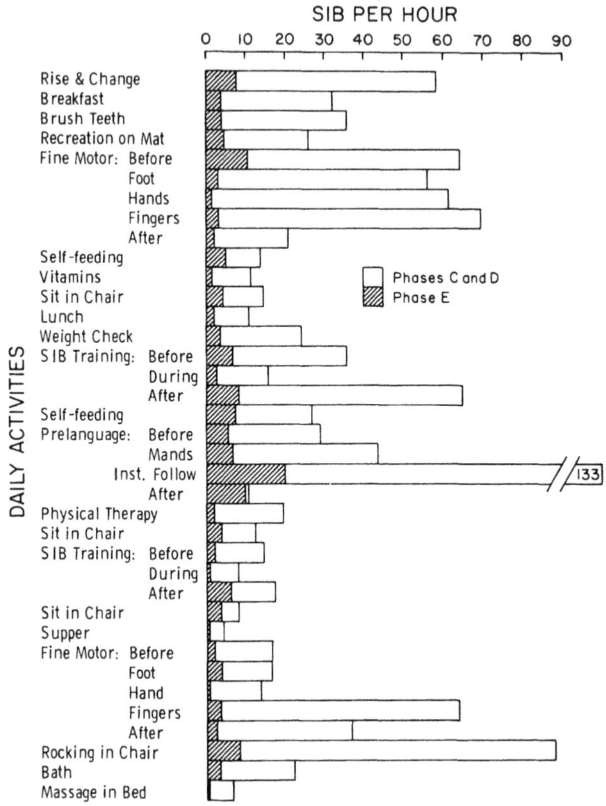

FIGURE 1. SIB per hour as a function of activities in which Pearl was involved. Phases *C* and *D* are the mean of the first eight weeks of intensive intervention. Phase *E* is the mean of the next 14 weeks of controlled intervention and fading out of physical restraints.

motor training in the morning was accompanied by much higher SIB than right after supper in the evening. A time-out procedure based on this ecobehavioral assessment, together with providing appropriate alternative behaviors for the client, very effectively decreased her SIB, whereas previous very arduous attempts at intervention had failed.

Interaction of Environmental Conditions with Effectiveness of Intervention

When we analyze the functional relationship of aberrant behaviors and the conditions under which they occur, our primary concern is the control and deceleration of these behaviors. In the past, however, functional analysis has usually focused exclusively on the immediate consequences of such responses. This practice has led to the application of management procedures without taking into account other variables that are often powerful determinants in the natural environment. This neglect becomes evident when we look at problems like the often encountered lack of generalization across settings, response generalization to other behaviors, substitution, etc. Even with perfectly executed management procedures, therapeutic interventions have to be designed not only to be adapted to the target behavior and its controlling conditions, but also to fit into the ecology of the client's habitat. Some procedures may be superior to others according to the prevailing conditions of the environment. Some environments are undoubtedly detrimental to the success of almost any therapeutic intervention.

Background Setting

Solnick, Rincover, and Peterson (1977) were emphasizing just this point when they investigated the importance of the background setting on the effectiveness of time-out. Their setting was either impoverished or enriched. In the impoverished setting, the client was presented with a discrimination task in which the correct response was either performed by the client or prompted by the experimenter. Edibles and praise plus a toy were given after each trial. The enriched setting involved the addition of music, new toys, and frequent prompting to play with the toys instead of engaging in the discrimination procedure. The time-out procedure involved a 90-sec period during which the experimenter left the room. This contingency was applied to one and then two behaviors (headbanging and spitting) in both types of setting. The context within which time-out occurred was found to be important. In the impoverished setting, the consequated target behaviors either increased or remained unchanged in frequency. In the enriched setting, the consequated target behaviors decreased tn frequency. Time-out was effective only when time-in was enriched.

A subsequent study by Williams, Schroeder, and Rojahn (1978) was an attempt to assess the generality of the results of Solnick *et al.* (1977) in a group setting with four clients instead of one. The experiment evaluated which factors of the time-in environment were important. The findings lend partial support to the results of Solnick *et al.* (1977). Although suppression was seen in all settings with all four subjects, time-out was even more effective in the enriched environment for two clients. The clients met first in a custodial setting where no toys were present and minimal supervision was offered; then in another setting where toys, but only minimal supervision, were offered; then in a third setting where the supervisor involved them in play, but without toys in the room; and finally in a setting where there were toys as well as a supervisor actively involving them in play. The room was rearranged to create the four settings. Results showed that the four settings established different amounts of toy contact and interaction, and differentially effective time-outs. However, the rates of SIB and stereotypic behaviors were not greatly different during baselines. The latter result is interesting in regard to previously reviewed hypotheses, in that the escape-from-demands hypothesis of SIB was not supported strongly with these subjects. Escape is still a possible explanation, however. Since the study took place in a novel setting for the subjects, an answer cannot be given about the differential effects of the four experimental settings *per se* on the development of new problem behaviors. SIB and stereotyped responses that were already present were unaffected in frequency by noncontingently changing the environmental conditions of the setting.

Availability of Alternative Behaviors

Another variable that interacts with the effectiveness of interventions is the availability of alternative behaviors that can be reinforced. This interaction was demonstrated in the study by Mulick *et al.* (1978). The subject was a 22-year-old, ambulatory, profoundly retarded man with impaired vision because of bilateral cataracts. He was referred for treatment of excessive nail-biting and fingerpicking. Screening observations revealed that the client spent most of his time sitting in his unit's large open dayroom. During unstructured periods, he remained seated, rocking back and forth, and intermittently biting small amounts of tissue from his fingertips, or he used his remaining fingernails to scratch at the tips of the fingers of the opposing hand until they were inflamed and infected. Nailbiting and fingerpicking did not occur during structured fine-motor and tabletop activities. The client was extremely compliant with staff, and he readily had engaged in fine-motor tasks, such as stringing beads.

The intervention program was based on the simple assumption that if a variety of toys was located centrally and the client was taught to exchange old materials for new ones by a system of gradually faded prompts, then a rudimentary form of independent play might come to be substituted for hand-related SIB. Preliminary observations provided information about toy preference in the client. Relatively little investment of staff time and minor alterations in the environment resulted in dramatic increases in reinforced independent toy play and concomitant decreases in target behaviors.

Environmental Conditions and Response Selection

There is very little research in this area. As Sidman (1978) has pointed out, the focus of the experimental analysis of behavior has been the investigation of reinforcement contingencies in controlled environments. We know much less about the technology of stimulus control in the environment. Naturalistic observational studies serve as a model for future research.

Sequential Relationships

MacLean and Baumeister (1979) used interactive analysis to study explicit sequential relationships among a variety of stereotyped topographies exhibited by a moderately retarded child as a function of environmental activities in an experimental preschool setting. They found that stereotypy was less frequent in settings where the child was more actively engaged and closely supervised by the teacher. There was a significant suppression in one stereotyped topography (headshaking), but not in others, which was correlated with the teacher's approach and "negative contact" with the child. It is important to note that the teacher's behavior was *not* sequentially dependent on the child's stereotyped behavior, but that the child's headshaking was temporarily decreased whenever any negative contact with the teacher occurred.

Complex Stimulus–Response Relationships

SIB is most prevalent among severely and profoundly retarded and autistic persons who also tend to have a high incidence of organic dysfunction, long history of performing SIB, and frequent communication handicaps (Schroeder, Schroeder, Smith, & Dalldorf, 1978). Their SIB topographies, however, tend to be highly discriminated operants. In the study by Schroeder and Humphrey (1977), the client reliably exhibited higher rates before and after unpleasant activities than after pleasant activities such as meals or snacks. Similarly, the selection of topography of SIB shifted dramatically, depending on the activity in which she was engaged.

Response–Response Relationships

It is necessary to study carefully not only complex stimulus–response relationships such as seen in the study by Schroeder and Humphrey (1977), but also simple response–response functions such as seen in the study by MacLean and Baumeister (1979). Studies of such response–response relationships have shown the intra-individual ecobehavioral dynamics of response classes, hierarchical response chains, contrast effects, and natural covariations among responses. In the MacLean and Baumeister (1979) study, the interrelatedness of two stereotyped behaviors was demonstrated. Stereotyped handflapping exhibited a relatively stable and significant sequential dependency with headshaking. The sequential analysis provided insight into the response complexity of these stereotypies of the subject. A similar result was achieved with the second subject of the study. Interactive analysis indicated that, given one form of stereotyped behavior, there were significant probabilities that another topography would follow immediately and continue. The results suggested a functional relationship between these two topographically different behaviors.

Response-response relationships were also found with multiple SIB topographies in a profoundly retarded man (Rojahn *et al.* 1978) through a *substitution effect.* The subject was a 30-year-old, nonambulatory, blind, profoundly retarded male with a long history of SIB. At the time he was referred for treatment the subject was demonstrating four different SIBs—two topographically related (headslapping with the palm of the hand and hitting the forehead with the knuckles of his fist) and two topographically unrelated (whipping his head toward his shoulder and wrapping his arms in his clothing until circulation of his blood was cut off). Treatment procedures consisted of a series of stimulus control procedures using a jacket with large sidepockets and/or a 10 cm foam rubber neckbrace in systematic combinations. The results showed an interdependent pattern of headwhipping and headbanging or slapping, as a result of which a prosthetic device was being worn.

Pearson correlation coefficients between headwhipping and each of the two headhitting behaviors across all treatments were $-.30$. Headbanging and slapping were uncorrelated ($r = .01$). The internal relationship between the three SIB topographies was such that both headslapping and headbanging, which were topographically similar, tended to preclude headwhip-

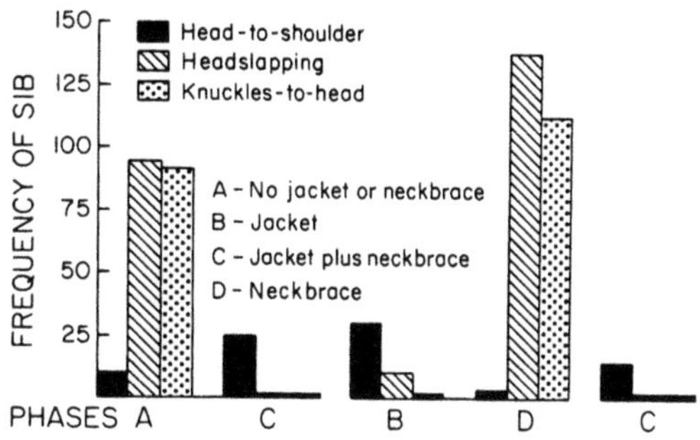

FIGURE 2. Mean percentage of intervals per session in which self-restraint occurred as a function of phases (A,B,C,D).

ping. But there was no functional dependency between headslapping and knuckles-to-forehead hitting, even though they were controlled by the same stimuli (see Figure 2).

Armwrapping precluded headslapping and headbanging. Substitution occurred when the neckbrace was worn: headwhipping decreased and headbanging increased. The converse occurred when the neckbrace was removed and the jacket was worn. Findings of this nature are important for estimating prognosis of intervention and its long-term appropriateness for the client in his natural setting.

Summary

Antecedent conditions affect the occurrence of SIB in a variety of ways. Ecological conditions such as territorial restriction, dietary control procedures, ambient noise, and the dominance hierarchy set the occasion for maladaptive behaviors. SIB can come under differential stimulus control of situational demands, physical self-restraint, and daily routine activities. The client's habitat, the background setting, and the availability of alternative reinforcers all affect the success of behavioral interventions with SIB. Environmental conditions affect the development of multiple SIB topographies, their sequential interrelationships, and their natural covariation. This information on the occurrence and management of SIB is a rich array of new findings. The challenge of future SIB research will be to elucidate the functional relationships among these antecedent conditions and relate them to treatment effectiveness.

Response-Contingent Techniques for Managing SIB

A variety of procedure options for treating SIB is well documented, and these are illustrated in the familiar operant contingency table in Figure 3.

The pervasiveness of this sort of classification scheme is shown by the frequent organization of review papers according to the response-reinforcement relation characterized within each cell (e.g.,Forehand & Baumeister, 1976; Schroeder, Mulick, & Schroeder, 1979). The reader is referred to several reviews and analyses of the various intervention techniques with SIB (Baumeister & Rollings, 1976; Frankel & Simmons, 1976; Harris & Ersner-Hershfield, 1978; Johnson & Baumeister, 1978; Schroeder, Mulick, & Schroeder, 1979). Few major new results have been reported since these data were published. In this section, we shall first summarize and update what has been done in connection with each intervention technique, and then make a detailed analysis of the research on each technique with each of the different SIB topographies.

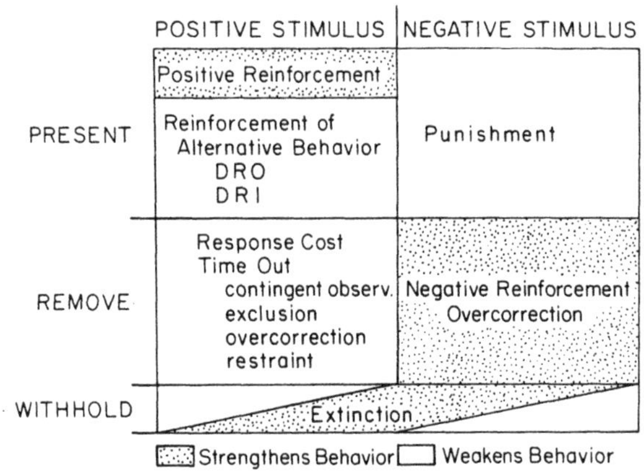

FIGURE 3. Contingency table showing the methods and consequences of strengthening and weakening behavior which have been used with self-injurious behavior.

Intervention Techniques for SIB

Punishment

Punishment consists of delivering an intense stimulus immediately contingent on occurrence of SIB, to suppress SIB. We emphasize that, according to Azrin and Holz (1966), the stimulus need not be aversive, but its presence must result in response suppression. If an aversive stimulus, when presented, results in an increase in the target response, it is, by definition, not a punisher. This point is often confused in the literature, where aversive stimulation and punishment are considered synonymous. No stimulation is inherently aversive or punishing, but is so only in relation to its basic parameters—intensity, duration, and frequency, and their consequences on behavior.

Punishment of SIB has taken several forms: lemon juice (Sajwaj, Libet, & Agras, 1974); slapping (Duker, 1975a); tickling (Greene & Hoats, 1971); loud noises (Sajwaj & Hedges, 1971); noxious odors (Tanner & Zeiler, 1975); hairpulling (Griffin, Locke, & Landers, 1975); restraint (Saposnek & Watson, 1974) and electrical stimulation (Tate & Baroff, 1966a). Verbal reprimands have been ineffective except when used in conjunction with physical or electrical stimuli. Most punishment studies involve the use of electrical stimulation. However, the parameters of punishment of SIB have not yet been researched carefully.

The suppressive effect of immediate contingent punishment is rapid and dramatic. When it occurs, it tends to be highly discriminated by the subject, and therefore generalization across settings is difficult to achieve. In Johnson and Baumeister's (1978) methodological review of 60 of the best-known studies of SIB, punishment procedures were used in 35, but failure was reported in only one study. The authors note that this effect probably reflects editorial bias in journals. In practice, punishment often fails to work. If it does work, it often loses its effectiveness (Birnbrauer, 1968). There have been reports of suppression beyond a year with training of parents and teachers in the generalized setting (Merbaum, 1973). However, it is unlikely that SIB would be eliminated with punishment unless there were naturally reinforced alternative behaviors readily available in the client's environment and continued surveillance of SIB.

Harris and Ersner-Hershfield (1978) have thoroughly reviewed the side effects of punishment of SIB, such as generalized anxiety, withdrawal, counteraggression, escape behaviors, and symptom substitution, and concluded that they do not outweigh the positive effects, such as compliance, eye contact, and prosocial behaviors. These results are difficult to interpret, since few of the punishment studies were designed to evaluate carefully side effects, positive or negative. The main point is that many of the vaunted fears about the negative side effects of a properly administered punishment procedure are generally unfounded. Nevertheless, due to the natural repugnance of caretakers and the general reluctance of administrators to approve punishment of SIB, an increase in research on the other techniques has occurred.

Avoidance Conditioning

Avoidance conditioning has not received much attention in SIB research, but it can be useful. For instance, Lovaas and Simmons (1969), after a number of SIB suppression trials in which "no" was paired with shock, found that "no" became sufficient to maintain suppression. Similarly, Tate and Baroff (1966b) noted that the buzz of the inductorium was enough to get a headbanger to eat again after SIB had been suppressed and he was refusing to eat. Duker (1975a) compared punishment and avoidance conditioning on two SIB topographies of a mentally retarded woman. Both procedures were effective; however, though suppression of the punished behavior was lost, the SIB on the avoidance schedule continued to be suppressed.

Overcorrection

Overcorrection is a complex punishment procedure designed by Foxx and Azrin in 1973 that attempts to capitalize on the suppressive effects of punishment while minimizing its negative side effects. Foxx (1978) has recently provided an excellent overview of overcorrection. The general rationale is "to require the misbehaving individual (a) to overcorrect the environmental effects of the inappropriate act, and (b) to practice overly correct forms of relevant behavior in those situations where the misbehavior commonly occurs" (p. 97). These two components are called restitution and positive practice. Epstein, Doke, Sajwaj, Sorell, and Rimmer (1974) have identified several components in overcorrection: (1) negative feedback; (2) time-out from positive reinforcement; (3) verbal reeducative instructions; (4) compliance training, such as gradual guidance or shadowing; and (5) negative reinforcement. Characteristics related to the success of acts are that they should (1) be directly related to the misbehaviors; (2) require effort; (3) be applied immediately following the misbehavior; (4) have a lengthy duration; and (5) be performed in a rapid, continued manner, so as to be inhibiting.

Overcorrection is a good example of the often found advantage of combining the effective components of several of the procedures outlined in Figure 3. But, like other forms of punishment, it is subject to both the same advantages (rapid, dramatic, and relatively enduring suppression of rate of SIB) and the same disadvantages (negative modeling, emotional conditioning, counteraggression, reinforcement of escape behavior, and substitution): (Harris & Ersner-Hershfield, 1978). The latter is especially true with strong, combative, noncompliant individuals. Foxx (1978) offers the guideline that if the overcorrection requires the involvement of two trainers instead of one, the danger of physical injury is greatly increased, and the procedure will not be feasible.

A recent bibliography by Matson and Ollendick (1977) on studies of overcorrection from 1971–1977 contains 77 items, of which only 10 studies are on SIB. The technique appears to hold a great deal of promise, but analysis of the effective ingredients remains to be performed (Ollendick & Matson, 1978). For instance, it is not always clear (1) when and how much restitution is necessary (Foxx, 1978); (2) how long the duration of positive practice needs to be: ranging from 40 sec (Doleys, McWhorter, Williams, & Gentry, 1977) up to 30 min (Foxx & Azrin, 1973); (3) what the degree and topography of gradual guidance should be (Harris & Romanczyk, 1976; Ollendick & Matson, 1978); and (4) how overcorrection should be combined with other procedures, such as rewarding alternative behaviors (i.e., differential reinforcement of other behavior [DRO]) (Azrin, Gottlieb, Hughart, Wesolowski, & Rahn, 1975). Hopefully, future research will help to sort out these issues.

Contingent Restraint

Prolonged noncontingent physical restraint is a relatively sure way to prevent SIB, but, as Favell *et al.* (1978) have noted, it may also become reinforcing for the SIB client. Often release from restraints is a high-risk occasion for serious SIB. Favell *et al.* (1978) have shown that such clients will even perform other operant tasks for the opportunity to be returned to restraints.

However, brief contingent physical restraints have been used successfully to suppress headbanging as time-out from positive reinforcement (Hamilton, Stephens, & Allen, 1967; Williams *et al.*, 1978), as a punishment for pica (Bucher, Reykdal, & Albin, 1976), and in conjunction with biofeedback relaxation training (Schroeder, Peterson, Solomon, & Artley, 1977). In the latter case, the therapist applied and withdrew very brief periods of restraints with the clients contingent upon their level of muscle tension. Relaxation, a state incompatible with SIB, was reinforced. The therapist effectively faded out physical control when the client relaxed. This technique was very similar to the graduated guidance and shadowing techniques reported with overcorrection. Brief contingent restraint periods run less risk of becoming reinforcing than prolonged "safe" periods provided by noncontingent restraint as conventionally used.

Withdrawal of Positive Reinforcement

Withdrawal of positive reinforcement is another technique that has been used extensively to control SIB. The major forms are *extinction* (e.g., Bucher & Lovaas, 1968; Corte *et al.*, 1971; Lovaas & Simmons, 1969) and *time-out* (e.g., Hamilton *et al.*, (1967).

It is important to remember that extinction presupposes a history of rewarding of patients of SIB, for example, with differential attention, physical contact, etc. Ignoring SIB of itself has little effect on frequency of SIB. In the Lovaas and Simmons (1969) study, the patient was released from restraint, and all attention to SIB was simply withdrawn. After 10 sessions and more than 9,000 instances of SIB, the behavior gradually disappeared. But in the Lovaas, Freitag, Gold, and Kassorla study (1965), continued noncontingent attention to or ignoring of the SIB did not change its rate significantly. The possibility of adventitious reinforcement can be controlled by what Jones, Simmons, and Frankel (1974) call noncontingent isolation—that is, removal to a special room. This procedure probably aided in controlling the number of stimuli that occasioned SIB, and also helped observers and therapists to control their own reactions to SIB. Indeed, the subject in this experiment hit herself 34,000 times before SIB was suppressed.

Extinction, though effective, often poses great risks, since the patient may seriously injure him or herself during treatment. In addition, the initial withdrawal of reward may lead to an increase in SIB before a decrease occurs (Lovaas, Freitag, Gold, & Kassorla, 1965). Extinction also depends greatly on the context in which reward for SIB has previously been delivered (Jones *et al.*, 1974). Thus, it has not always proven effective (Corte *et al.*, 1971). Studies with animals have shown that rate of extinction depends on conditioning history. Therefore, the longer the history of SIB, the longer it should take to extinguish. There has been no research with SIB on this latter point. Finally, as with punishment, problems with generalization, durability, and substitution have been observed with extinction (Duker, 1975a; Jones *et al.*, 1974; Miron, 1971).

Time-out—the withdrawal of reinforcement contingent on SIB—has been used much more successfully than extinction. A detailed analysis of the various forms of time-out is given in Schroeder, Mulick, and Schroeder (1979). Essentially they are: contingent observation; withdrawal time-out; exclusion time-out; seclusion time-out; contingent restraint time-out; and response cost. All these forms vary on dimensions of intrusiveness of intervention, environmental demands, etc. A recently developed technique, "facial screening," has shown promise as well (Lutzker, 1978; Zegiob, Alford, & House, 1978). In this instance, time-out consists of covering the client's face with a cloth bib or some other opaque material as a visual screen.

MacDonough and Forehand (1973) have reviewed several of the parameters of time-out, most of which have not been investigated at all, let alone among SIB cases. Lucero, Frieman, Spoering, and Fehrenbacher (1976) compared the effects of food withdrawal and attention on SIB at mealtime in three profoundly retarded girls and found food withdrawal more effective. Whether this effect held beyond mealtime was not mentioned. Effective time-out durations have varied from 90 sec to 30 min (White, Nielsen, & Johnson, 1972; Williams *et al.*, 1978). Investigation of optimal durations appears to be based on the interpretation of time-out as punishment, rather than a choice by the cltent of time-out or time-in so as to maximize reinforcement (Leitenberg, 1965). It appears that time-out parameters cannot be isolated from time-in parameters. Probably elements of both punishment and maximization of reinforcement are involved in most time-out procedures. Birnbrauer (1976) has suggested that a main effect of time-out may be disruption of an ongoing chain of inappropriate behavior, and that the effective duration may interact with other parameters, such as inhibition of responses during time-out, contingent release, and the reinforcing nature of the time-on environment. (See discussion in previous section on ecology.)

Rewarding Alternative Behaviors (DRO)

The term *DRO* was coined in operant animal research (Reynolds, 1961) to reflect the pigeon's withholding of a pecking response for a criterion period that was followed by reinforcement. It has occasionally been known in the behavior therapy literature as omission training (Weihar & Harman, 1975).

Presumably, whatever "other" response was occurring at the time of reinforcement was strengthened. Thus, an SIB client may be rewarded for other non-SIB behaviors for longer and longer periods of time (DRO). If SIB occurs before a specific time period is completed, the time period is recycled, and reward is withheld until the criterion time period has elapsed. Good examples of this technique are described by Brawley, Harris, Allen, Fleming, and Peterson (1969), Lovaas, Freitag, Gold, and Kassorla (1965), Peterson and Peterson (1968), and Weihar and Harman (1975). DRO procedures are typically used in conjunction with other methods, such as extinction or time-out from positive reinforcement (Repp & Dietz, 1974). This technique makes an evaluation of the DRO contingency alone difficult to assess because of the confounding effects of time-out (Baumeister & Rollings, 1976).

The mere reinforcement of alternative behaviors may not be sufficient to suppress SIB (Young & Wincze, 1974). Tarpley and Schroeder (1979) performed an experiment with three profoundly retarded headbangers, comparing extinction, DRO, and DRI (differential reinforcement of incompatible behavior) in a multiple-schedule design. Another dimension of this study was that three forms of prompting incompatible behavior were used: manual guidance, manual and verbal prompts, and verbal prompts only. DRI suppressed SIB more than DRO, which suppressed SIB more than extinction. The degree of prompting incompatible behavior affected clients differently. For a compliant subject, verbal prompts were sufficient to make DRI effective. In another experiment, involving biofeedback, Schroeder *et al.* (1977) showed that relaxation training with two severe headbangers resulted in a physiological state that was incompatible with the performance of SIB. Thus, receptive state of the client and degree of incompatibility of the alternative behavior are probably related to effectiveness of reinforcement for alternative behavior.

As with punishment, generalizability and substitution with differential reinforcement procedures seem to be a problem, although there is not as much research available here. Durability seems to be a little better, but again not enough is known about the relevant parameters to make a conclusive statement.

Satiation

Techniques based on *reinforcement alone* have not been very effective in suppressing SIB. However, there have been three case reports of headbanging in nonretarded persons (Mogel & Schiff, 1967; Wooden, 1974). In Wooden

(1974), a nocturnal headbanger was reinforced for negative practice of SIB, which resulted in quick, permanent suppression. Every night before sleeping he was told to grind his head into his pillow until he could no longer stand the pain. SIB stopped after four nights. An attempt at satiation in a severely mentally retarded girl (Duker, 1975b), was unsuccessful. However, Jackson, Johnson, Ackron, and Crowley (1975), and Libby and Phillips (1979) have used food satiation very successfully to decelerate rumination. In the Jackson *et al.* study, the client was given a thick milkshake about 90 min after mealtime. Presumably this method averted the initial link in the chain of regurgitation leading to rumination and reconsumption of the vomitus. This study is one of a few demonstrations (see also Kohlenberg, 1970; Lang & Melamed, 1969) that shows that intervention early in the chained sequence can prevent SIB. It would be important to research prevention procedures with other SIB topographies.

Relating Interventions to Types of SIB Topographies

Frankel and Simmons (1976) in their review of 49 studies of SIB noted that in 35 studies decelerating a single response topography occurred. However, in those same 35 studies only six reported headbanging by itself. Hamilton *et al.* (1967) suggested two types of SIB clients: those who use one topography exclusively, and those who exhibit a variety of topographies. Azrin *et al.* (1975) have suggested that seven of the 11 cases in their study who were "cured" of their SIB with overcorrection were "outer-directed"—that is, their behavior was maintained by interaction with the environment, as opposed to "inner-directed," self-stimulating behaviors. Schroeder, Mulick, and Rojahn (1980) have suggested a similar distinction between social SIB —such as headbanging, biting, gouging, and hairpulling—and nonsocial SIB—consummatory topographies as pica, ruminative vomiting, copraphagy, and aerophagia. The social consequences of the latter behaviors are less obvious to persons in the immediate environment, unless they become socially obnoxious. Therefore, such responses are less likely to be maintained by the social consequences.

Whether any of these classifications has utility for differential analysis and management effectiveness remains to be seen. In an effort to discover whether the published literature could provide data to suggest answers to any of the above questions, a detailed analysis of 75 research studies covering 140 SIB clients was performed. The criteria for inclusion were: (1) direct observational data were reported; (2) observer agreement was calculated; (3) a statistically significant or an 80% reduction from baseline SIB levels was demonstrated. (The studies in the sample are marked with an asterisk in the reference section.)

The demographic characteristics of the 140 subjects were: (1) their average age was 15 years; (2) average length of institutionalization was 12 years; (3) average age chronicity of SIB was 6.7 years; (4) 51% were males; (5) 88% were severely or profoundly retarded; (6) 37 of 52 reported had severe organic syndromes; (7) 29 of 30 reported had no expressive language; (8) 15 of 17 reported had severe visual or hearing impairments; (9) 14 of 19 reported were on behavior-control medication; (10) 30 of 40 reported exhibited "outer-directed" SIB. Even though there were obvious reporting biases, the overall characteristics of the population are very similar to those reported by Maisto and Baumeister (1978) and Schroeder, Schroeder, Smith, and Dalldorf (1978) in prevalence surveys of SIB in institutions. The above research sample is, therefore, apparently representative of severe SIB topographies.

The frequencies of SIB topographies and combinations with associated misbehaviors are shown in Table I. Frequency of topographies occurring alone is given on the diagonal. Combinations of two topographies are seen in the matrix. Multiple topographies of three or more are shown in the row labelled "Mult." Analysis of the results suggests that behaviors to the left of the vertical perforated line are social forms of "outer-directed" SIB. These responses occur in many combinations, and they do not overlap with nonsocial consummatory SIB topographies. Unlike social SIB, other forms of antisocial behavior, such as aggression and tantrum, were observed infrequently in combination with nonsocial SIB. The most prevalent social SIB was self-hitting, in combination with biting, scratching, and other antisocial behaviors. These results are similar to the results of a survey with 208 SIB cases observed at a state facility for the mentally retarded over a 3-year period (Schroeder, Mulick, & Rojahn, 1980).

Table II gives a breakdown of success ratios—number of clients whose SIB level was reduced divided by the total number of clients reported—for each intervention technique with eight SIB topographies. Although few failures were reported, probably because of editorial reviewing policies that were biased toward reporting positive results (Johnson & Baumeister, 1978), several interesting results are still apparent.

Self-Hitting, Scratching, Gouging, and Hairpulling

Self-hitting includes headbanging, headslapping, body-to-object con-

TABLE I
Associated Topographies of SIB and Related Behaviors

Self-injurious behaviors	H	Bi	Scr	Gou	Pin	PH	Pica	Mou	RV	Copro	Aero	Poly
Hitting self (H)	49											
Biting self (Bi)	11	2										
Scratching self (Scr)	5		3									
Gouging self (Gou)	3			0								
Pinching self (Pin)	2				1							
Pulling out own hair (PH)	2				1	2						
Stuffing orifices (Pica)							10					
Mouthing & sucking (Mou)								1				
Ruminative vomiting (RV)							1		10			
Coprophagy (Copro)	1						3		2	0		
Aerophagia (Aero)											1	
Polydipsia (Poly)												0
Multiples of three or more	13	9	6	6	4	1		1		1		1
Stereotyped behaviors	23											
Aggression & destruction	12	6				1	1					
Emotional behavior	16	7										
Tantrums & screaming	23	7				1						
Other	14		1				1					
Self-restraint	11		1									

TABLE II
Ratio of Success of Response-Contingent Procedures (at Least 80% Reduction from Baseline Levels) as a Function of Different SIB Topographies (Based on 75 Published Studies Using 140 Subjects)

Response-contingent procedures	Self-injurious behaviors: Hitting	Biting	Gouging, scratching	Hairpulling	Scavenge, pica	Ruminate, vomit	Copro	Aero
Punishment	21/22	1/6	1/1	1/1	2/3	3/3		1/1
Overcorrection	23/25	1/1	1/1	1/1	7/7	2/2	3/3	
Time-out	32/33	5/5			0/1	0/1		
Contingent restraint	6/6				2/2		1/1	
Reward alternative behavior	12/15	1/2		1/1	0/1	4/5		
Extinction	3/3	2/2			0/1	0/1		
Satiation	0/1					3/3		

TABLE III
Success Ratios for Seven Response-Contingent Procedures with SIB on Four Criteria of Effectiveness

Effectiveness criteria	Behavior management techniques: Punishment	Overcorrection	Contingent restraint	Time-out	Reinforcing alternative Rs	Extinction	Satiation
Maintenance	9/15 (8)[a]	23/24 (7)	3/3 (7)	9/11 (15)	4/5 (3)	3/3 (10)	2/2 (1)
Stimulus generalization	0/4	2/5	0/4	5/5	4/5	3/3	2/2
Positive covariation	—	—	1/1	3/3	1/1	—	—
Negative covariation	2/2	3/3	1/1	1/4	1/3	1/1	—

[a] — Numbers in parentheses indicate average months for which maintenance was reported.

tact, body-to-body contact, kicking self, slapping other parts of the body, thrusting knuckles or fingers forcefully against the roof of the mouth, etc. The success ratios in the different response-contingent procedures for the above topographies is suprisingly similar, except for rewarding alternative behaviors and satiation. However, when *rate of reduction* rather than *level of reduction* of SIB frequency is the measure of effectiveness, punishment has usually been found to reduce SIB rates more rapidly than other procedures.

If four other commonly used criteria (Schroeder, Mulick, & Schroeder, 1979) are compared with rate reduction of self-hitting (Table III), it appears that the effects of punishment were not maintained well, showed poor stimulus generalization, little positive covariation (e.g., response generalization), and occasional negative covariation (e.g.,response substitution). The results in Table III were taken only from studies that presented data, and not from studies presenting anecdotal accounts of side effects alone.

Biting Self

Biting self appears to be handled best with time-out. This success ratio, depicted in Table II, reflects behavior management studies with the Lesch–Nyhan syndrome (Anderson, Dancis, & Alpert, 1978; Bull & Lavecchio, 1978; Duker, 1975b). It was found that punishment increased self-biting, whereas time-out and extinction reduced it. The reason for this result is unclear. However, Nyhan (1976) has pointed out that these children differ from other SIB clients in many ways: (1) they tend not to be severely retarded; (2) they exhibit idiosyncratic stereotypies related to the motor sequelae of the Lesch–Nyhan syndrome, for example, neck-whipping; and (3) there is some evidence that their behavior management can be improved by 5-hydroxytryptophan (Mizuno & Yugari, 1974). Therefore, whether time-out is the intervention of choice for patients other than Lesch–Nyhan patients is still a question open to research.

Pica, Scavenging, Mouthing, and Coprophagy

The woeful lack of research in this area might appear to be surprising. However, when one considers the risk involved in any type of experimentation with persons who swallow rocks, razor blades, towels, screws, safety pins, etc., it is clear why only procedures and settings where risks can be minimized have been investigated. Overcorrection (Table II) appears to have been the most successful management procedure with these behaviors (Foxx & Martin, 1975; Matson, Stephens, & Smith, 1978; Rojahn *et al.*, 1979;

Rusch, Close, Hops, & Agosta, 1976). It seems likely that the effectiveness of the overcorrection procedure was related to the fact that the subjects of these experiments were fairly compliant with the oral-hygiene positive practice methods used (except for the woman in the Matson *et al.* study). From Table III, it appears that maintenance, but not generalization, is good with overcorrection for pica.

Albin (1977) has criticized the practice of the baiting of the treatment environment in order to increase an artificial frequency of scavenging and pica, which may then be overcorrected and suppressed. This practice, and the consequation of every response during treatment, may account for the lack of generalization to the natural setting. Albin raises the interesting speculation that pica is an aberrant generalization of fingerfeeding, beyond which pica clients have not progressed. Thus far, such speculation has not been tested experimentally.

Chronic Ruminative Vomiting.

Chronic ruminative vomiting consists of repeated vomiting, chewing, and reingestion of vomitus. It is often considered self-injurious, especially when it is related to severe weight loss, dehydration, respiratory complications, infections, and possible esophageal lesions (Richmond, Eddy, & Green, 1958). It also has antisocial components, since ruminators tend to be socially ostracized because of foul odor and appearance.

The prevalence of ruminative vomiting among normal children is unknown, although a number of treatment studies in psychiatric and pediatric settings have been published on young, normal, autistic, or mentally retarded (Schroeder, Schroeder, Smith, & Dalldorf, 1978) revealed ruminative vomiting in .1% of that population. This finding is probably a conservative estimate, since many ruminators are cosmetically clean and are clever in concealing the behavior. The problem comes to the attention of staff in institutional settings only when ruminating becomes a health hazard, or is socially obnoxious.

Vomiting is an adaptive reflex. Although it can reportedly be attenuated by antiemetics (Carter, 1961), brain lesion (Borison, 1959), and surgery (Randolph, Lilly, & Anderson, 1974) ruminative vomiting has not been so successfully treated medically or pharmacologically (Carter, 1961).

The psychoanalytic interpretation of rumination (Richmond & Eddy, 1957; Richmond *et al.*, 1958) is that it is a symptom of disrupted mother–child relationships. The prescribed treatment is hospitalization and copious noncontingent attention to the child by staff to establish a surrogate mother relationship. This procedure has proven successful for young-normal and retarded children (Berlin, McCullough, Lisha, & Szurek, 1957; Wright & Menolascino, 1970). In the latter study, a 6-month follow-up in the home with mothers who had been trained showed maintenance of treatment gains. Thus, it seems that modifying eating habits and improving the environment in which eating occurs may have a significant effect on rumination (Ball, Hendrickson, & Clayton, 1974). How much of this is owing to improved mother–child relationships as opposed to social approval the child receives for eating appropriately is not clear.

Vomiting has been demonstrated to be a conditioned reflex (Collins & Tatum, 1925; Kleitman & Crisler, 1927; Pavlov, 1927). In this context, treatment of ruminative vomiting has been based on operant conditioning procedures: extinction (Wolf, Birnbauer, Lawler, & Williams, 1970) and punishment, such as electrical or other aversive stimulation contingent on a prevomiting response (Kohlenberg, 1970; Lang & Melamed, 1969; Luckey, Watson, & Musick, 1968; Sajwaj *et al.*, 1974; White & Taylor, 1967). Jackson *et al.* (1975) successfully applied a satiation technique to treat two severely retarded chronic ruminators. Two experiments were modestly successful in preventing rumination by reinforcing alternative play (Mulick, Schroeder, & Rojahn, 1977; Smith & Lyon, 1976).

From Tables II and III it would appear that satiation is the treatment of choice. However, it is difficult to compare the effectiveness of the above-mentioned procedures. The psychodynamically based studies were poorly controlled. Only one operant study compared different procedures on the same subjects. The older studies did not present generalization of follow-up data. The punishment studies with normal children reported dramatic and permanent results (Lang & Melamed, 1969). However, in none of the studies with mentally retarded subjects was durability of effects beyond six months reported.

Generally, the impression is left that total suppression of ruminative vomiting is difficult. This result may be because several factors may be involved in maintaining the behavior, that is, social reinforcers, consummatory behaviors, and primary reinforcers related to deprivation. These factors may be highly individual from one subject to another. Any procedure designed to suppress rumination should probably take all these factors into account.

Summary of Response-Contingent Techniques for Reducing SIB

There now exist at least 75 studies with 140 SIB clients using several intervention techniques. The most frequently used techniques have incorporated punishment. This procedure has been used effectively with nearly all SIB topographies, except biting among Lesch–Nyhan patients, for whom it has aggravated SIB. Most punishment techniques do not generalize and maintain treatment effects as well as overcorrection. The latter method has been used effectively with nearly all SIB topographies, particularly self-hitting and pica. Time-out can be used effectively to suppress self-hitting and especially self-biting; but it is probably less advised for nonsocial consummatory types of SIB, such as pica, ruminative vomiting, and coprophagy, since its effectiveness depends primarily on the preexistence of a reinforcing time-in environment. Brief contingent restraint has been used effectively with self hitting and pica. A caution with a contingent restraint is necessary, lest the restraint provide "safe" periods that themselves become reinforcing for the SIB client. Rewarding alternative behaviors has been used primarily with self-hitting and ruminative vomiting. DRI is likely to be more effective when it differentially provides reinforcement of alternative behaviors that are specifically incompatible with topographies of SIB and/or the contingencies reinforcing SIB. Though extinction has been used successfully with self-hitting, it is generally considered risky. The technique occasionally has been successful when punishment has failed, for instance, with self-biting among Lesch–Nyhan syndrome patients or as noncontingent social isolation for self-hitting. Satiation has been used effectively only with chronic ruminative vomiting.

Our analysis of the response-contingent techniques illustrated in Figure 3 may convey a false sense of simplicity with regard to the clinical decision to apply them to the individual case. The application of these techniques never occurs in a vacuum. Therefore, the choice of technique must be mitigated by several qualifiers.

Response-dependent decelerative procedures may temporarily remove a reinforcer, as in response cost and time-out, or provide a negative stimulus following each response, as in punishment. Both procedures lead to direct reductions in the rate of target behaviors. The other two cells represent response-dependent procedures that lead to an increase in the rate of the target behavior. Treatment procedures that derive from such *strengthening effects* on behavior depend on substitution of a new behavior for an old one. Thus, differential positive reinforcement may be provided for topographically incompatible behaviors, or for the absence of SIB itself as in Differential Reinforcement of Other Behavior (or DRO). Negative reinforcement may also be used to strengthen competing behavior, as Lovaas, Schaeffer, and Simmons (1965) have shown, by increasing the social approach in autistic children through the use of contingent termination of electrical stimulation. Similarly, it is believed that the overcorrection procedure, as described by Foxx and Azrin in 1973, utilizes negative reinforcement to strengthen competing behavior, but also involves a period of time-out from other reinforcers, and is, therefore, classified in more than one cell (Epstein *et al.*, 1974; Wells, Forehand, & Hickey, 1977). However, since these relationships have not yet been clearly demonstrated, this classification in Figure 3 must be viewed with caution.

The effects of noncontingently withholding a stimulus—or using an extinction procedure—will depend on whether the self-injurious behavior was dependent on the presentation or the removal of the stimulus (Carr, 1977). In practice the use of extinction to treat SIB usually involves withholding positive consequences thought to maintain the behavior. But the difficulty of identifying and controlling all sources of positive reinforcement, and the gradual decrease in responding characteristic of extinction (Lovaas & Simmons, 1969), precludes its use in many cases.

An overall treatment strategy is beginning to emerge that stems in part from an analysis of what happens when procedures from more than one cell are combined. As already alluded to in the case of overcorrection, it is recognized that immediate suppressive effects and their long-run durability are enhanced when decelerative procedures are combined with attempts to increase systematically, and ultimately substitute, setting-appropriate behaviors. The goal is then to arrange conditions so that appropriate behaviors come to occupy functional positions in the individual's habitual repertoire of daily activities.

The strategy is sound enough. The difficulty comes in actually selecting the components of an individualized treatment plan. One problem is that decelerative procedures differ in their intrusiveness and aversiveness, and no experimental analysis of these procedures as they relate to client characteristics or the severity and nature of the problem behavior yet exists. Because of ethical considerations, outside consultants representing various concerned interest groups are often employed to help set limits in the treatment programs. In practice, treatment options are simply arranged on a continuum of restrictiveness, with positive reinforcement procedures and less obvious negative consequences at one end and severe restrictions on freedom of movement and contingent aversive stimulation at the other. This arrangement, however, is not necessarily related to treatment effectiveness or appropriateness.

Similarly, appropriate target behaviors are selected partly on the basis of response topography and partly on the basis of the likelihood that the new behaviors will continue to be reinforced in the natural environment. The absolute availability of human and material resources in the treatment and posttreatment environments, and prevailing social expectations for what appropriate behavior should be, set practical limits on treatment objectives. Treatment objectives are also limited by the need for staff or caretaker training and the need for additional environmental enrichment—that is, specific activity schedules, toys and educational materials, and changes in physical or social environment. Many clients exhibiting SIB have extremely limited, undifferentiated repertoires of behavior, and many also suffer from multiply handicapping sensory and motor impairments and, therefore, require extensive shaping and high rates of reinforcement to establish even simple appropriate behaviors like eye contact, simple communication skills, self-help skills, fine-motor exploration, and toy play.

EVALUATION OF TREATMENT EFFECTS

Criteria for Successful Interventions

Warren (1977) has identified five criteria for successful behavioral intervention. Essentially, these criteria have been viewed as a means of quantitatively assessing the quality of a behavioral intervention. The dimensions are: (1) response rate; (2) stimulus and response generalization; (3) response durability (maintenance); (4) response diversity (whether suppressed behaviors are supplanted with appropriate alternative prosocial behaviors); and (5) consumer satisfaction.

Not all of these criteria are equally relevant to the management of SIB, but they are all interrelated. It is difficult to evaluate rate reduction without taking into account maintenance, since they are both segments of the same time-frequency continuum. Frequency can be reduced to time allocation, and vice-versa. However, as Albin (1977) has shown for pica management, a rigid adherence to the rate measure does not take into account severe, but low-rate, SIB. As an alternative, Rojahn *et al.* (1979) successfully used latency-to-first-pica response following contingent release as an alternative measure. Measures of SIB severity are also needed.

Another case where Warren's criteria may give a spurious estimate of effectiveness is with severe very high-rate headbanging, where tempo and the cumulative effects of SIB are of concern. It appears that punishment has often been chosen in order to achieve a rate reduction quickly. However, this may not necessarily be a satisfactory long-range objective for behavior management of SIB. When there is an imminent danger of death or serious injury due to SIB—which is not the usual case, according to Nyhan (1976)—rapid reduction in rate by punishment may be very important. But once this reduction is accomplished, provision for generalization and maintenance may be achieved more expeditiously by fading to some other management procedure.

There are many factors other than rate reduction, maintenance, generalization, response diversity, and consumer satisfaction that enter into the equation by which the effectiveness and timeliness of an intervention is judged. Most often additional questions, such as (1) the restrictiveness of the procedure and the treatment environment, (2) what constitutes a success or failure, or (3) what procedures fit the capabilities of the response system where the treatment will be used and maintained, are the province of Human Rights Committees and Internal Review Boards. These issues center around the reaction of the environment to behavior changes of the client before, during, and after intervention. To evaluate such factors, an ecobehavioral assessment of the treatment is needed.

Ecobehavioral Assessment

Ecobehavioral analysis extends traditional views of behavior-modification tactics from the unidimensional to the multidimensional aspects of intervention. It reflects the complexity of behavior changes by observing behaviors of one person as he or she interacts with the group, rather than by being preoccupied with the behavior of one person who is not adapting to the environment. Perhaps environments could be altered on several levels to fit the needs of their inhabitants, and thereby reduce occasions for SIB. Interventions in such environments are also more likely to be successful.

Environmental Organization

Environmental organization should also be based on objective behavior analysis (Risley, 1977; Schroeder, Rojahn, & Mulick, 1978a). For example, Rojahn *et al.* (1979) showed that the use of self-protective devices with SIB residents decreased not only SIB, but also social interactions with caretakers. This finding is an important consideration, since such clients depend so heavily on caretakers for the development of their adaptive skills. An unintended side effect of the noncontingent prevention of SIB may be the reinforcement of using more physical restraints by caretakers, simply because they require less effort than arduous surveillance and behavior management of a severe case of SIB.

Effects of Medication

Another important area of ecobehavioral assessment is evaluation of the effects of medication on SIB. Lipman (1970) and Sprague and Baxley (1978) have estimated that over half the residents in state facilities across the U.S. receive regular psychotropic drugs, 58% of which are large doses of the neuroleptic tranquillizers sustained over long periods of time—for example, thioridazine and chlorpromazine—for behavioral control. Schroeder, Rojahn, and Mulick (1978a) demonstrated how ecobehavioral assessment can be used to study caretaker reactivity in drug treatment of SIB. Although a client's SIB and tantrums were being modified by a time-out procedure, his medication was changed independently in double-blind fashion. As the client improved, caretakers' positive responses to him increased. The course of improvement followed the time-out intervention, whereas the change in medication had a suppressive effect on all behaviors. If multiple behaviors of client and caretakers had not been recorded, a false conclusion might have been reached that thioridazine had brought tantrum behavior under control.

Side Effects

Ecobehavioral assessments have proven useful for examining covariation among collateral behaviors when intervention with target behaviors occurs. The problem of unwanted "side effects" became an issue with the use of intrusive punishment for the management of SIB. A second type of covariation is transitional change in target behaviors as a function of changes in stimulus conditions, for instance, behavioral contrast (Reynolds, 1961). A change in behavior is called a contrast when the change in the rate of responding during the presentation of one stimulus is in a direction away from the rate of responding generated during the presentation of a different stimulus, for example, as in baseline rebound effects following a reinforcing intervention. When a new undesirable behavior emerges as a function of suppression of other behaviors, this type of covariation is called response substitution (Baumeister & Rollings, 1976). Originally found mainly with punishment of SIB, substitution has been observed with nearly every suppression technique (Schroeder, Mulick, & Schroeder, 1979), even stimulus-control procedures (Rojahn *et al.*, 1978). The multicategory system used in ecobehavioral assessment is designed to detect such "side effects."

Site Specificity

In addition to environment and medication, another area of stimulus control with SIB that could be investigated successfully with ecobehavioral technology is site specificity (Schoggen, 1978). This term refers to the notion that certain place-behavior systems are rather strictly organized and fixed, so that behaviors and environmental demands remain fairly constant within and across individuals. Examples would be school behaviors, home behaviors, ward behaviors, church behaviors, mealtime etiquette, etc. Questions of interest from an ecological standpoint would be: (1) Are certain SIB topographies for specific to certain places? (2) What are the antecedents and consequences for SIB in different sites? (3) Do different sites promote different degrees of adaptive behavior, communication, etc., that affect occasions for SIB? Some of the pertinent literature has been reviewed in previous sections, but this is a vastly unresearched area in behavior management of SIB.

Summary

Ecobehavioral analysis attempts to look at not only SIB target behaviors, but also their covariants and setting characteristics, their patterns, sequential dependencies, and so forth, over extended periods of an intervention program. In the future research is likely to focus on complex organism–environment interactions. A substantial technology already exists, and has developed greatly in the past decade. It is hoped that such technology will improve the quality of treatment and the prevention of SIB among the retarded.

Some Programmatic Considerations with SIB

The reader is warned that the present section lacks the firm data base of the previous sections. The system of service delivery with which behavior-management specialists must interface is at least as important as the intervention itself if a program is to be carried out and successfully maintained. Behavior management is usually only part of a treatment package (e.g., the Individualized Educational Plan [IEP]). Behaviorists often consider behavior analysis the "bottom line" in an IEP; but, if they are honest, they recognize that behavior-analysis data must go through several transformations, such as defining behaviors, getting interobserver agreement, and choosing units of measurement and validating them before the data can be adapted for use in a particular setting (Cone & Hawkins, 1977). They also make use of other sources of information besides direct observations, for example, self-reports, daily logs, subjective impressions, etc. (Hersen, 1978). The need for a systems model for clinical decision making has been recognized repeatedly by behavior analysts (Baer, 1977; Gaylord-Ross, 1978; Rogers-Warren & Warren, 1977). Recent reviews about SIB (Carr, 1977; Harris & Ersner-Hershfield, 1978) contain a series of questions for selecting particular interventions. Most of these schemes address broader programming issues of which behavior management is a component. In this section we address these issues more from a perspective of pointing out the need for research in the future than with a view toward answering any of the difficult questions posed.

Legal and Ethical Issues

Because of the high-risk nature of SIB, and because it is managed most frequently in restrictive settings like residential institutions or among persons who are usually severely or profoundly intellectually handicapped, program review committees play a vital role in deciding what, when, where, and how to modify behavior. Program review committees are basically legally mandated, so that no behavior analyst can independently specify the most effective or least restrictive treatment. It should also be remembered that program decisions should be shared with clients to the fullest extent possible, and with their families and their support systems.

The most common mechanism for program review is the internal review board composed primarily of members of the institution (Cooke, Tannenbaum, & Gray, 1977). Although internal review boards serve an important function in protecting human rights, it must be recognized that they also have a vested interest in self-protection. Thus, a treatment strategy can be chosen out of caution, and not necessarily because of effectiveness. As a consequence, external review boards composed of persons employed outside the institution have come into vogue.

External review boards are also very important to delivery of services. However, their role and impact on service systems have rarely been the subject of research. In many states they are now mandated by law for residential facilities. The same type of monitoring should be mandated for other service settings, such as school programs and developmental day care, as well. Schroeder, Rojahn, and Mulick (1978b) have outlined a behavioral analysis of the roles of members on an external review board in a program for managing SIB in a state residential facility. The service professionals on the board acted mainly as problem solvers, whereas administrators dealt primarily with administrative or political matters, and legal professionals were interested in detecting abuse of rights. Although all these roles are useful for a good program review, their balanced representation on the review board can be important to the success of the behavior management specialist. For instance, if the primary mandate of the review board is to prevent abuse, and if there is little apparent danger of abuse in the program, members' attendance at meetings will extinguish, the board's mandate will be compromised, and programming will be impeded. However, if the primary mandate is the enhancement of patients' rights, the review board can be another resource for improving development, implementation, and maintenance of programs as well.

Service Delivery Systems

There are few behavior management programs that require more arduous, continuous, and direct "hands-on" intervention than SIB. This means that the demands on any service system will be a severe drain on manpower and financial resources. For an inefficient service delivery system, managing SIB may be impossible. The need for a vertically organized administration with adequate accountability seems to be recognized in the current trend to institutionalize SIB clients in "high control" units in residential facilities. There are many risks involved in such a programming strategy, for instance, modeling others' inappropriate behaviors, aperiodic reward and punishment of SIB, and lack of generalization beyond that specialized setting, to say nothing of the increased danger of physical injury. However, accountability in the community, in our experience, is often far worse than in the institution. There are some exceptions, of course, but most community programs do not consider severe behavior management problems like SIB a part of their mandate of training and rehabilitation. Rather, SIB clients are recommended for institutionalization. Therefore, the nature of the service delivery system can have a profound effect on whether a behavior management program for SIB will be implemented competently in one setting, regardless of its proven effectiveness in another setting.

Programming Structures

Nearly all service delivery systems require that each client have an individualized program plan. Yet the program structures under which this mandate is implemented may vary tremendously. In an organization whose habilitation plans are strongly influenced by the medical model, the accepted methods of managing SIB may be psychotropic medication and self-protective restraint devices like camisoles, helmets, and fencing masks. In a behaviorally oriented establishment, just the opposite extreme may be in effect. Perhaps the so-called lack of generalization among SIB clients may really be adaptive discrimination of programming structures in different settings. Whatever the case, the role of the behavior analyst in both structures is usually that of a consultant.

The role of the behavioral consultant on a treatment team is primarily that of the ecobehavioral analyst. Not only is his or her task the management of the client's SIB, but also the management of the primary caretakers' behavior. Therefore, the behavioral consultants' primary client is usually the caretaker, not the SIB client. Unfortunately, a behavioral analysis of consultation is a rarely researched area, and thus poorly understood.

The beginnings of a behavioral analysis of consultation have been made by Schroeder (1978), Schroeder and Miller (1975), and Schroeder and Schroeder (1979). This model is adapted from the familiar behavior-analysis cycle of defining behavior, gathering baseline, planning programs, doing follow-up, and giving feedback—but to caretakers instead of the clients themselves. Each step in this cycle contains important issues for the consultant. The first step is consultant entry. The primary issue here is to define the consultee. Schroeder and Miller (1975) discuss several entry patterns and their relative advantages for developing with the consultee a joint ownership of the consulting problem. The next step is taking baseline on the consultee to discover skill levels, strengths, and weaknesses. Often a consultee may begin by requesting a simple information- or task-oriented consultation and end up really wanting training consultation (e.g., workshops and courses, or collaborative long-term consultation). Each type of consultation requires different contingencies and different levels of effort by the consultant. The consultant's role in planning interventions, doing follow-up, and giving feedback occurs only in collaborative consultation. The best contingencies in collaborative consultation are written contingency contracts with the consultee and written consultant reports. Schroeder and Schroeder (1979) have given a brief outline and analysis of the contingencies in using consultant reports.

The vicissitudes of the consultant's role on a team managing SIB are striking. Often consultees change because of staff turnover. Very often referral agents look upon the behavior management specialist as simply another resource to solve their staffing problems. If the consultant gives in to the pressure to "take over" noncontingently, rather than share ownership of the problem, the intervention program will be transferred later with even greater difficulty. More than likely, it will be discontinued once the consultant withdraws, regardless of whether it has been effective or not.

Staffing Considerations

Little is known about the proper selection, entering competencies, motivation, skills, and reasons for rapid turnover of direct caretakers for the severely and profoundly handicapped. Only recently has this area become of interest to behavioral researchers (Zaharia & Baumeister, 1978). Obviously, staff development must be a continuing operation for caretakers dealing with SIB, because (1) a continued high level of competence in behavior management is required to deal effectively with SIB; (2) staff support to maintain focus on program objectives and new techniques is necessary because of the risky nature of SIB and the "high-pressure" circumstances under which behavioral intervention takes place; and (3) the arduous nature of the daily regimens required for effective management is emotionally draining. The latter factor leads to sickness, absenteeism, and eventually turnover if some respite for staff is not periodically arranged.

Staff Training

After several years of experience with the formal education of direct caretaking staff in certification programs, continuing-education programs, and so forth, we have concluded that most formal training, such as lectures, coursework, and demonstration workshops, are good public relations but are relatively useless for creating new skills. An analysis of the contingencies affecting staff performance makes the reasons apparent: (1) state personnel policies often fail to provide the necessary financial incentives for direct-care staff to undergo the hardships of continuing education; (2) the level of expertise required to develop and implement adequate programs to manage problems as severe as SIB requires extensive education and training. Although most direct-care staff have skills in patient care, they are not qualified to design programs or exert quality control of behavior intervention programs.

The only staff training that has been effective in our work with SIB has been where direct caretakers referred a client with SIB to us, and then the client's program was developed jointly with them to meet a specific need that they had. Once this bridge was crossed, more general topics related to intervention tactics could be addressed with a view toward further training. This approach is more difficult for the consultant than traditional staff-training models, but it is also more efficient, because it concentrates only on those staff persons who have strong incentives to participate and use their training.

CONCLUDING REMARKS

What has happened to Suzie, the girl in Tate's (1972) study mentioned in the introduction? A brief update of Suzie's SIB history is very informative. Suzie was 18 when Tate and Baroff (1966b) first began working with her. She had been restrained to her bed by her wrists and ankles for 7½ years, except for periods during which custodial care, such as changing sheets, was performed; she was blinded with cataracts, probably from headbanging; she had had all her teeth removed because of severe self-biting. Tate used an arduous combination of time-out, contingent restraint, and electrical stimulation to suppress her SIB, while at the same time keeping her free from restraints. Seven months after the therapists had left the institution, direct-care staff were still carrying out the program, and Suzie was free of restraints, drugs, and SIB. Three years later (1969), however, Tate learned that Suzie had performed some SIB for which she was noncontingently restrained in a chair by direct-care staff. Six years later (1975), the senior author was called back to consult with direct-care staff because Suzie was again a severe SIB case. Two trainers worked with Suzie, reinstating Tate's (1972) time-out and contingent-restraint procedures. Once again, these methods were effective, and Suzie was "not a problem." Two years later (1977), Suzie had been changed to another residential unit at the same institution, and, once more, she was restrained to a chair because her SIB was "a bad problem." This time a program involving DRO and time-out proved effective. In 1979, Suzie was observed restrained to a chair once again. Meanwhile, there had been turnover in key professional and direct-care staff. Suzie's SIB is being managed currently with an overcorrection procedure.

What can be said about 13 years of Suzie's behavior management? Which program was most effective? The criteria that are most often used, as outlined in previous sections, are problematic for Suzie. Nearly every behavior modification program attempted was successful. Yet she still has a serious SIB problem. The concluding comments of Tate (1972) are indeed sobering:

> The goal of reducing self-injury to a point where Suzie could begin to live in the institution free of restraints, padding, or medication was achieved. This demonstration lends support to the growing body of evidence that conditioning techniques are effective in the control of chronic self-injurious behavior. An effective and economical program whereby the initial benefits of conditioning can be maintained is now much needed. We never enjoyed the illusion that Suzie's self-injury had been permanently eliminated. After all, some of the responses had been in her repertoire for roughly 14 years, and many of her self-injurious acts probably had been reinforced hundreds of times on lean schedules of both positive and negative reinforcement. Obviously, causes of the return of Suzie's self-injury sometime between seven months and three years after therapy cannot be determined. Most probably, spontaneous recovery occurred one day and a new attendant on the ward, or possibly another patient, unfortunately reinforced it with attention and misguided "loving kindness." (p. 83)

Tate's analysis makes a fitting conclusion to the present chapter. Dealing effectively with Suzie's case required careful consideration of the complexity of her multiple SIB topographies, the settings, and the contingencies which maintained them. The management programs were only effective within their ecobehavioral context. Her SIB was not eliminated or cured, but only controlled through a long and arduous series of interventions under circumstances that permitted a high level of consistent contingency management. The behavioral technology for such programming is time-consuming and expensive. However, no alternative is feasible at present.

ACKNOWLEDGMENT

Thanks are due to Martin Wilcox for critically reading the manuscript.

REFERENCES

ALBIN, J. The treatment of pica (scavenging) behavior in the retarded: A critical analysis and implications for research. *Mental Retardation*, 1977, *15*, 14–18.

*ALTMAN, K., HAAVIK, S., & COOK, J. Punishment of SIB in natural settings using contingent aromatic ammonia. *Behavior Research and Therapy*, 1978, *16*, 85–96.

*ANDERSON, L., DANCIS, J., & ALPERT, M. Behavioral contingencies and self mutilation in Lesch-Nyhan Diseased. *Journal of Consulting and Clinical Psychology*, 1978, *46*, 529–536.

*AUSMAN, J., BALL, T. S., & ALEXANDER, D. Behavior therapy of pica with a profoundly retarded adolescent. *Mental Retardation*, 1974, *12*, 16–18.

AYLLON, T., & AZRIN, N. Punishment as a discriminative conditioned reinforcer with humans. *Journal of the Experimental Analysis of Behavior*, 1966, *9*, 411–419.

AZRIN, N. H., & HOLZ, W. C. Punishment. In W. K. Honig, (Ed.), *Operant behavior: Areas of research and application*. New York: Appleton-Century-Crofts, 1966.

*AZRIN, N. H., & WESOLOWSKI, M. Theft reversal: An overcorrection procedure for eliminating stealing by retarded persons. *Journal of Applied Behavior Analysis*, 1974, *7*, 577–581.

*AZRIN, N. H., GOTTLIEB, L. H., HUGHART, L., WESOLOWSKI, M. D., & RAHN, T. Eliminating self-injurious behavior by educative procedures. *Behaviour Research and Therapy*, 1975, *13*, 101–111.

BACHMAN, J. A. Self-injurious behavior: A behavioral analysis. *Journal of Abnormal Psychology*, 1972, *80*, 211–224.

BAER, D. M. Some comments on the structure of the intersection of ecology and applied behavior analysis. In A. Rogers-Warren & S. Warren (Eds.), *Ecological perspectives in behavior analysis*. Baltimore: University Park Press, 1977.

BAER, D. M., WOLF, M. M., & RISLEY, T. Some current dimensions of applied behavior analysis. *Journal of Applied Behavior Analysis*, 1968, *1*, 91–97.

*BALL, T. S., HENDRICKSON, H., & CLAYTON, J. A special feeding technique for chronic regurgitation. *American Journal of Mental Deficiency*, 1974, *78*, 486–493.

*BALL, T. S., SIBBACH, L., JONES, R., STEELE, B., & FRAZIER, L. An accelerometer activated device to control assaultive and self-destructive behaviors in retardates. *Journal of Behavior Therapy and Experimental Psychiatry*, 1975, *6*, 223–228.

*BARNARD, J. D., CHRISTOPHERSON, E. R., ALTMAN, K., & WOLF, M. M. Parent mediated treatment of self-injurious behavior using overcorrection. *Journal of Pediatric Psychology*, 1976, *1*, 56–62.

BAUMEISTER, A. A. Origins and control of stereotyped movements. In C. E. Meyers (Ed.) *Quality of life in severely and profoundly mentally retarded people: Research foundations for improvement*. Washington: AAMD Monograph, No. 3, 1978.

*BAUMEISTER, A. A., & BAUMEISTER, A. A. Suppression of repetitive self-injurious behavior by contingent inhalation of aromatic ammonia. *Journal of Autism and Childhood Schizophrenia*, 1978, *8*, 71–77.

BAUMEISTER, A. A., & FOREHAND, R. Stereotyped acts. In N. R. Ellis (Ed.), *International review of research in mental retardation* (Vol. 6). New York: Academic Press, 1973.

BAUMEISTER, A. A., & ROLLINGS, P. Self-injurious behavior. In N. R. Ellis (Ed.), *International review of research in mental retardation* (Vol. 9). New York: Academic Press, 1976.

BERKSON, G. Abnormal stereotyped acts. In J. Zubin & H. Hunt (Eds.), *Comparative psychopathology*. New York: Grune & Stratton, 1967.

BERKSON, G., & LANDESMAN-DWYER, S. Behavioral research on severe and profound retardation (1955–1974). *American Journal of Mental Deficiency*, 1977, *81*, 428–454.

BERKSON, G., & MASON, W. A. Stereotyped movements of mental defectives: III. Situational effects. *Perceptual and Motor Skills*, 1964, *19*, 635–652.

BERKSON, G., & MASON, W. A. Stereotyped movements of mental defectives: IV. The effects of toys and the character of the acts. *American Journal of Mental Deficiency*, 1964, *68*, 511–524.

*BERLIN, I., MCCULLOUGH, G., LISHA, E., & SZUREK, S. Intractable episodicvomiting in a three-year-old child. *Psychiatric Quarterly*, 1957, *31*, 228–249.

BIRNBRAUER, J. S. Generalization of punishment effects: A case study. *Journal of Applied Behavior Analysis*, 1968, *1*, 201–211.

BIRNBRAUER, J.S. Mental retardation. In H. Leitenberg (Ed.), *Handbook of behavior modification and behavior therapy*. New York: Appleton-Century-Crofts, 1976.

BITTICK, K., FLEEMAN, W., & BRIGHT, T. *Reduction of self-injurious behavior utilizing sensory integration techniques*. Paper presented at the Gatlinburg Conference on Mental Retardation, Gatlinburg, Tennessee, March 1978.

BORISON, H. L. Effect of ablation of medullary emetic chemoreceptor trigger zone on vomiting responses to cerebral intraventricular injection of adrenaline, apomorphine, and pilocarpine in the cat. *Journal of Physiology*, 1959, *147*, 172–177.

*BRAWLEY, E., HARRIS, F., ALLEN, K., FLEMING, R., & PETERSON, R. Behavior modification of an autistic child. *Behavioral Science*, 1969, *4*, 87–97.

BROWN, J. S., MARTIN, R., & MORROW, M. Self-punitive behavior in the rat: Facilitative effects of punishment on resistance to extinction. *Journal of Comparative and Physiological Psychology*, 1964, *57*, 127–133.

*BRYSON, Y., SAKATI, N., NYHAN, W., & FISH, C. Self-mutilative behavior in the Cornelia de Lange Syndrome. *American Journal of Mental Deficiency*. 1971, *76*, 319–324.

*BUCHER, B., & LOVAAS, O. I. Use of aversive stimulation in behavior modification in mental retardation. In M. R. Jones (Ed.), *Miami symposium on the prediction of behavior: Aversive stimulation*. Coral Gables, Fl: University of Miami Press, 1968, pp. 77–145.

*BUCHER, B., REYKDAL, B., & ALBIN, J. Brief physical restraint to control pica. *Journal of Behavior Therapy and Experimental Psychiatry*, 1976, *1*, 137–140.

*BULL, M., & LAVECCHIO, F. Behavior therapy of a child with Lesch-Nyhan Syndrome. *Developmental Medicine and Child Neurology*, 1978, *20*, 368–375.

BYRD, L. Responding in the rat maintained under response-independent electric shock and response-produced electric shock. *Journal of the Experimental Analysis of Behavior*, 1969, *12*, 1–10.

CARR, E. G. The motivation of self-injurious behavior. *Psychological Bulletin*, 1977, *84*, 800–816.

CARR, E. G., NEWSOM, C. D., & BINKOFF, J. A. Stimulus control of selfdestructive behavior in a psychotic child. *Journal of Abnormal Child Psychology*, 1976, *4*, 139–153.

CARTER, C. Carphenazine in mental defective: A specific antiemetic. *Archives of Pediatrics*, 1961, *78*, 349–356.

CLARK, D., KREUTZBERG, J. R., & CHEE, F. Vestibular stimulation influence on motor development in infants. *Science*, 1977, *196*, 1228.

COLLINS, K. H., & TATUM, A. L. A conditioned salivary reflex established by chronic morphine poisoning. *American Journal of Physiology*, 1925, *74*, 14–15.

CONE, J., & HAWKINS, R. Current status and future directions in behavioral assessment. In J. Cone & R. Hawkins (Eds.), *Behavioral assessment*. New York: Bruner Mazel, 1977.

COOKE, R., TANNENBAUM, A., & GRAY, B. A survey of institutional review boards and research involving human subjects. Final grant report on contract No. NO 1-HU-6-2110, Institute for Social Research, University of Michigan, 1977..

*CORTE, H. E., WOLF, M. M., & LOCKE, B. J. A comparison of procedures for eliminating self-injurious behavior of retarded adolescents. *Journal of Applied Behavior Analysis*, 1971, *4*, 201–213.

CRABTREE, L. H. A psychotherapeutic encounter with a self-multilating patient. *Psychiatry*, 1967 *30*(1), 91–100.

DAVENPORT, R., & BERKSON, G. Stereotyped movements of mental defectives. II: Effects of novel objects. *American Journal of Mental Deficiency*, 1963, *67*, 879–882.

*DECATANZARO, D., & BALDWIN, G. Effective treatment of self-injurious behavior through a forced arm exercise. *American Journal of Mental Deficiency*, 1978, *82*, 433–439.

*DIZMANG, L., & CHEATHAM, C. The Lesch-Nyhan Syndrome. *American Journal of Psychiatry*, 1970, *127*, 671–677.

DOLEYS, D., MCWHORTER, A., WILLIAMS, S., & GENTRY, W. Encopresis: Its treatment and relation to nocturnal enuresis. *Behavior Therapy*, 1977, *8*, 77–82.

*DUKER, P. C. Behavior therapy for self-injurious behavior: Two case studies. *Research Exchange and Practice in Mental Retardation*, 1975, *1*(4), 223–232.(a)

*DUKER, P. C. Behavior control of self-biting in a Lesch-Nyhan patient. *Journal of Mental Deficiency Research*, 1975, *19*(11), 11–19.(b)

*DUKER, P. C., & GATHERCOLE, S. Remotely applied punishment vs. avoidance conditioning in the treatment of self-injurious behaviors. *Behavior Analysis and Modification*, 1976, *3*, 179–188.

*DUKER, P. C., & SEYS, D. Elimination of vomiting in a retarded female using restitutional overcorrection. *Behavior Therapy*, 1977, *8*, 255–257.

EPSTEIN, H., DOKE, L., SAJWAJ, T., SORELL, S., & RIMMER, B. Generality and side effects of overcorrection. *Journal of Applied Behavior Analysis*, 1974, *7*, 385–390.

ERWIN, J., MITCHELL, G., & MAPLE, T. Abnormal behavior in non-isolate reared monkeys. *Psychological Reports*, 1973, *33*, 515–523.

*FAVELL, J., MCGIMSEY, J., & JONES, M. The use of physical restraint in the treatment of self-injury and as positive reinforcement. *Journal of Applied Behavior Analysis*, 1978, *11*, 225–241.

FITZHERBERT, J. The origin of headbanging: A suggested explanation with an illustrative case history. *Journal of Mental Science*, 1950, *96*, 793–795.

FOREHAND, R., & BAUMEISTER, A. A. Deceleration of aberrant behavior among retarded individuals. In M. Hersen, R. M. Eisler, & P. M. Miller (Eds.), *Progress in behavior modification* (Vol. 2). New York: Academic Press, 1976..

FOXX, R. An overview of overcorrection. *Journal of Pediatric Psychology*, 1978, *3*, 97–101.

FOXX, R. M., & AZRIN, N. H. The elimination of self-stimulatory behavior of autistic and retarded children by overcorrection. *Journal of Applied Behavior Analysis*, 1973, *6*, 1–14.

*FOXX, R. M., & MARTIN, E. D. Treatment of scavenging behavior (coprophagy and pica) by overcorrection. *Behaviour Research and Therapy*, 1975, *13*, 153–162.

FRANKEL, F., & SIMMONS, J. Q. Self-injurious behavior in schizophrenic and retarded children. *American Journal of Mental Deficiency*, 1976, *80*, 512–522.

FRANKEL, F., FREEMAN, B., RITVO, E., CHIKAMI, B., & CARR, E. Effects of frequency of photic stimulation upon autistic and retarded children. *American Journal of Mental Deficiency*, 1976, *81*, 32–40.

FREDERICK, C., & RESNIK, H. How suicidal behaviors are learned. *American Journal of Psychotherapy*, 1971, *25*, 37–55.

*Freeman, B., Graham, V., & Ritvo, E. Reduction of self-destruction by overcorrection. *Psychological Reports*, 1975, *37*, 446.
Freud, A. Self-mutilative behavior. *The Psychoanalytic Study of the Child*, 1954, *8*, 9–19.
Gaylord-Ross, R. *A decision model for the treatment of aberrant behaviors in applied settings.* Unpublished Manuscript, 1978.
Gluck, J., & Sackett, G. Frustrations and self-aggression in social isolate rhesus monkeys. *Journal of Abnormal Psychology*, 1974, *83*, 331–334.
Green, A. Self-mutilation in schizophrenic children. *Archives of General Psychiatry*, 1967, *17*, 234–244.
Green, A. Self-destructive behavior in physically abused schizophrenic children. *Archives of General Psychiatry*, 1968, *19*, 171–179.
Greenacre, P. Certain relationships between fetishism and faulty development of the body image. *The Psychoanalytic Study of the Child*, 1954, *8*, 78–98.
Greene, R., & Hoats, D. Aversive Tickling: A simple conditioning technique. *Behavior Therapy*, 1971, *2*, 389–393.
Gregg, C., Haffner, M., & Korner, A. The relative efficacy of vestibular-proprioceptive stimulation and the upright position in enhancing visual pursuit in neonates. *Child Development*, 1976, *40*, 309.
*Griffin, J. C., Locke, B. J., & Landers, W. Manipulation of potential punishment parameters in the treatment of self-injury. *Journal of Applied Behavior Analysis*, 1975, *8*, 458–464.
*Hamilton, H., Stephens, L., & Allen, P. Controlling aggressive and destructive behavior in severely retarded institutionalized residents. *American Journal of Mental Deficiency*, 1967, *71*, 852–856.
*Harris, S., & Ersner-Hershfield, R. Behavioral suppression of seriously disruptive behavior in psychotic and retarded patients: A review of punishment and its alternatives. *Psychological Bulletin*, 1978, *85*, 1352–1375.
Harris, S., & Romanczyk, R. Treating self-injurious behavior of a retarded child by overcorrection. *Behavior Therapy*, 1976, *7*, 235–239.
Hereford, S. M., Cleland, C. C., & Fellner, M. Territoriality and scent-marking: A study of profoundly retarded enuretics and encopretics. *American Journal of Mental Deficiency*, 1973, *77*, 426–430.
Hersen, M. Do behavior therapists use self-reports as major criteria? *Behavior Analysis and Modification*, 1978, *2*, 328–334.
Holz, W., & Azrin, N. Discriminative properties of punishment. *Journal of the Experimental Analysis of Behavior*, 1961, *4*, 225–232.
Holz, W., & Azrin, N. Interactions between the discriminative and adversive properties of punishment. *Journal of the Experimental Analysis of Behavior*, 1962, *5*, 229–234.
*Jackson, G. M., Johnson, C. R., Ackron, G. S., & Crowley, R. Food satiation as a procedure to decelerate vomiting. *American Journal of Mental Deficiency*, 1975, *80*, 223–227.
Johnson, W. & Baumeister, A. A self-injurious behavior: A review and analysis of methodological details of published studies. *Behavior Modification*, 1978, *2*, 465–484.
*Jones, F. H., Simmons, J. G., & Frankel, F. Case study: An extinction procedure for eliminating self-destructive behavior in a 9-year-old autistic girl. *Journal of Autism and Childhood Schizophrenia*, 1974, *4*, 241–250.
Kanner, L. *Child psychiatry*. Springfield, Ill: Charles C Thomas, 1957.
Kelleher, R., Riddle, W., & Cook, L. Persistence of behavior maintained by unavoidable shocks. *Journal of the Experimental Analysis of Behavior*, 1963, *6*, 507–517.
Kleitman, N., & Crisler, G. A quantitative study of the conditioned salivary reflex. *American Journal of Physiology*, 1927, *79*, 571–614.

*KOHLENBERG, R. The punishment of persisting vomiting: A case study. *Journal of Applied Behavior Analysis*, 1970, *3*, 241–245.
*KOHLENBERG, R., LEVIN, M., & BELCHER, S. Skin conductance changes and the punishment of self-destructive behavior. *Mental Retardation*, 1973, *11*, 11–13.
LANE, R. G., & DOMRATH, R. P. Behavior Therapy: A case history. *Hospital and Community Psychiatry*, 1970, *21*, 150–153.
*LANG, P., & MELAMED, B. Case report: Avoidance conditional therapy of an infant with chronic ruminative vomiting. *Journal of Abnormal Psychology*, 1969, *74*, 1–8.
LEITENBERG, H. Is time-out from positive reinforcement an aversive event? A review of the experimental evidence. *Psychological Bulletin*, 1965, *64*, 428–441.
LEMKE, H., & MITCHELL, R. Controlling the behavior of a profoundly retarded child. *The American Journal of Occupational Therapy*, 1972, *26*, 261–264.
LESCH, M., & NYHAN, W. A familial disorder of uric acid metabolism and central nervous system function. *American Journal of Medicine*, 1964, *36*, 561–570.
LESTER, D. Self-mutilating behavior. *Psychological Bulletin*, 1972, *78*, 119–128.
*LIBBY, D., & PHILLIPS, E. Eliminating rumination behavior in a profoundly retarded adolescent: An exploratory study. *Mental Retardation*, 1979, *17*, 94–95.
LICHTSTEIN, K., & WAHLER, R. The ecological assessment of an autistic child. *Journal of Abnormal Child Psychology*, 1976, *4*, 31–54.
LIPMAN, R. The use of psychopharmacological agents in residential facilities for the retarded. In F. Menolascino (Ed.), *Psychiatric approaches to mental retardation*. New York: Basic Books, 1970.
LOURIE, R. The role of rhythmic patterns in childhood. *American Journal of Psychiatry*, 1949, *105*, 653–660.
*LOVAAS, O. I. & SIMMONS, J. Q. Manipulation of self-destruction in three retarded children. *Journal of Applied Behavior Analysis*, 1969, *2*, 143–159.
*LOVAAS, O. I. FREITAG, G., GOLD, V., & KASSORLA, I. Experimental studies in childhood schizophrenia: Analysis of self-destructive behavior. *Journal of Experimental Child Psychology*, 1965, *2*, 67–84.
LOVAAS, O. I., SCHAEFFER, R., & SIMMONS, J. Q. Experimental studies in childhood schizophrenia: Building a social behavior in autistic children by the use of electric shock. *Journal of Experimental Research in Personality*, 1965, *1*, 99–109.
LUCERO, W., FRIEMAN, G., SPOERING, K., & FEHRENBACHER, J. A comparison of three procedures in reducing self-injurious behavior. *American Journal of Mental Deficiency*, 1976, *80*, 548–554.
*LUCKEY, R. E., WATSON, C., & MUSICK, C. Aversive conditioning as a means of inhibiting vomiting and rumination. *American Journal of Mental Deficiency*, 1968, *73*, 139–147.
*LUISELLI, J., HELFEN, C., COLOZZI, G., DONELLON, S. & PEMBERTON, B. Controlling self-inflicted biting of a retarded child by the differential reinforcement of other behavior. *Psychological Reports*, 1978, *42*, 435–438.
*LUTZKER, J. R. Reducing self-injurious behavior by facial screening. *American Journal of Mental Deficiency*, 1978, *82*, 510–513.
MACDONOUGH, T., & FOREHAND, R. Response-contingent time-out: Important parameters in behavior modification with children. *Journal of Behavior Therapy and Experimental Psychiatry*, 1973, *4*, 231–236.
MACLEAN, W., & BAUMEISTER, A. A. *An environmental analysis of sterotyped behavior of developmentally delayed children*. Paper presented at the Twelfth Annual Gatlinburg Conference on Research in Mental Retardation, Gulf Shores, Alabama, April 1979.
MAISTO, C., & BAUMEISTER, A. An analysis of variables related to self-injurious behavior among institutionalized retarded persons. *Journal of Mental Deficiency Research*, 1978, *12*, 27–36.

MARIE, C., ROYER, P., & RAPPAPORT, R. Congenital hypercicimia with neurological renal and hematologic problems. *Archives Francaises de Pediatric*, 1967, *24*(5), 501–510.

MATSON, J. I., & OLLENDICK, T. Overcorrection: A Bibliography, 1971–1977. Unpublished manuscript, 1977.

MATSON, J. L., STEPHENS, R. L., & SMITH, C. Treatment of self-injurious behavior with overcorrection. *Journal of Mental Deficiency Research*, 1978, *22*, 175–178.

*MCPHERSON, L., & JOACHIM, R. The use of electric shock to reduce headbanging in a mentally retarded boy—a case study. *Australian Journal of Mental Deficiency*, 1974, *3*, 20–24.

*MEASEL, J., & ALFIERI, P. A. Treatment of self-injurious behavior by a combination of reinforcement for incompatible behavior and overcorrection. *American Journal of Mental Deficiency*, 1976, *81*, 147–153.

MERBAUM, M. The modification of self-destructive behavior by a mother-therapist using aversive stimulation. *Behavior Therapy*, 1973, *4*, *442*, 447.

MIRON, N. Behavior modification techniques in the treatment of self-injurious behavior in institutionalized retardates. *Bulletin of Suicidology*, 1971, *8*, 64–69.

*MIZUNO, T., & YUGARI, Y. Self-mutilation in Lesch-Nyhan Syndrome. *Lancet*, 1974 1, *761*.

MOGEL, S., & SCHIFF, W. Extinction of a head bumping symptom of eight years duration in 2 minutes: A case reports. *Behaviour Research and Therapy*, 1967, *5*(2), 131–132.

*MULICK, J. A., SCHROEDER, S. R., & ROJAHN, J. *A comparison of four procedures for the treatment of chronic ruminative vomiting*. Paper presented at the Gatlinburg Conference on Mental Retardation, Gatlinburg, Tennessee, March 1977.

MULICK, J., HOYT, R., ROJAHN, J., & SCHROEDER, S. Reduction of a "nervous habit" in a profoundly retarded youth by increasing toy play: A case study. *Journal of Behavior Therapy and Experimental Psychiatry*, 1978, *9*, 381–385.

MURRAY, M., & NEVIN, J. Some effects of correlation between response-contingent shock and reinforcement. *Journal of the Experimental Analysis of Behavior*, 1967, *10*, 301–309.

*MYERS, J., & DIEBERT, A. Reduction of self-abusive behavior in a blind child by using a feeding response. *Journal of Behavior Therapy and Experimental Psychiatry*, 1971, *2*, 141–144.

*NUNES, D., MURPHY, R., & RUPRECHT, M. L. Reducing self-injurious behavior of severely retarded individuals through withdrawal of reinforcement procedures. *Behavior Modification*, 1977, *1*, 499–516.

NYHAN, W. L. The Lesch-Nyhan Syndrome: Self-destructive biting, mental retardation, neurological disorder and hyperuricaemia. *Developmental Medicine and Child Neurology*, 1967, *9*, 563–572.

NYHAN, W. L. Clinical features of the Lesch-Nyhan syndrome: Introduction—Clinical and genetic features. *Federation Proceedings*, 1968, *27*(4), 1027–1033. (a)

NYHAN, W. L. Summary of clinical features. *Federation Proceedings*, 1968, *27*(4), 1034–1041. (b)

NYHAN, W. L. Behavior in the Lesch-Nyhan Syndrome. *Journal of Autism and Childhood Schizophrenia*, 1976, *6*, 235–252.

NYHAN, W. L., PESEK, J., SWEETMAN, L., CARPENTER, D. G., & CARTER, C. H. Genetics of an X-linked disorder of uric acid metabolism and cerebral function. *Pediatric Research*, 1967, *1*(1), 5–13..

OLLENDICK, T., & MATSON, J. Effectiveness of hand overcorrection for topographically similar and dissimilar self-stimulatory behavior. *Journal of Experimental Child Psychology*, 1978, *25*, 396–403.

PALUCK, R. J., & ESSER, A. H. Controlled experimental modification of aggressive behavior in territories of severely retarded boys. *American Journal of Mental Deficiency*, 1971, *76*, 23–290. (a)

PALUCK, R. J., & ESSER, A. H. Territorial behavior as an indicator of changes in clinical behavioral conditioning of severely retarded boys. *American Journal of Mental Deficiency*, 1971, *76*, 284-290. (b)

PAVLOV, I. P. *Conditioned reflexes: An investigation of the physiological activity of the cerebral cortex. Lecture III.* Oxford: Oxford University Press, 1927.

*PEINE, H. The elimination of a child's self-injurious behavior at home and school. *School Applications of Learning Theory*, 1972, *4*, 1-11.

*PETERSON, R., & PETERSON, L. The use of positive reinforcement in the control of self-destructive behavior in a retarded boy. *Journal of Experimental Child Psychology*, 1968, *6*, 351-360.

*PROCHASKA, J., NELSON, S., MARZILLI, R., COLBY, J., & DONOVAN, W. Remote-control aversive stimulation in the treatment of head-banging in a retarded child. *Journal of Behavior Therapy and Experimental Psychiatry*, 1974, *5*, 285-289.

*RAGAIN, R., & ANSON, J. The control of self-mutilating behavior with positive reinforcement. *Mental Retardation*, 1976, *14*, 22-25.

RAGO, W. V. Identifying profoundly mentally retarded subtypes as a means of institutional grouping. *American Journal of Mental Deficiency*, 1977, *81*, 470-473.

RAGO, W., PARKER, R., & CLELAND, C. H. Effect of increased space on the social behavior of institutionalized profoundly retarded male adults. *American Journal of Mental Deficiency*, 1978, *82*, 554-558.

*RAMEY, G. Use of electric shock in the classroom: The remediation of self-abusive behavior of a retarded child. *Behavioral Engineering*, 1973-1974, *1*, 4-9.

RANDOLPH, J., LILLY, J., & ANDERSON, W. Surgical treatment of gastroesophageal reflux in infants. *Annals of Surgery*, 1974, *180*, 479-486.

REPP, A. C., & DEITZ, S. M. Reducing aggressive and self-injurious behavior of institutionalized retarded children through reinforcement of other behavior. *Journal of Applied Behavior Analysis*, 1974, *7*, 313-325.

REYNOLDS, G. S. Behavioral contrast. *Journal of the Experimental Analysis of Behavior*, 1961, *4*, *57*, 71.

*RICHMOND, J., & EDDY, E. Rumination: A psychosomatic syndrome. *Psychiatric Research Reports*, 1957, *8*, 1-11.

RICHMOND, J., EDDY, E., & GREEN, M. Rumination: A psychosomatic syndrome in infancy. *Pediatrics*, 1958, *22*, 49-55.

*RINN, R., & JACKSON, J. The treatment of aeurophagia with self-administered response-contigent shock. *Behavioral Engineering*, 1974, *2*, 7-8.

RISLEY, T. The ecology of applied behavior analysis. In A. Rogers-Warren & S. Warren (Eds.), *Ecological perspectives in behavior analysis.* Baltimore: University Park Press, 1977..

ROGERS-WARREN, A., & WARREN, S. *Ecological perspectives in behavior analysis.* Baltimore: University Park Press, 1977.

ROJAHN, J., MULICK, J. A., MCCOY, D. & SCHROEDER, S. R. Setting effects, adaptive clothing, and the modification of head banging and self-restraint in two profoundly retarded adults. *Behavioral Analysis and Modification*, 1978, *2*, 185-196.

*ROJAHN, J., MULICK, J., & SCHROEDER, S. R. *Analysis of generalization and setting effects during overcorrection to control pica in two retarded adults.* Paper presented at the Twelfth Annual Gatlinburg Conference on Mental Retardation, Gulf Shores, Alabama, April 1979.

*ROLLINGS, J. P., BAUMEISTER, A., & BAUMEISTER, A. The use of overcorrection procedures to eliminate stereotyped behaviors in retarded individuals. *Behavior Modification*, 1977, *1*, 29-46.

*ROMANCZYK, R., & GOREN, E. Severe self-injurious behavior: The problem of clinical control. *Journal of Clinical Psychology*, 1975, *43*, 730-739.

*Rusch, F., Close, D., Hops, H., & Agosta, J. Overcorrection: Generalization and maintenance. *Journal of Applied Behavior Analysis*, 1976, *9*, 498.

Sajwaj, T., & Hedges, D. *"Side-effects" of a punishment procedure in an oppositional retarded child.* Paper presented at Western Psychological Association, San Francisco, April 1971.

*Sajwaj, T., Libet, J., & Agras, S. Lemon juice therapy: The control of life-threatening rumination in a six-month-old infant. *Journal of Applied Behavior Analysis*, 1974, *1*, 557–566.

Sallustro, F., & Atwell, C. Body rocking, head banging, and head rolling in normal children. *Journal of Pediatrics*, 1978, *93*, 704–708.

Sandler, J Masochism: An empirical analysis. *Psychological Bulletin*, 1964, *62 197*, 204.

*Saposnek, D. T., & Watson, L. S. The elimination of the self-destructive behavior of a psychotic child: A case study. *Behavior Therapy*, 1974, *5*, 79–89.

Schoggen, P. Ecological psychology and mental retardation. In G. Sackett (Ed.), *Observing Behavior* (Vol. I). Baltimore: University Park Press, 1978.

Schroeder, C. *The psychologist's role in P.L. 94–142: Consultation strategies with peer groups of handicapped children.* Paper presented at the Annual Convention of the American Psychological Association, Toronto, September 1978.

Schroeder, C., & Miller, F. T. Entry patterns and strategies in consultation. *Professional Psychology*, 1975, *2*, 182–186.

Schroeder, C., & Schroeder, S. *A behavioral model to school consultation.* Paper presented at the annual convention of the American Association on Mental Deficiency, Miami, May 1979.

Schroeder, S. Usage of stereotypy as a descriptive term. *The Psychological Record*, 1970, *29*, 457–464.

*Schroeder, S. R., & Humphrey, R. H. *Environmental context effects and contingent restraint time-out of self-injurious behavior in a deaf-blind profoundly retarded woman.* Paper presented at the 101st Annual Meeting of the American Association on Mental Deficiency, New Orleans, 1977.

*Schroeder, S. R., Peterson, C., Solomon, L., & Artley, J. EMG feedback and the contingent restraint of self-injurious behavior among the severely retarded: Two case illustrations. *Behavior Therapy*, 1977, *8*, 738–741.

Schroeder, S. R., Rojahn, J., & Mulick, J. Eco-behavioral organization of developmental day care for the chronically self-injurious. *Journal of Pediatric Psychology*, 1978, *3*, 81–88. (a)

Schroeder, S. R., Rojahn, J., & Mulick, J. A behavioral analysis of consent committee performance. *North Carolina Journal of Mental Health*, 1978, *8*, 25–30. (b)

Schroeder, S. R., Schroeder, C., Smith, B., & Dalldorf, J. Prevalence of self-injurious behavior in a large state facility for the retarded. *Journal of Autism and Childhood Schizophrenia*, 1978, *8*, 261–269.

Schroeder, S., Mulick, J., & Schroeder, C. Management of severe behavior problems of the retarded. In N. Ellis (Ed.), *Handbook of mental deficiency*, (2nd ed.). New York: Erlbaum, 1979.

Schroeder, S., Mulick, J., & Rojahn, J. The definition, taxonomy, epidemiology, and ecology of self-injurious behavior. *Journal of Autism and Developmental Disorders*, 1980, *10*, 417–432.

Sidman, M. Remarks. *Behaviorism*, 1978, *6*, 265–268..

Sidman, M., Hernstein, R., & Conrad, D. Maintenance of avoidance behavior by unavoidable shocks. *Journal of Comparative and Physiologica Psychology*, 1957, *50*, 558–562.

Skinner, B. F. Science and human behavior. New York: Macmillan, 1953.

Slawson, P. F., & Davidson, P. W. Hysterical self-mutilation of the tongue. *Archives of General Psychiatry*, 1964, *11*(6), 581–588.

*SMITH, D., & LYON, R. Eliminating vomiting behavior in a profoundly retarded resident. *Research and the Retarded*, 1976, *3*, 24–27.

*SOLNICK, J. V., RINCOVER, A., & PETERSON, C. R. Some determinants of the reinforcing and punishing effects of time out. *Journal of Applied Behavior Analysis*, 1977, *10*, 415–424.

SPRAGUE, R. L., & BAXLEY, G. B. Drugs used for the management of behavior in mental retardation, with comments on some legal aspects. In J. Wortis (Ed.), *Mental retardation* (Vol. 10). New York: Bruner/Mazel, 1978.

STINNETT, J. L., & HOLLANDER, J. H. Compulsive self-mbtilation. *Journal of Mental and Nervous Diseases*, 1970, *150*, 371–375.

STRETCH, R., ORLOFF, E., & DALRYMPLE, S. Maintenance of responding by fixed-interval schedules of electric shock presentation in squirrel monkeys. *Science*, 1968, *162*, 583–586.

STUBBS, D., & SILVERMAN, P. Second-order schedules: Brief shock at the completion of each component. *Journal of the Experimental Analysis of Behavior*, 1972, *17*, 201–212.

TALKINGTON, L., & HALL, S. Hearing impairment and aggressiveness in mentally retarded. *Perceptual and Motor Skills*, 1969, *28*, 303–306.

TALKINGTON, L., & RILEY, J. Reduction diets and aggression in institutionalized MR. *Mental retardation research series* (No. 1). Austin, Texas: Austin State School, 1970.

TALKINGTON, L. W., HALL, S. M., & ALTMAN, R. Communication deficits and aggression in the mentally retarded. *American Journal of Mental Deficiency*, 1971, *76*, 235–237.

*TANNER, B. A., & ZEILER, M. D. Punishment of self-injurious behavior using aromatic ammonia as the aversive stimulus. *Journal of Applied Behavior Analysis*, 1975, *8*, 53–57.

*TARPLEY, H., & SCHROEDER, S. A comparison of DRO and DRI procedures in the treatment of self-injurious behavior. *American Journal of Mental Deficiency*, 1979, *84*, 188–194.

*TATE, B. Case study: Control of chronic self-injurious behavior by conditioning procedures. *Behavior Therapy*, 1972, *3*, 72–83.

*TATE, B., & BAROFF, G. Aversive control of self-injurious behavior in a psychotic boy. *Behavior Research and Therapy*, 1966, *4*(4), 281–287. (a)

TATE, B., & BAROFF, G. *The application of reinforcement theory to modification of self-mutilative behavior.* Paper presented at the meeting of the Southeastern Psychological Association, New Orleans, March 1966. (b)

*THOMAS, R. L., & HOWARD, G. A. A treatment program for a self-destructive child. *Mental Retardation*, 1971, *9*, 16–18.

WAHLER, R. Some ecological problems in child behavior modification. In S. Bijou & E. Ribes-Inesta (Eds.), *Behavior modification: Issues and extensions.* New York: Academic Press, 1970.

WAHLER, R. G., HOUSE, A. E., & STAMBAUGH, E. E. *Ecological assessment of child problem behavior.* New York: Pergamon, 1976.

WALLER, M., & WALLER, P. The effects of unavoidable shocks on a multiple schedule having an avoidance component. *Journal of the Experimental Analysis of Behavior*, 1963, *6*, 29–37.

*WARD, E. *Overcorrection: A component analysis of its effects and side effects on the appropriate and inappropriate behavior of retarded children and adults.* Paper presented at the Gatlinburg Conference on Mental Retardation, Gatlinburg, Tennessee, March 1977.

WARREN, S. A useful ecobehavioral perspective for applied behavior banalysis. In A. Rogers-Warren & S. Warren (Eds.), *Ecological perspectives in behavior analysis.* Baltimore: University Park Press, 1977.

*WEBSTER, O. R., & AZRIN, N. H. Required relaxation: A method of inhibiting agitative-disruptive behavior of retardates. *Behavior Research and Therapy*, 1973, *11*, 67–78.

*WEIHAR, R., & HARMAN, R. The use of ommission training to reduce self-injurious behavior in a retarded child. *Behavior Therapy*, 1975, *6*, 261–268.

WELLS, K., FOREHAND, R., & HICKEY, K. Effects of a verbal warning and overcorrection on stereotyped and appropriate behaviors. *Journal of Abnormal Child Psychology,* 1977, *5,* 387–403.

*WHITE, G., NIELSEN, G., & JOHNSON, S. Time-out duration and the suppression of deviant behavior in children. *Journal of Applied Behavior Analysis,* 1972, *5,* 111–120.

WHITE, J. C., & TAYLOR, D. J. Noxious conditioning as a treatment for rumination. *Mental Retardation,* 1967, *5,* 30–33.

*WILLIAMS, J., SCHROEDER, S. R., & ROJAHN, J. *Effects of environmental enrichment and contingent teacher interaction on the effectiveness of time-out for self-injurious behavior.* Paper presented at the Gatlinburg Conference on Mental Retardation, Gatlinburg, Tennessee, April 1978.

*WOLF, M., RISLEY, T., & MEES, P. Application of operant conditioning procedures to the behavior problems of an autistic child. *Behavior Research and Therapy,* 1964, *1,* 305–312.

WOLF, M., RISLEY, T., JOHNSON, M., HARRIS, F., & ALLEN, E. Application of operant conditioning procedures to the behavior problems of an autistic child. A follow-up and extension. *Behavior Research and Therapy,* 1967, *5,* 103–111.

WOLF, M. M., BIRNBRAUER, J., LAWLER, J., & WILLIAMS, T. The operant, extinction, reinstatement, and re-extinction of vomiting behavior in a retarded child. In R. Ulrich, T. Stachik, & J. Mabry (eds.), *Control of human behavior: From cure to prevention* (Vol. 2). Glenview, Ill: Scott, Foresman, 1970.

WOODEN, H. Use of negative practice to eliminate nocturnal headbanging. *Journal of Behavior Therapy and Experimental Psychiatry,* 1974, *5,* 81–82.

WRIGHT, M., & MENOLASCINO, F. Rumination, mental retardation, and interventive therapeutic nursing. In F. Menolascino (Ed.), *Psychiatric approaches to mental retardation.* New York: Basic Books, 1970.

*YOUNG, J. A., & WINCZE, J. P. The effects of the reinforcement of compatible and incompatible alternative behaviors of the self-injurious and related behaviors of a profoundly retarded female adults. *Behavior Therapy,* 1974, *5,* 614–623.

ZAHARIA, E., & BAUMEISTER, A. Technician turnover and absenteeism in public residential facilities. *American Journal of Mental Deficiency,* 1978, *82,* 580–593.

*ZEGIOB, L., ALFORD, G., & HOUSE, A. Response suppressive and generalization effects of facial screening on multiple self-injurious behavior in a retarded boy. *Behavior Therapy,* 1978, *9,* 688.

4 *Treating Self-Stimulatory Behavior*

FLOYD O'BRIEN

THE SELF-STIMULATORY CLASS OF BEHAVIOR

Common Forms

Mentally retarded and other developmentally disabled people perform repetitious motor behavior to such an excess that they are readily distinguished from developmentally normal people. They may rock their bodies in a stereotypic manner, wave their hands in front of their faces, weave their hands from side to side, rub their fingers together, grind their teeth, twirl their hair around their fingers, repeatedly make stereotypic sounds, grimace, tap their feet, etc. Some developmentally disabled people perform repetitious behaviors that produce physical injury to themselves (e.g., bang their heads against objects, bite their arms, slap their faces), a class of repetitious acts generally called "self-injurious behavior." (For a discussion, see Chapter 3.) In the present chapter, the discussion will be confined to those repetitious acts generally referred to as "self-stimulatory behavior"—behaviors that are stereotyped and performed repetitiously, and that fail to produce any apparent positive environmental consequences or physical injury.

Prevalence

About two-thirds of the mentally retarded clients that live in large institutional settings perform self-stimulatory behaviors (Berkson & Davenport, 1962). Kaufman and Levitt (1965) observed bodyrocking in 69% of a sample of residents in such a facility. Similarly, in a survey of teachers who work with severely delayed students, Wehman and McLaughlin (1979)

FLOYD O'BRIEN • Department of Psychology, University of the Pacific, Stockton, California 95204.

found self-stimulatory behavior second only to noncompliance as the most frequently identified problem. Autistic persons, who are functionally mentally retarded (i.e., developmentally disabled), perform self-stimulatory behaviors to the extent that these are an identifying characteristic of the label "autism" (Rimland, 1964; Rincover & Koegel, 1977). Thus, people with autism and mental retardation engage in self-stimulation to the extent that it is viewed by treatment personnel as a major problem. As Whitman and Scibak (1979) concluded, "[Self-stimulation] is one of the more serious and widespread problems manifested by the severely and profoundly retarded" (p. 313).

Labels

Several different labels are used when referring to repetitious, stereotyped behavior. "Self-stimulatory behavior" was selected for this review because it is the most prevalent term. When authors use the label "self-stimulation," they implicitly assume that people perform these acts to increase stimulation for themselves, be the stimulation visual, auditory, proprioceptive, kinesthetic, or tactile. Other labels similarly contain implied assumptions as to why the behaviors are performed. The label "inward-directed" similarly implies that the behaviors are performed to produce internal stimulation. By calling these behaviors "nonfunctional," authors are assuming that the behavior has no environmental function, that is, no positive effects from the environment as a consequence. In so doing, these authors also imply that the behaviors are performed to produce an internal function. The same can be said of the labels "purposeless" and "unrewarded." A similar internal function is implied when authors use the label "autisms," since dictionaries (e.g., Webster's Seventh New Collegiate Dictionary, 1972) define this term as an internal function. Finally, we find one label that is without inference and purely descriptive, "stereotyped movements."

By providing any one label for all these different behaviors (e.g., rocking, handflapping, fingerflipping), we are categorizing them together in one class, presumably because these behaviors have something in common that differentiates them from other behaviors. One common characteristic of these behaviors is their stereotypical nature; that is, the behaviors are performed in the same, almost mechanical way each time they occur. In addition, the individuals perform the stereotyped acts repetitiously, doing them again and again, or maintaining the same posture for long periods (e.g., keeping a hand in the mouth, an arm entangled in a blouse, maintaining both hands in a tight grasp on the collar of a shirt). Other stereotyped acts commonly occur in the community both on the job (e.g., fastening a nut to a bolt in an assembly line) and at play (e.g., dancing, playing tennis). The difference between classifying these activities as normal versus "self-stimulatory" is that normal behaviors are functional in (i.e., reinforced by) the environment, whereas self-stimulatory behaviors are ignored or punished.

The discussion in this chapter will be limited to behaviors that are stereotypical and performed repetitiously, and that fail to produce any apparent positive environmental consequences or physical injury. The discussion will focus on treatment of the problem, and, with that focus, will present theoretical explanations, review treatment studies, and conclude with guidelines to follow for treating self-stimulation.

THEORETICAL EXPLANATIONS

Several explanations have been provided as to why mentally retarded people perform self-stimulatory behavior. In his chapter on the "Origins and Control of Stereotyped Movements," Baumeister (1978) concluded that each of the major theoretical explanations is, in part, correct. Conclusions were based on evidence which partially validates most of the widely held theoretical explanations. In the present review, an attempt will be made to choose a theoretical explanation that best advances the goal of treating self-stimulatory behavior.

Psychodynamic Explanations

Theorists of the psychodynamic orientation have offered two popular explanations or hypotheses. One is that some people have problems discriminating between their bodies and the surrounding environment, and perform self-stimulatory behaviors to test the boundary (Bychowski, 1954; Greenacre, 1954; Hartmann, Kris, & Loewenstein, 1949). As Baumeister concluded, this interpretation is without value in science, because the constructs (e.g., hysteria, body reality, ego boundary) used to explain the phenomenon are so poorly defined.

A second popular psychodynamic explanation is that self-stimulatory behaviors result from severe disruptions in normal mother–infant interactions. The best evidence to support this explanation is the finding that nonhuman primates develop self-stimulatory behavior when they are reared alone, without mothers (Baumeister, 1978; Baumeister & Forehand, 1973; Berkson, 1967, 1973; Davenport & Menzel, 1963; Harlow, 1960; Hollis, 1978). Further supporting evidence is the fact that self-stimulation is often performed by people who reside in large, barren, and understaffed institutions, settings with too few mother surrogates. But, being reared alone in a small laboratory cubicle includes an absence of many other variables besides mother–infant interactions (Hollis, 1978). And, as Baumeister (1978) notes, many of the people who live in institutions performed self-stimulatory behavior before they were admitted to that setting. Further, maternal deprivation is so broad a construct that one feels compelled to ask what specific interactions between the mother and the infant account for the problem (Yarrow, 1961). From a treatment perspective, this explanation suggests that self-stimulatory behavior can be decreased by preventing maternal deprivation, something already attempted in the community. When confronted with clients who perform self-stimulatory behavior, this mother–infant interaction explanation provides no guidelines on how to treat the problem. Thus, neither of these popular psychodynamic explanations is particularly useful for treating self-stimulatory behavior.

Organic Explanations

Some authors suggest that self-stimulatory behavior is a result of disturbed physiological processes. Baumeister (1978) presents several arguments supporting this organic explanation. He notes that self-stimulatory behaviors are more likely to be performed by persons with lower scores on intelligence tests, and these are the people who have more physiological disturbances. One such problem, PKU, was frequently accompanied by self-stimulatory behavior when not under dietary control. (Fortunately, this problem seldom occurs now, since mandatory screening for this disorder has been initiated.) That this disorder is accompanied by self-stimulation is weak evidence to support the physiological-disturbance explanation, however, because PKU results in lower IQ scores (greater developmental delay), and research has shown that the lower the IQ, the greater the prevalence of self-stimulation (Berkson & Davenport, 1962). This same argument can be used to explain why other physiological syndromes (e.g., Lesh–Nyhan, de Lange, and Down's syndromes) produce self-stimulatory behaviors; that is, they produce lower IQ scores, which is correlated with self-stimulatory behaviors. Thus, although various physiological processes and structures (e.g., brain, spinal cord) can produce lower IQ scores when disturbed, this fact does not explain why mentally retarded people perform self-stimulatory behaviors, or what should be done to treat it.

Other physiological-disturbance explanations cannot similarly be dismissed because a lower IQ score is a correlate of the disorder. One of these is that self-stimulation is a method for obtaining pain relief. This explanation was first used to explain self-injurious behavior, but has since been applied to self-stimulation. The explanation is based on findings by de Lissovoy (1963) of a greater proportion of ear infections among a group of headbangers than among a matched group of subjects that did not bang their heads, and findings by Harkness and Wagner (1975) of a greater proportion of ear infections among scratchers than nonscratchers. Carr (1977) tempered the importance of De Lissovoy's findings by noting that most of the subjects in the headbanger group had no ear infections. Similarly, Carr noted that, in the Harkness and Wagner study, some subjects with ear infections did not scratch themselves. Yet, even if the findings were more solid, the pain-relief explanation would be valuable to a treatment perspective only if it were demonstrated that reducing the pain eliminated the self-stimulation.

Two other physiological disturbance explanations may similarly be dismissed for lack of utility in a treatment perspective. One of these is that self-stimulation may be a result of brain lesions. Baumeister (1978) suggests that we retain this explanation by noting that an increase in self-stimulation has occurred as a result of experimentally producing lesions in the brains of laboratory animals. He also implies that we retain an explanation regarding chemical disturbance as a cause of self-stimulation because studies have shown that self-stimulation increases when animals are subjected to injection of some drugs, for example, caffeine (Baumeister, 1978). From a treatment perspective, however, these physiological disturbance explanations will remain without value until it is demonstrated that remediation of these disorders is associated with a decrease in self-stimulation.

The argument presented does not reject physiological phenomena as possible agents effecting self-stimulation. All behavior is performed with physiological structures (e.g., muscle, brain, nerve tissue) and processes (e.g., chemical, electrical); therefore, a change in physiology may effect behavior. One general physiological process is maturation, and its relevance to the emergence of self-stimulation will be presented next.

Normal Development Explanation

In the last section, we reviewed explanations that suggested disturbed physiological structures and processes as agents effecting self-stimulation. The normal-development explanation asserts that disturbance is unnecessary, and that self-stimulatory behaviors emerge within the normal development of humans. Authors expressing this normal-development explanation for the emergence of self-stimulation are numerous (Bakwin & Bakwin, 1960; Berkson, 1967; Brody, 1960; Gesell & Amatruda, 1947; Hollis, 1978; Nissen, 1956; Provence & Lipton, 1962). Baumeister (1978) concludes that the earlier development of some forms of self-stimulation (e.g., rocking) may be essential to the later development of adaptive behaviors. Berkson (1973) further hypothesizes that humans are preprogrammed to perform self-stimulatory behaviors during normal development. Such arguments are supported by developmental studies finding forms of self-stimulation emerging within the normal development of children who are without pathology (e.g., Bakwin & Bakwin, 1960; Gesell & Amatruda, 1947). Such studies generally pinpoint the emergence as occurring at a period of transition from one stage to another, such as rocking emerging between sitting and standing (Hollis, 1978).

Thus, the normal-development explanation asserts that self-stimulation emerges during the normal development of humans. Unfortunately, the explanation alone is insufficient to explain why most people cease performing self-stimulation, whereas many mentally retarded people continue with self-stimulation as their dominant behavior pattern. A sufficient explanation is available, however, that may be viewed as an extention of the normal-development explanation. It is covered in the next section.

Competition between Self-Stimulation and Adaptive Behavior

Berkson (1967) extends the normal-development explanation by declaring that self-stimulation emerges and becomes dominant within normal development, but is later displaced by more mature forms of behavior (i.e., adaptive behavior). Berkson's notion that self-stimulation will remain dominant until adaptive behaviors develop is one basis of the explanation provided by Foxx and Azrin (1973). These authors further suggest that mentally retarded persons perform a higher frequency of self-stimulation than other people because they have learned to perform fewer adaptive behaviors. Thus, self-stimulation remains dominant, and adaptive behavior seldom occurs. In agreement with Berkson (1967), Foxx and Azrin (1973) conclude that self-stimulation competes with adaptive behavior—increasing one decreases the other.

To expand further on why mentally retarded people continue performing self-stimulation, Foxx and Azrin (1973) declared that self-stimulation is reinforced by tactile, proprioceptive, and sensory stimulation. (The notion that self-stimulatory behavior is maintained by intrinsic reinforcement from tactile, proprioceptive, and sensory stimulation had been earlier hypothesized by others—[e.g., Lovaas, Schaeffer, & Simmons, 1965]—but has only recently been verified by Rincover, 1978, who decreased self-stimulation by removing or blocking the consequent auditory, visual, or proprioceptive stimulation.) Foxx and Azrin (1973) note that this intrinsic reinforcement maintains such a high frequency of self-stimulation that mentally retarded clients have little time remaining to learn adaptive behaviors. Presumably, people decrease self-stimulating as it is displaced by adaptive behaviors, but because mentally retarded clients learn fewer adaptive behaviors, they continue performing self-stimulation, and this further decreases their opportunity to learn adaptive behaviors.

The theoretical explanation regarding the competition between adaptive and self-stimulatory behaviors appears to be the most fruitful from a treatment perspective. First, it can encompass the emergence of self-stimulation by the normal-development, organic, or psychodynamic explanations. Second, the explanation answers why mentally retarded people continue self-stimulating when others of us do not. Third, by specifying a competition between self-stimulation and adaptive behaviors, the explanation ensures that treatment personnel attend to the essence of the mental retardation problem, the deficit in adaptive behaviors. Finally, the explanation provides sufficient information to generate treatment prescriptions.

Using this theoretical explanation, Foxx and Azrin (1973) generated the following treatment prescriptions:

1. Decrease the reinforcement for self-stimulatory behavior by interrupting the behavior when it occurs.
2. Prevent the continued practice of the self-stimulatory behavior by prompting the client to perform adaptive behavior.
3. Punish self-stimulatory behavior by arranging annoying consequences to follow such.
4. Teach adaptive behavior.
5. Reinforce adaptive behavior.

An added benefit of Foxx and Azrin's explanation is that it can be encompassed within a theoretical model that provides an abundance of theoretical explanations based on basic and applied research findings. The relevant issues in the explanation fit the philosophical endeavor of behaviorism, and the applied paradigms known as behavior modification, behavior therapy, and applied behavior analysis.

The issue of competition between self-stimulatory behavior and adaptive behavior relates well to the issues of concurrent schedules of reinforcement (e.g., Catania, 1966), in which affecting one behavior by manipulating its reinforcement contingency affects another behavior with unchanged contingencies.

Several applied studies have shown such concurrent effects. When Risley (1968) placed a child on food deprivation, and used food as a reinforcer to teach language skills, the child's constant climbing and rocking behaviors so interfered that learning language skills could not occur. Yet, when climbing was reduced by punishment, the child began to perform the instructional behaviors required to learn language skills even though the reinforcement contingency was unchanged. When O'Brien, Bugle, and Azrin (1972) taught a child to eat with a spoon, the child continued eating with her fingers instead. When they changed the contingency for fingerfeeding from reinforcement to extinction (i.e., no food in mouth for fingerfeeding), she began to use her spoon even though the reinforcement contingency for spoonfeeding was unchanged. Similarly, O'Brien, Azrin, and Bugle (1972) increased walking by profoundly mentally retarded children without changing the reinforcement contingency for walking; instead, they changed the contingency for and thereby reduced crawling. These studies showed concurrent effects on behaviors that were physically incompatible (e.g., one cannot eat with and without a spoon at the same time). O'Brien and Azrin (1972) also showed concurrent effects on behaviors that could be performed at the same time when they reduced a woman's screaming by increasing her adaptive skills (e.g., grooming, cooking, cleaning) with positive reinforcement.

Further treatment studies will be reviewed in the next section, and will be related to the theoretical explanation regarding competition between self-stimulation and adaptive behavior as presented by Foxx and Azrin (1973). In closing this survey of theoretical explanations, it should be remembered that an attempt was made to select the explanation that seemed most fruitful in the treatment of self-stimulatory behavior. The Foxx and Azrin (1973) explanation appears to be the best for our purpose; yet, only treatment studies can substantiate the wisdom of this choice. Studies of this nature will be discussed in the following pages.

Treatment by Reinforcing Other Behavior

Foxx and Azrin (1973) recommend increasing adaptive behavior as one method for decreasing self-stimulatory behavior. Laboratory studies with primates and mentally retarded people showed a decrease in self-stimulatory behavior when subjects were given objects to play with (e.g., Berkson & Mason, 1963, 1964; Davenport & Berkson, 1963; Guess & Rutherford, 1967; Menzel, 1963; Menzel, Davenport, & Rogers, 1963; Tizard, 1968; Warren & Burns, 1970). Unfortunately, the reductions in self-stimulatory behavior were small and transient (Baumeister, 1978). Presumably, reductions were short lived because subjects became habituated to the novelty of the objects and, consequently, stopped playing with them. Hollis (1978) overcame this habituation phenomenon by reinforcing mentally retarded youths for ball-pulling, and maintained an almost complete absence of bodyrocking. He concluded that bodyrocking can be displaced ("blocked") by rewarding clients for performing an alternative behavior.

Further support for the Foxx and Azrin recommendation to decrease self-stimulatory behavior by increasing adaptive behavior comes from studies in applied settings. Cuvo (1976) decreased repetitive dawdling in a 66-year-old mentally retarded woman by reinforcing promptness in returning to her dormitory. Flavell (1973) decreased self-stimulatory behavior in three mentally retarded clients by reinforcing playing with toys; as toy play increased, self-stimulatory behavior decreased. Azrin, Kaplan, and Foxx (1973) provided training and reinforcement for clients' use of recreational and educational materials (e.g., pointing to pictures of objects; separating blocks on the basis of size, shape, color; stringing beads). Five of the nine hospitalized adults reduced self-stimulating by 75% or more. These findings also lend support to the recommendation that adaptive behaviors be taught and reinforced.

Other studies lend support to this recommendation by rewarding clients for going periods of time without performing self-stimulatory behaviors. This procedure is called differential reinforcement of other behavior (DRO), and, as implied by its name, is presumed to decrease self-stimulation by increasing other behavior that is adaptive. Repp, Deitz, and Speir (1974) virtually eliminated self-stimulation by three clients when they provided hugs and praise to clients for going periods of time without self-stimulating. (Unfortunately, because they also reprimanded clients for self-stimulating, we cannot conclude that the reduction was totally due to reinforcing other behaviors.) Polvinale and Lutzker (1980) reduced genital self-stimulation by providing praise in a DRO schedule of reinforcement. Harris and Wolchik (1979) produced a marginal reduction in handpatting by an autistic child using a DRO procedure, but found no effect with two other children, and an increase in self-stimulation with a fourth child. Differential reinforcement of other behavior was concluded by Baumeister (1978) to have demonstrated mixed results, with some studies reporting no effectiveness (e.g., Luiselli, 1975), and others reporting marginal success (e.g., Mulhern & Baumeister, 1969).

When Risley (1968) tried to teach language skills to a developmentally disabled child, he used a powerful positive reinforcement contingency (i.e., continuous food reinforcement for a food-deprived child) to increase modeling behaviors. Yet, the child's climbing on chairs and furniture occurred so frequently that Risley got little increase in the desired behaviors. These findings suggest an explanation for the failures to reduce self-stimulation by differential reinforcement of other behavior. The failures at decreasing self-stimulation are likely due to the failure of the reinforcement contingency to increase adaptive behavior sufficiently. Foxx and Azrin (1973) mention that developmentally disabled clients have few adaptive behaviors to compete with self-stimulation. Consequently, clients continue performing self-stimulation, and the self-stimulation continues to be intrinsically reinforced until it becomes so pervasive that it almost eliminates the opportunity for adaptive behaviors to emerge. Under these conditions, even the most powerful positive reinforcement contingency for adaptive behaviors may fail. Therefore, treatment procedures (e.g., punishment) for directly decreasing self-stimulatory behaviors should be strongly considered.

TREATMENT BY PUNISHING SELF-STIMULATION

The Need for Punishment

Foxx and Azrin (1973) suggest that we punish self-stimulatory behavior by arranging annoying consequences to follow instances of self-stimulation. In the previous discussion, studies were reviewed in which self-stimulation was decreased by increasing adaptive behavior. Some of these studies showed only marginal success at decreasing self-stimulation, presumably because the reinforcement contingency failed sufficiently to increase adaptive behavior. This matter was exemplified by Risley's (1968) study, in which a powerful reinforcement contingency (i.e., continuous food reinforcement for a food-deprived child) failed to increase adaptive behavior. With the reinforcement contingency remaining, Risley introduced punishment for self-stimulatory climbing behavior by applying painful electric shock as the annoying consequence for climbing. The client increased adaptive behavior when climbing decreased by punishment, but further increases ceased when punishment was discontinued and climbing was allowed to resume.

Prior to using electric shock as the annoying consequence, Risley tried to decrease climbing by less punitive methods. He tried ignoring the behavior to ensure that his interactions were not reinforcing climbing. No effects were noted. He tried having the child's mother decrease climbing in the home by giving the child 10 min of isolation in her bedroom as an annoying consequence for climbing, once again without effect. Only after these less punitive methods were found to fail did Risley introduce electric shock. This latter method proved to be the most effective.

Risley (1968) later tried to teach this autistic child to imitate handclapping. Little progress was made, however, and Risley presumed that this occurred because the child spent so much time weaving her head from side to side. To decrease this self-stimulation, Risley used a shake–startle procedure as an annoying consequence. It consisted of his telling the child to stop, holding her about the shoulders, and briefly shaking her. This punishment contingency reduced her frequency of head-weaving by 50%, and reduced the total time she engaged in this self-stimulation from 25% to 1% of each treatment session. With this reduction in self-stimulation, the child increased her imitative handclapping from about 5 to 25 per 10-min session. Because this progress occurred immediately after self-stimulation decreased, Risley concluded that the reduction in self-stimulation facilitated improvements in adaptive behaviors, and suggested that the elimination of self-stimulation may be a prerequisite to establishing adaptive behaviors.

Time-Out as an Annoying Consequence

Researchers have also used "time-out" as an annoying consequence for self-stimulation. When using time-out, the researchers removed positive reinforcers (or the opportunity to earn positive reinforcement) from the clients after self-stimulation. Baer (1962) used a form of time-out on thumbsucking while children watched cartoons. He decreased this type of self-stimulation by withdrawing the sound and picture as a consequence for thumbsucking. Greene, Hoats, and Hornick (1970) distorted the sound of music as a consequence for bodyrocking, and completely eliminated this behavior. Music was also used by Mattos (1969) to decrease facial ticks and finger sucking by stopping the music as a consequence for self-stimulation. Laws, Brown, Epstein, and Hocking (1971) decreased handgesturing and headbobbing in two clients who were earning reinforcement during language training by looking away from the client until self-stimulation stopped. Using a similar time-out procedure with four autistic boys, Harris and Wolchik (1979) produced a partial reduction in self-stimulation with two clients, no change with a third, and a marginal increase with the fourth.

Isolation as an Annoying Consequence

Several researchers have used isolation as an annoying consequence to suppress self-stimulatory behavior (e.g., Hamilton, Stephens, & Allen, 1967; Miron & Rooney, 1973; Pendergrass, 1972; Wolf, Risley, Johnston, Harris, & Allen, 1967). Baumeister (1978) reported that when he used noncontingent isolation—isolation occurring regardless of the client's behaviors at the time—bodyrocking and handwaving decreased somewhat during isolation, but then stabilized at a rate that was still too high. Because isolation suppresses self-stimulation when used contingently, but does not do so when used noncontingently, we may infer that isolation is a punisher. Yet, this finding does not justify the often expressed conclusion that its suppressive effects are owing to time-out from positive reinforcement. Regardless, contingent isolation has been demonstrated to be an effective annoying consequence (i.e., punisher) to suppress self-stimulation.

Other Annoying Consequences

Researchers have used other annoying consequences to decrease self-stimulation. Koegel, Firestone, Kramme, and Dunlap (1974) decreased self-stimulation in two autistic children who each displayed a wide variety of such behaviors (e.g., grimacing, handwaving, lip rubbing, handflapping, foottapping). These researchers used a verbal reprimand ("No") and a brisk slap or a short manual restraint of the relevant body part as annoying consequences. They found that these procedures reduced self-stimulation and generated an increase in spontaneous play. A brisk slap was also used by Foxx and Azrin (1973) with two children for mouthing behaviors, but this decreased self-stimulation with only one of them. Baumeister and Forehand (1972) used a loud verbal reprimand ("Stop Rocking") to decrease body rocking in six clients known to respond to verbal commands. Finally, Lutzker (1978) virtually eliminated hand-to-head behaviors that were frequently self-injurious by using facial screening as an annoying consequence (i.e., covering the client's face with a cloth until the behavior stopped for three seconds).

Overcorrection as an Annoying Consequence

Description of Overcorrection

Since the Foxx and Azrin article of 1973, researchers have frequently used overcorrection as the annoying consequence. Overcorrection is a treatment strategy for decreasing behavior that requires clients to perform adaptive behaviors as a consequence of undesirable acts. The adaptive behaviors required by the overcorrection rationale are of two types: restitution and positive practice. In restitution overcorrection, the client is required to restore the environment to a state improved over what existed before the client performed the undesirable act. An example would be to require a client who vomits and rubs the material on her clothing and chair to bathe, rinse her mouth, change her clothing, and clean several chairs. In positive-practice overcorrection, the client is required to practice performing a behavior that is incompatible with the undesirable act. An example of positive-practice overcorrection would be to require clients who dangle shoe laces in front of their eyes to lace several shoes properly. Caution must be used to ensure that the performance requirement be done in a manner that is annoying and not reinforcing (e.g., giving verbal commands in a matter-of-fact style, providing as little physical contact as necessary to get the client to complete the performance requirement, and not reinforcing the client during the overcorrection period). When applied in this manner, overcorrection has been shown to be an effective treatment strategy for decreasing self-stimulation.

Foxx and Azrin (1973) tested the efficacy of overcorrection on several self-stimulatory behaviors displayed by four profoundly retarded children who were seven and eight years old. Mouthing of objects was virtually eliminated in two children when overcorrection was used as the annoying consequence. In these cases, overcorrection consisted of saying "No" in a firm voice, brushing the child's mouth with a toothbrush immersed in an oral antiseptic, and wiping the child's lips with a wash cloth. Foxx and Azrin (1973) demonstrated this overcorrection to be more effective than reinforcement for nonmouthing and noncontingent reinforcement for both children. With one child, they also found overcorrection to be more effective at suppressing mouthing of a hand than was painting a distasteful solution on the hand.

To decrease headweaving, Foxx and Azrin (1973) designed the following overcorrection procedure: the trainer restrained the client's head, instructed the client to hold her head in one of three positions, up, down, or straight ahead for 15 sec, and randomly changed among the three positions for 5 min, providing only as little manual guidance as necessary to get the client to perform as indicated. This overcorrection requirement virtually eliminated the child's headweaving in about 10 days (although the procedure was modified by increasing the time devoted to positive practice from 5 to 20 min on day 7, and decreasing to 2 min after 10 days). To decrease handclapping, Foxx and Azrin (1973) designed an overcorrection requirement similar to the one for headweaving, in which five hand positions were used: above the head, straight out in front, in pockets, held together, and behind the back. Handclapping decreased from about 100 to 20 the first day, 3 the second day, and virtually zero by the third.

Azrin, Kaplan, and Foxx (1973) used an overcorrection requirement similar to that mentioned above for headweaving after reprimanding the client (e.g., "No, Sally, don't move your head like that"), and requiring the client to move to a different area of the room. In this study, nine severely mentally retarded, hospitalized adults were required to practice 20 min after each instance of self-stimulation. For bodyrocking, clients practiced maintaining their shoulders in two positions: away from and against the back of the chair. For handgazing and flipping paper with the fingers, clients practiced three hand positions: above the head, outstretched from the sides of the body, and against the sides of the body. For fingering movements (i.e., clothrolling, stringthreading, and pillrolling), clients practiced maintaining two hand positions with the thumbs in an upright position: hands held together and hands held apart. Trainers required clients to maintain these positions for 30 sec, and chose positions at random, or alternated for practice requirements with only two positions. The nine clients originally spent from 70% to 85% of the time engaging in self-stimulation. When trainers taught them adaptive behaviors and reinforced these skills, the clients reduced self-stimulation to between 15% and 35% of the time. (The authors note, however, that this reduction was found in only half the group; the other clients were unaffected.) When overcorrection was added to the reinforcement program, self-stimulation was virtually eliminated in about 10 days (i.e., two episodes of self-stimulation per client per week). Table I lists a number of other studies in which positive effects were found using overcorrection.

Problems Noted Using Overcorrection

Several reviewers have discussed a variety of concerns regarding the use of overcorrection as an annoying consequence to decrease self-stimulation (e.g., Baumeister, 1978; Hobbs, 1967a,b; Hobbs & Goswick, 1977; Judkins, 1976; Rollings, Baumeister & Baumeister, 1977). The concerns discussed included methodological, theoretical, and treatment issues. Four such issues dominate the discussion: collateral side effects of decreasing self-stimulation with overcorrection, the generalization of the suppressive effects, failures to reduce self-stimulation with overcorrection, and the "educative" effects of positive practice. A brief discussion of these four issues follows.

Side Effects. Epstein, Doke, Sajwaj, Sorrell, and Rimmer (1974) noted that self-stimulation of feet increased when overcorrection decreased self-

TABLE I
Sample of Studies Finding Positive Effects with Overcorrection

Author(s)	Target behavior(s)
Barnard, Christopherson, Altman, & Wolf (1974)	Mouthing
Matson & Stephens (in press)	Wallpatting, headrubbing, hairflipping, facepatting
Herendeen, Jeffrey, & Graham (1974)	Mouthing, rocking
Rollings, Baumeister, & Baumeister (1977	Rocking
Epstein, Doke, Sajwaj, Sorrell, & Rimmer (1974)	Improper vocalizations, hand and foot movements
Ollendick, Matson, & Martin (1978)	Nosetouching, headweaving, handshaking, inappropriate laughter
Polvindale & Lutzker (1980)	Genital self-stimulation
Harris & Wolchik (1979)	Handpatting, handstroking, handtapping
Wells, Forehand, Hickey, & Green (1977)	Object manipulation, hand movements, mouthing
Martin, Weller, & Matson (1977)	Repetitive object transfer between hands
Azrin & Wesolowski (1975)	Repetitive vomiting
Doke & Epstein (1975)	Mouthing
Roberts, Iwata, McSween, & Desmond (1979)	Mouthing, growling, tablehitting

stimulatory vocalizations. Herendeen, Jeffrey, and Graham, (1974) noted an increase in mouthing when body rocking was decreased, and Roberts, Iwata, McSween, and Desmond (1979) found grabbing to increase when mouthing decreased. Rollings (1975) and Doke and Epstein (1975) similarly noted an increase in other maladaptive behaviors when self-stimulatory behaviors were reduced with overcorrection, or with a warning that overcorrection would be used. Harris and Wolchik (1979) noted the emergence of headbobbing after overcorrection had largely suppressed self-stimulatory behaviors performed with the hands. Rollings *et al.* (1977) noted increases in other forms of self-stimulation when targeted self-stimulation was reduced with overcorrection. More importantly, however, they noted the emergence of behaviors not previously seen, including self-pinching, headbanging, and self-scratching. These self-injurious behaviors emerged after a less critical self-stimulatory behavior (i.e., headweaving) had been reduced.

On the other hand, Epstein *et al.* (1974) and Harris and Wolchik (1979) reported an increase in appropriate toy play as self-stimulatory hand movements decreased with overcorrection. Roberts *et al.* (1979) reported that mouthing decreased when growling was reduced with overcorrection. Martin, Weller, and Matson (1977) noted that smiling and on-task behaviors increased when self-stimulatory object manipulation was decreased with overcorrection. Ollendick, Matson, and Martin (1978) noted that when they used overcorrection to reduce the self-stimulation of students in a classroom, the teacher reported an increase in attending and learning. Matson and Stephens (in press) recorded an increase in smiling and verbal communications when they decreased wallpatting with overcorrection. Finally, Doke and Epstein (1975) reported that one child decreased thumbsucking when the child observed overcorrection being applied to another child for thumbsucking.

Thus, studies that decreased self-stimulation with overcorrection have reported both negative and positive side effects on other behaviors. Although collateral behavior changes should be expected whenever a behavior is modified (cf. Catania, 1966), these studies serve us well as reminders to stay alert to these changes when decreasing self-stimulatory behavior. Should the change include developing more critical behaviors (e.g., Rollings *et al.*, 1977), treatment personnel would be well-advised to institute treatment strategies for decreasing them. Should the change include an emergence of even more appropriate behaviors (e.g., Matson & Stephens, in press), treatment personnel would be well advised to institute strategies for reinforcing them. Nonetheless, that overcorrection has been shown to produce collateral behavior change is a fact which should neither be used for overselling nor for condemning the use of this type of treatment.

Generalization of Suppression. Studies concerning the extent to which the suppressive effects of punishment transfer to nonpunishment situations conclude that suppression is unlikely to transfer without adding deliberate procedures to promote transfer (e.g., Azrin & Holtz, 1966; Gardner, 1969; Lovaas & Simmons, 1969; Risley, 1968; Weisberg, 1971). Yet, Martin *et al.* (1977) reported that object manipulation that was suppressed with overcorrection in the classroom also decreased in the client's home (i.e., hospital ward). Similarly, Barnard *et al.* (1974) reported that the suppression of mouthing by overcorrection in a client's home transferred to the client's school.

Conversely, some studies in which self-stimulation decreased with overcorrection demonstrated little transfer of suppression. Foxx and Azrin (1973) noted that, although overcorrection virtually eliminated mouthing of objects by one client in a day-care program, parents reported that mouthing increased in the home. Rollings *et al.* (1977) demonstrated a client's ability to discriminate between safe and punishment conditions on the basis of the proximity of the trainer to the client—the closer the trainer, the greater the suppression. In one ingenious study, Matson and Stephens (in press) recorded the frequency of wallpatting in three hallways. In a multiple baseline design, they introduced overcorrection for wallpatting at different times in the different hallways. As wallpatting decreased in the first hallway by overcorrection, no decreases occurred in the other two. Similarly, though overcorrection proved successful for suppressing wallpatting in the second hallway, the suppression did not generalize to the remaining "safe" hallway. Suppression occurred there only when overcorrection was applied. Treatment personnel would be well advised to adhere to the recommendations of Matson and Stephens, that treatment be applied in a manner that minimizes the clients' ability to discriminate between "safe" and treatment situations.

Failures with Overcorrection. If there were many reported studies that showed overcorrection to be ineffective, reviewers could determine which forms of self-stimulation or what characteristics of clients or overcorrection procedures are likely to result in failure. Furthermore, a study in which overcorrection was tried with, let us say, 100 clients randomly selected from a hospital population would be useful for discovering the percentage of clients that fail. Such information would better allow us to determine the extent to which we can generalize the efficacy of overcorrection across the mentally retarded population. As Baumeister (1978) notes, the problem of generalizing across individuals remains because most behavior analysis studies report the effects of treatments on one or only a few clients, and when failures occur in small sample studies the results are unlikely to be reported.

Foxx and Azrin (1973) originally designed an overcorrection consequence that was to require positive practice for 5 min, but during treatment they increased the time to 20 min. Presumably, they did so because the suppression resulting from 5 min was initially insufficient. Rollings *et al.* (1977) developed little suppression of headweaving in a laboratory study after 22 sessions of overcorrection. They concluded that the failure was owing to the many within-session reversals to "safe" time periods—periods during which overcorrection was not used—and the obvious stimulus conditions that signaled the difference (i.e., trainer present or absent). Accordingly, they avoided this failure when they next used overcorrection to decrease rocking of another client by making these "safe" signals less obvious. In this case, rocking was eliminated in seven sessions.

These two brief notes regarding "failures" seem to concur with the experience of others with whom the author has consulted, as well as personal experience in using overcorrection since the early 1970s. In many cases, the original design of the overcorrection consequence seemed ineffective. However, with some minor adjustments (e.g., increase the time devoted to positive practice, reduce the verbalizations of the trainer during positive practice, choose a positive-practice topography that is more annoying, decrease the safe periods, eliminate "safe" signals), overcorrection significantly suppressed self-stimulation.

Overcorrection—Educative or Punitive. Foxx and Azrin (1973) mentioned that, in addition to decreasing self-stimulation, overcorrection serves to teach the adaptive behaviors included in the positive practice or restitution requirement. This assertion stimulated an enormous amount of discussion. For example, Hobbs (1976a) found little data to justify this assertion, and mentioned that "overcorrection may be nothing more than a complex punishment procedure " (p.3) Similarly, Doke and Epstein (1975) cautioned practicioners to alert themselves to the difference between the specifics required to make overcorrection effective and the "rational 'packaging' that makes overcorrection easier to sell " (p. 510). The easier-to-sell attribute of overcorrection is the assertion that it teaches adaptive behaviors, rather than simply function as a punishment procedure. The question often raised is whether the educative attribute is necessary or beneficial.

Epstein *et al.* (1974) designed a study to determine whether the educative attribute is necessary. They did so by designing a positive-practice requirement for a form of self-stimulation performed with the hands, and applied it to a form of self-stimulation performed with the feet. They hypothesized that, should the education of an adaptive behavior performed with the feet prove necessary for the overcorrection to suppress self-stimulation, then this postive-practice requirement should fail. However, should positive practice prove successful simply because it is annoying, this positive-practice requirement would serve to suppress self-stimulation.

When the positive-practice requirement for self-stimulation with hands was applied to self-stimulation with feet, the behavior decreased significantly. Similarly, when they applied it to a form of vocal self-stimulation, that behavior also decreased. Later, Doke and Epstein (1975) suppressed object manipulation and body movements with a positive-practice requirement designed for handmouthing. These studies suggest that the punitive attribute of overcorrection may be sufficient to produce the suppression of self-stimulation.

On the other hand, some findings suggest the additive value of the educative attribute. When Wells *et al.* (1976) incorporated appropriate playing with toys in the positive-practice requirement for decreasing object manipulation, hand movements, and mouthing, they noted an increase in appropriate toy play for one of their two autistic clients. When Roberts *et al.* (1979) applied a positive-practice requirement designed for handclapping to mouthing, mouthing decreased. However, handclapping also decreased, even though it was not consequated in any way. Similarly, when they decreased tablehitting with overcorrection designed for grimacing, their client reduced grimacing, although very little. (However, no change occurred in fingering when overcorrection designed for fingering was applied to and decreased growling and mouthing.) Finally, Ollendick *et al.* (1978) used hand overcorrection to reduce two hand-stimulation behaviors (i.e., handshaking and nosetouching) and two behaviors not involving hands (i.e., laughing and headweaving). All four self-stimulatory behaviors decreased; however, the two hand behaviors were reduced more quickly and remained lower after treatment than the two behaviors that were dissimilar to the hand overcorrection. Thus, although the punitive attribute of overcorrection may be sufficient to reduce self-stimulation, the educative attribute may produce improved treatment.

Interruption as an Annoying Consequence

Overcorrection can be extremely annoying to the client as well as the trainers who must frequently use manual guidance to get the client to perform the overcorrection, often for as long as 20 min each time self-stimulation occurs. (In many settings, the number of trainers is already so limited that applying overcorrection requires interrupting another treatment for lack of sufficient numbers of staff to continue both.) Also, when overcorrection is aversive to the clients, they attempt to avoid or escape from the annoying consequence, thereby increasing the aversiveness for the trainers (Baumeister, 1978; Azrin & Wesolowski, 1980).

Possibilities for decreasing the aversiveness of an annoying consequence can be generated from the studies previously reviewed. Those studies that demonstrated the efficacy of using overcorrection requirements that were topographically dissimilar to the self-stimulation suggest the possibility that one standard annoying consequence could be used for all types of self-stimulation. The previous discussion mentioned the efficacy of one very simple, mildly aversive consequence, that is, telling the client to stop self-stimulating (Baumeister & Forehand, 1972). It must be noted, however, that these authors selected clients known to have complied with similar commands. If all clients could learn to comply with commands in a similar fashion, this less aversive and more feasible annoying consequence could be used.

Azrin and Wesolowski (1980) designed an annoying consequence in such a fashion. After intensive training, the annoying consequence consisted of reprimanding clients for self-stimulating, "No, don't. . . ," and guiding the clients' hands to their laps or table tops, typically requiring one sec. Initially, they recorded the frequency of self-stimulation that occurred in a classroom situation with about 10 students per class and one trainer. They selected 7 of the 30 clients they observed who performed self-stimulation 40% or more of the time they were engaged in instruction. They provided these clients with intensive individual training in adaptive behaviors outside these classes. When clients self-stimulated, trainers interrupted the behavior and required the clients to place their hands in their laps or on the edge of the table for 2 min. Clients remained in this intensive training until they went 30 consecutive minutes without self-stimulating.

After completing the requirement of 30 consecutive minutes without self-stimulating, each client advanced to a special class in which they received praise and snacks as reinforcers for adaptive behaviors from two trainers. The special class progressively increased from 1 to 7 clients as each met the 30-min criterion for entry. Initially, each client received the 2-min interruption for self-stimulation, but when they went 30 min without self-stimulating, the time of interruption was reduced by half progressively, until the trainer simply said, "No, don't . . . ," and required the clients momentarily to place their hands on their laps or on the table. (However, when clients self-stimulated more than once in any 30-min period, the duration was returned to 2 min, and the process of reducing the time began again.) Within this special class, the 7 clients reduced self-stimulating from an average of 1½ times per hour during the first 3 class sessions to virtually zero during the remaining 12.

After completing the requirement of 30 consecutive minutes without self-stimulating during the intensive individual training, each client also returned to the ongoing class, in which they received praise and physical contact for adaptive behaviors from only one trainer. The one trainer used only the 1-sec interruption procedure for self-stimulation. In this ongoing class, the seven clients self-stimulated about 12 times per hour in the first class session, about 6 in the fifth session, and virtually none from class sessions 11 to 15.

Thus, Azrin and Wesolowski began with an ongoing class of about 10 clients with one trainer using praise and physical contact as reinforcers for adaptive behavior, then provided intensive individual training, and advanced the clients to a special class with a progressively decreasing duration of the interruption procedure. At the same time, the clients also returned to the ongoing class. During the intensive individual training and special class, edibles were used as reinforcers for adaptive behaviors. Also, two trainers were available during the special class. The use of edibles as reinforcers and the improved trainer density which allowed for using the 2-min interruption may account for the fact that self-stimulation was suppressed over twice as fast in the special class and individual training than in the ongoing class. Regardless, with only one trainer using social reinforcers and the 1-sec interruption procedure, the mean percent of class time per student devoted to self-stimulation decreased from 75 to 80% during baseline to zero over the last 10 ongoing class sessions. Thus, with special training, Azrin and Wesolowski were able to use a less annoying consequence effectively to decrease self-stimulation.

Treatment by Sensory Extinction

The theoretical explanation presented by Foxx and Azrin (1973) includes the notion that self-stimulation is intrinsically reinforced by tactile, proprioceptive, and sensory stimulation. Consequently, they recommended decreasing this reinforcement by interrupting self-stimulation when it occurs.

Rincover (1978) similarly recommends decreasing the intrinsic reinforcement, but recommends doing so while allowing the self-stimulation to occur. Presumably, this process would be more effective because it would directly weaken the response strength of self-stimulation through the process of extinction. In line with this rationale, he called the principle "sensory extinction," and developed treatments based on this principle which involve removing the sensory stimulation that normally occurs as a consequence of the inappropriate behavior. For example, he tested the efficacy of this procedure on an autistic child who spun objects on a table repetitively. He assumed that the major mode of stimulation was auditory, and removed it by carpeting the top of the table. The child consequently stopped twirling objects.

Rincover, Cook, Peoples, and Packard (1979) further extended this treatment procedure by introducing toys that provided sensory stimulation after applying sensory extinction. Four autistic children, 8 to 10 years old, were treated. Each displayed a high rate of self-stimulation and little appropriate play. Proprioceptive stimulation was masked for two clients' finger and arm movements by taping a small vibrator to the backs of their hands. Auditory stimulation was removed for a client's platespinning by carpeting the top of the table. Visual stimulation was decreased for finger and hand movements with a blindfold for one child, and by decreasing the room lighting for another.

For three of the clients, self-stimulation was eliminated by the second session of sensory extinction. This reduction is remarkable, because baseline recordings showed the clients performing self-stimulation from 65% to 100% of the time. For the fourth client, however, the removal of visual stimulation for handflapping only decreased its occurrence from an average of 93% during baseline sessions to about 75%, with a range of 17% to 85% across sessions. After returning to baseline conditions and recovering a rate of self-stimulation at 100%, Rincover *et al.* (1979) applied a vibrator to mask the proprioceptive stimulation for handflapping, and produced a marginal decrease to about 75% in three sessions. Again, they returned to baseline conditions and recovered a high rate of self-stimulation (i.e., 90% to 95%). Finally, they introduced both the blocking of the proprioceptive and the visual stimulation together. This combined sensory extinction procedure reduced the handflapping to about 30% across six sessions, with a range 5-50% of the time per session.

The sensory extinction procedures demonstrated that proprioceptive, auditory, and visual stimulation had served as reinforcers for maintaining self-stimulation, Rincover *et al.* (1979) used this information to establish appropriate toy play by selecting toys that provided the stimulation demonstrated as reinforcers for each client. They selected a music box for auditory stimulation (and, later, an autoharp), building blocks and stringing beads for proprioception, and a bubble-blowing kit for visual stimulation. When they simply introduced these items to the clients for play, no play occurred, and self-stimulation occurred from 60% to 100% of the time. Then, therapists trained the clients to play with the toys until each spontaneously played correctly. Next, they reintroduced the toys without sensory extinction or external reinforcement, and recorded the clients' self-stimulation and appropriate toy play. Three of the clients virtually stopped self-stimulating within four sessions, and began appropriate play with toys over 80% of the time. After four sessions, the fourth client was self-stimulating about 75% of the time, and playing appropriately only 20% of the time. When clients were tested again 1, 6, 9, and 13 months later, their percentages of time spent self-stimulating and playing with toys remained at that level (i.e., little self-stimulating and much appropriate toy play for three of the four clients).

SUMMARY OF TREATMENT STUDIES

The previous review demonstrates that self-stimulation has been suppressed by a variety of different procedures based on the principles of extinction, displacement by increasing other behaviors, and punishment, including interruption, verbal reprimands, time-out, isolation, overcorrection, slaps, and electric shock. However, it was also demonstrated that self-stimulation was not sufficiently suppressed in a few cases applying similar principles. With this in mind, one feels compelled to join other reviewers (e.g., Hobbs, 1976 a,b) in recommending more studies that compare the efficacy of applying different principles.

Risley (1968) demonstrated that electric shock was more effective than isolation, social extinction, and reinforcing other behaviors. Foxx and Azrin (1973) found overcorrection more effective than slapping the client, painting a distasteful solution on a client's hand, social extinction, and differential reinforcement of other behavior. Harris and Wolchik (1979) got a rapid and significant suppression of self-stimulation with four autistic boys using overcorrection, but less significant suppression with three of the four using time-out, and a modest suppression with only one of the four using differential reinforcement of other behavior. These studies suggest that punishment is more effective than reinforcing other behaviors, social extinction, and differential reinforcement of other behavior. However, Risley (1968), Foxx and

Azrin (1973), and Harris and Wolchik (1979) used positive reinforcement for alternative behaviors when they applied punishment to self-stimulation, as did Azrin, Kaplan, and Foxx (1973), Azrin and Wesolowski (1980), and others. Thus, the summary that punishment has proved most effective must be tempered with the qualifier that positive reinforcement be available for alternative behaviors.

That punishment produces rapid suppression of behavior when alternative behaviors are reinforced has previously been demonstrated in laboratory studies (Azrin & Holtz, 1966; Herman & Azrin, 1964). In applied studies with mentally retarded individuals, it has similarly been demonstrated that effective treatment occurs when applying a suppression procedure for undesired behaviors in conjunction with a facilitation procedure for desired behaviors (O'Brien, Azrin, & Bugle, 1972; O'Brien, Bugle, & Azrin, 1972). In these studies, it was also demonstrated that neither the facilitation nor the suppression procedures were effective alone, but that they were effective only when applied simultaneously.

Thus, comparing the efficacy of punishment for self-stimulation with positive reinforcement for alternative behaviors requires a qualifier that makes the comparison fruitless. For many clients, it is probable that reinforcement for alternative behaviors will be ineffective alone, but when applied in conjunction with punishment will demonstrate significant efficacy (e.g., Azrin, Kaplan, & Foxx, 1973; Risley, 1968). The converse may also be true, but has yet to be demonstrated; that is, that for many clients punishment will be ineffective alone. The studies reviewed, however, do demonstrate that punishment for self-stimulation along with positive reinforcement for alternate behaviors is an effective treatment.

The practitioner might benefit from knowing what manner of punishment (e.g., overcorrection, time-out) and reinforcement is most effective. Harris and Wolchik (1979), for example, concluded that overcorrection was more effective than time-out and differential reinforcement of other behavior, But their time-out procedure consisted of the trainers' reprimanding the clients and turning away from them for 10 sec. Would time-out have been as ineffective if the clients had been deprived of food and the time-out procedure included 30 min of their watching other clients eat chocolate ice cream? Had food deprivation been the case, would differential reinforcement of other behavior have proved so ineffective if food had been used as the reinforcer instead of praise? The problem in determining the relative efficacy of applying different principles (e.g., punishment, differential reinforcement of other behaviors) is that there is an infinite number of procedures that could be referred to as examples of each principle, varying from dramatic to ineffective in their effects on target behaviors. This fact may account for the contradiction between the studies reviewed, generally demonstrating overcorrection to be the most effective principle, and the study by Lambert, Bruwier, and Cobben (1975) reported by Rollings, Baumeister, and Baumeister (1977) that found overcorrection to be the least efficient of five principles tested. The problem is that each principle or treatment strategy can be applied in varying degrees of power. Consequently, assessing the efficacy of two or more procedures should not be mistaken as demonstrating the comparative efficacy between different principles or treatment strategies. For this reason, it is unlikely that one could design a definitive study comparing the efficacy of applying different principles or treatment strategies.

Many of the studies included in this review have serious investigative weaknesses. Some have no independent observations to demonstrate the reliability of their recordings. Some used frequency measures of self-stimulation such that a lower frequency count could occur when the proportion of time the client self-stimulated actually increased. Some studies using overcorrection may not have separated the time the client was in positive practice from the time of the session, so that no change in self-stimulation would appear as a decrease (e.g., if a client self-stimulated 10 times in a 10-min session during baseline, but only 5 times when a 1-min overcorrection was used, the decrease from 10 to 5 might have occurred because the client was still self-stimulating at once each minute but was in overcorrection for 5 min of a 10-min session). Some studies made comparisons between procedures without controlling for order effects. Some included inadequate descriptions of the clients, duration of time the clients had self-stimulated, extent of self-stimulation before introducing treatment, methods of recording, methods of treatment, collateral effects on other behaviors, and too few short sessions in laboratory situations, little follow-up, and no mention of transfer effects or maintenance of suppression. In addition to recommending that all future studies overcome these deficiencies, a reviewer might feel compelled to dismiss studies with these deficiencies before summarizing. However, I will not do so because most findings that occurred in a study with a major problem were replicated in a study without that problem.

Guidelines for Treating Self-Stimulation

Of the theoretical explanations reviewed, Foxx and Azrin (1973) provided one that seemed to be most fruitful in generating prescriptions for treatment. Their explanation ignores why self-stimulation emerges in the first place, but could incorporate the normal-development explanation which assumes the self-stimulation emerges in all people during normal development, and that most people cease self-stimulating as it is displaced by forms of adaptive behavior. Foxx and Azrin further explain why mentally retarded people continue performing self-stimulation—it is intrinsically reinforcing, and these people have learned few adaptive behaviors. Thus, mentally retarded and other developmentally disabled people continue self-stimulating at such an extreme rate as to dismiss the opportunity to learn the adaptive behaviors. Because they do not learn the adaptive behaviors that would displace self-stimulation, they continue performing these behaviors at a high rate.

With this theoretical explanation, Foxx and Azrin (1973) recommended that treatment include the following:

1. Decrease reinforcement for self-stimulation by interrupting it when it occurs.
2. Prevent further occurrence of self-stimulation by prompting the client to perform adaptive behavior.
3. Punish self-stimulation by providing annoying consequences.
4. Teach adaptive behavior.
5. Reinforce the client's performance of adaptive behavior.

The studies reviewed in this chapter support the wisdom of these recommendations.

This theoretical explanation and the treatment recommendations are behaviorally oriented. For this reason, a primary guideline to be followed is to have someone with adequate training and experience in behavior analysis assist in planning, implementing, and evaluating treatment. Although this chapter provides knowledge concerning the treatment of self-stimulation, that knowledge alone is insufficient for developing, implementing, monitoring, and evaluating treatment programs. Skills in defining and recording behavior, selecting and using reinforcers and punishers, evaluating treatment, and designing intervention strategies are generally mastered by behavior analysts, and these skills must be included to develop effective treatment programs.

Whether to Treat

When mentally retarded people perform self-stimulatory behaviors that cause physical injury, few would question the need to treat the problem (see Chapter 3). Even less extreme forms of self-stimulation may produce physical injury (e.g., tapping knuckles on hard surfaces, mouthing objects made of toxic substances, flipping fingers in front of eyes focused on the sun, keeping hands in a tight fist around the collar of a shirt). Under conditions in which the behavior may cause physical injury, the problem should be treated. Not doing so for a client under one's charge seems unethical, and is probably illegal (Repp & Deitz, 1978).

Another reason to treat self-stimulation is incorporated in the concern for providing clients with the least restrictive placement. When mentally retarded people are restricted from normal life experiences because of their self-stimulation, it should be treated. For instance, if it were determined that a client in the community be placed in a hospital because of the self-stimulation, then there is sufficient justification for treating it. Also, if the client is already in a hospital, (typically considered the most restrictive alternative), and restricted from some hospital services because of self-stimulation, treatment is justified. Baumeister (1978), for example, suggests that many clients in a hospital are restricted from training programs because they exhibit too much self-stimulation. When such is the case, it should be treated.

Should the clients' self-stimulation produce no physical injury or create any restrictions from normal life experiences or needed services, the decision as to whether to treat is more difficult to make. Some would decide to do so if treatment would increase reinforcement. The problem in making this decision is that self-stimulation is intrinsically reinforcing. As Baumeister (1978) notes, some forms of self-stimulation are normal under some conditions, and he further reminds us that the rocking chair was designed for such a purpose. Following this line of argument, one should allow a client to self-stimulate because the client obtains reinforcement for doing so. If the goal is to maximize reinforcement or minimize annoyance for the client, self-stimulation should be treated only if it is determined that doing so would increase reinforcement or decrease annoyance for the client.

Decreasing annoyance is a reason for treating self-stimulation. If parents, teachers, or peers reprimand, berate, or tease a client for self-stimulating, it should be treated. Similarly, treatment should be provided if clients are regularly required to accept less preferred sitting or sleeping arrangements because they self-stimulate. Requiring clients to sit in a position farthest from the television set, sit at the least preferred table in the dining room, sleep in a less-preferred bed, or sit in a less-preferred seat on the bus are examples of this. When these types of annoyance can be reduced, it seems reasonable to treat self-stimulation.

Similarly, increasing reinforcement in the clients' lives is justification for treating the problem. Two situations to look for are those in which clients receive less reinforcement because they self-stimulate, and those in which clients receive less reinforcement because they perform self-stimulation instead of another behavior that would be reinforced. Examples of the former are situations like snack time in which everybody gets a snack except the self-stimulators, grooming class in which everyone receives praise for their nicely combed hair except for clients who are self-stimulating (although their hair is combed, trainers do not want to reinforce the behavior accidentally). Treating self-stimulation is reasonable for clients who experience such situations.

Decreases in reinforcement also occur when clients perform self-stimulation instead of other behaviors that would be reinforced. Treating self-stimulation is justified in these cases, especially when the clients are able to perform the behavior that would be reinforced. In cases where the clients are incapable of performing the behavior, it would be justifiable to treat the self-stimulation if that were necessary to teach the skill that would ultimately be reinforced.

Thus, some guidelines on whether to treat self-stimulation as a problem include determining whether treatment will decrease physical injury (or deformity), decrease restrictions from normalized activities or needed services, decrease annoyance, or increase reinforcement. Should any of these be likely, treatment is justified. To the extent that none of these goals is likely, it may be inappropriate to treat self-stimulation as a problem; rather, it may be considered as a leisure time activity and a source of reinforcement for the client.

Designing a Treatment Plan

Should a decision be made to treat self-stimulation, a behavioral evaluation must be completed. The evaluation should determine the situations in which self-stimulation occurs, its topography, frequency, and duration, and its consequences. If during the evaluation it is found that self-stimulation occurred only under one condition (e.g., in front of a particular mirror, when wearing turtleneck sweaters), and it was reasonable to restrict the client from this condition, that might be the preferred treatment. Should it seem unreasonable to restrict the client from a particular situation in which self-stimulation occurred, it might be reasonable to apply sensory extinction (e.g., if self-stimulation occurs only at a wooden desk, the client could be seated in a soft-fabric chair).

Should a behavioral evaluation determine that people regularly provide a consequence for the self-stimulation, that consequence should be reviewed as a possible reinforcer. Throughout this chapter, discussion has been limited to behaviors that fail to produce any apparent, positive, environmental consequences. However, behaviors that are stereotyped and performed repetitiously may produce positive environmental consequences, and these may be reinforcing the behavior. Hollis (1978), for example, demonstrated that rocking behaviors could be established and modified like other behaviors (e.g., buttonpushing, knobpulling) by providing different schedules of reinforcement. Thus, should a behavioral evaluation determine that a client's self-stimulation regularly produces a consequence, initial treatment should include witholding that consequence. Should the behavior decrease, it is likely that the consequence was a reinforcer. Completing a behavioral evaluation is required before the utility of similar treatments can be determined.

Should the behavior evaluation determine that self-stimulation occurs in many different situations, that the sensory consequences would be difficult to modify, and that no other consequences are regularly provided, a program should be designed along the recommendations presented by Foxx and Azrin (1973), including teaching and reinforcing adaptive behaviors, interrupting self-stimulation, and scheduling an annoying consequence to follow such.

When designing a treatment based on these recommendations, planners must address themselves to two treatment concerns: providing the least restrictive (lease intrusive) plan and providing treatment that is effective. In some cases, these concerns seem to recommend opposite strategies. For instance, the concern for efficacy might suggest using a most-intrusive treatment. One example would include depriving a client of food and liquids, using these as reinforcers to teach and motivate adaptive behaviors, and using electric shock as an annoying consequence for every occurrence of self-stimulation.

The concern for using a less aversive treatment might suggest using procedures that would be ineffective. One example might include praising clients whenever they go 30 min without self-stimulating, when typically those clients perform few adaptive behaviors, are ignored when they do so, and spend much of their time self-stimulating in chairs on a barren ward of a state hospital. When planners address both concerns, however, the apparent contradiction is resolved by designing the least restrictive, but still effective, treatment. For some situations, a simple verbal reprimand or interruption may suffice. For others, edibles as reinforcers for adaptive behaviors and 20-min overcorrection consequences may be required.

The art of designing the least restrictive, effective plan requires thorough understanding of the clients, their daily activities, and the constraints (e.g., regulations, resources) of the caregivers, educators, and treatment personnel. Although a precise system to ensure adequate attention to these matters has not yet been specified, a general process can be recommended, namely, the transdisciplinary approach. As specified by the Accreditation Council for Services for Mentally Retarded and Other Developmentally Disabled Persons (1978), the transdisciplinary approach includes establishing a team for designing client plans, a team which consists of persons from professions, disciplines, or service areas that are relevant to the clients' needs, including those persons who most directly interact with the clients, families and advocates. As cumbersome as team decisions can be, the needed information is available to be shared in meetings with such teams. With such information and participation by a behavior analyst, teams are able to design treatments that are least restrictive and most effective in helping mentally retarded and other developmentally disabled people to decrease self-stimulatory behaviors.

REFERENCES

ACCREDITATION COUNCIL FOR SERVICES FOR MENTALLY RETARDED AND OTHER DEVELOPMENTALLY DISABLED PERSONS. *Standards for services for developmentally disabled individuals.* Chicago: Joint Commission on Accreditation of Hospitals, 1978.

AZRIN, N. H., & HOLTZ, W. C. Punishment. In W. K. Honig (Ed.), *Operant behavior: Areas of, research and application*. New York: Appleton-Century-Crofts, 1966.

AZRIN, N. H., & WESOLOWSKI, M. D. Eliminating habitual vomiting in a retarded adult by positive practice and self-correction. *Journal of Behavior Therapy and Experimental Psychiatry*, 1975, *6*, 145–148.

AZRIN, N. H., & WESOLOWSKI, M. D. A reinforcement plus interruption method of eliminating behavioral stereotypy of profoundly retarded persons. *Behavior Research and Therapy*, 1980, *18*, 113–120.

AZRIN, N. H., KAPLAN, S. J., & FOXX, R. M. Autism reversal: Eliminating stereotyped self-stimulation of retarded individuals. *American Journal of Mental Deficiency*, 1973, *78*, 241–248.

BAER, D. M. Laboratory control of thumbsucking by withdrawal and representation of reinforcement. *Journal of the Experimental Analysis of Behavior*, 1962, *5*, 522–528.

BAKWIN, H., & BAKWIN, R. M. *Behavior disorders in children*. New York: Saunders, 1960.

BARNARD, J. B., CHRISTOPHERSON, E. R., ALTMAN, K., & WOLF, M. M. *Parent mediated treatment of self-injurious behavior using overcorrection*. Paper presented at the 82nd Annual Convention of the American Psychological Association, New Orleans, 1974.

BAUMEISTER, A. A. Origins and control of stereotyped movements. In C. E. Meyers (Ed.), *Quality of life in severely and profoundly mentally retarded people: Research foundations for improvement*. Washington, D.C.: American Association on Mental Deficiency, 1978.

BAUMEISTER, A. A., & FOREHAND, R. Effects of contingent shock and verbal command on body rocking of retardates. *Journal of Clinical Psychology*, 1972, *28*, 586–590.

BAUMEISTER, A. A., & FOREHAND, R. Stereotyped acts. In N. R. Ellis (Ed.), *International review of research in mental retardation* (Vol. 6). New York: Academic Press, 1973.

BERKSON, G. Abnormal stereotyped motor acts. In J. Zubin & H. F. Hunt (Eds.), *Comparative psychopathology—animal and human*. New York: Grune & Stratton, 1967.

BERKSON, G. Visual defect does not produce stereotyped movements. *American Journal of Mental Deficiency*, 1973, *78*, 89–94.

BERKSON, G., & DAVENPORT, R. K. Stereotyped movements of mental defectives: Initial survey. *American Journal of Mental Deficiency*, 1962, *66*, 849–852.

BERKSON, G., & MASON, W. A. Stereotyped movements of mental defectives. III: Situation effects. *American Journal of Mental Deficiency*, 1963, *68*, 409–412.

BERKSON, G., & MASON, W. A. Stereotyped movements of mental defectives. IV: The effects of toys and the character of the acts. *American Journal of Mental Deficiency*, 1964, *68*, 511–524.

BRODY, S. Self rocking in infancy. *Journal of the American Psychoanalytic Association*, 1960, *8*, 464–491.

BYCHOWSKI, G. Problems of infantile neurosis: A discussion. In R. S. Eissler (Ed.), *The psychoanalytic study of the child* (Vol. 9). New York: International Universities Press, 1954.

CARR, E. G. The motivation of self-injurious behavior: A review of some hypotheses. *Psychological Bulletin*, 1977, *84*, 800–816.

CATANIA, A. C. Concurrent operants. In W. K. Honig (Ed.), *Operant behavior—areas of research and application*. New York: Appleton-Century-Crofts, 1966.

CUVO, A. J. Decreasing repetitive behavior in an institutionalized mentally retarded resident *Mental Retardation*, 1976, *14*, 22–25.

DAVENPORT, R. K., & BERKSON, G. Stereotyped movements of mental defectives. II: Effects of novel objects. *American Journal of Mental Deficiency*, 1963, *67*, 879–882.

DAVENPORT, R. K., & MENZEL, E. W. Stereotyped behavior of the infant chimpanzee. *Archives of General Psychiatry*, 1963, *8*, 99–104.

DE LISSOVOY, V. Head banging in early childhood: A suggested cause. *Journal of Genetic Psychology*, 1963, *102*, 109–114.

DOKE, L. A., & EPSTEIN, L. H. Oral overcorrection: Side effects and extended applications. *Journal of Experimental Child Psychology*, 1975, *20*, 496–511.

EPSTEIN, L., DOKE, L., SAJWAJ, T., SORRELL, S., & RIMMER B. Generality and side effects of overcorrection. *Journal of Applied Behavior Analysis*, 1974, *7*, 26–31.

FLAVELL, J. E. Reduction of stereotypes by reinforcement of toy play. *Mental Retardation*, 1973, *11*, 21–23.

FOXX, R. M., & AZRIN, N. H. The elimination of autistic self-stimulatory behavior by overcorrection. *Journal of Applied Behavior Analysis*, 1973, *6*, 1–14.

GARDNER, W. I. The use of punishment procedures with the severely retarded: A review. *American Journal of Mental Deficiency*, 1969, *74*, 86–103.

GESELL, A., & AMATRUDA, C. S. *Developmental diagnosis*. New York: Harper 1947.

GREENACRE, P. Problems of infantile neurosis: A discussion. In R. S. Eissler (Ed.) *The psychoanalytic study of the child* (Vol. 9). New York: International Universities Press, 1954.

GREENE, R. J., HOATS, D. L., & HORNICK, A. J. Music distortion: A new technique for behavior modification. *Psychological Record*, 1970, *20*, 107–109.

GUESS, D., & RUTHERFORD, G. Experimental attempts to reduce stereotyping among blind retardates. *American Journal of Mental Deficiency*, 1967, *71*, 984–986.

HAMILTON, J., STEPHENS, L., & ALLEN, P. Controlling aggressive and destructive behavior in severely retarded institutionalized residents. *American Journal of Mental Deficiency*, 1967, *71*, 852–856.

HARKNESS, J. E., & WAGNER, J. D. Self-mutilation in mice associated with otitis media. *Laboratory Animal Science*, 1975, *25*, 315–318.
HARLOW, H. F. Primary affectional patterns in primates. *American Journal of Orthopsychiatry*, 1960, *30*, 676–684.
HARRIS, S. L., & WOLCHIK, S. A. Suppression of self-stimulation: Three alternative strategies. *Journal of Applied Behavior Analysis*, 1979, *12*, 185–198.
HARTMANN, H., KRIS, E., & LOEWENSTEIN, R. M. Notes on the theory of aggression. In R. S. Eissler (Ed.), *The psychoanalytic study of the child* (Vols. 3 & 4). New York: International Universities Press, 1949.
HERENDEEN, D. L. JEFFREY, D. B. & GRAHAM, M. L. *Reduction of self-stimulation in institutionalized children: Overcorrection and reinforcement of nonresponding*. Paper presented at the 8th Annual Meeting of the Association for the Advancement of Behavior Therapy, Chicago, 1974.
HERMAN, R. L., & AZRIN, N. H. Punishment by noise in an alternative response situation. *Journal of the Experimental Analysis of Behavior*, 1964, *7*, 185–188.
HOBBS, S. A. Modifying stereotyped behaviors by overcorrection: A critical review. *Rehabilitation Psychology*, 1976, *23*, 1–11. (a)
HOBBS, S. A. Further comments on overcorrection and stereotyped behavior. *Rehabilitation Psychology*, 1976, *23*, 32–38. (b)
HOBBS, S. A. & GOSWICK, R. A. Behavioral treatment of self-stimulation: An examination of alternatives to physical punishment. *Journal of Clinical Child Psychology*, 1977, *6*, 20–23.
HOLLIS, J. H. Analysis of rocking behavior. In C. E. Meyers (Ed.), *Quality of life in severely and profoundly mentally retarded people: Research foundations for improvement*. Washington, D.C.: American Association on Mental Deficiency, 1978.
JUDKINS, J. D. Overcorrection procedures with the institutionalized retarded: An evaluative review. *Mental Retardation Bulletin*, 1976, *4*, 98–110.
KAUFMAN, M. E., & LEVITT, H. A study of three stereotyped behaviors in institutionalized mental defectives. *American Journal of Mental Deficiency*, 1965, *69*, 467–473.
KOEGEL, R. L., FIRESTONE, P. B., KRAMME, K. W., & DUNLAP, G. Increasing spontaneous play by suppressing self-stimulation in autistic children. *Journal of Applied Behavior Analysis*, 1974, *7*, 521–528.
LAMBERT, J. L., BRUWIER, D., & COBBEN, A. La réduction d'un comportement stéréotypé chez un enfant arrière mental profond: Comparison de cinq méthods. *Revue Suisse de Psychologie Pure et Appliquée*, 1975, *34*, 1–18.
LAWS, D. R., BROWN, R. A., EPSTEIN, J., & HOCKING, N. Reduction of inappropriate social behavior in disturbed children by an untrained paraprofessional therapist. *Behavior Therapy*, 1971, *2*, 519–533.
LOVAAS, O. I , SCHAEFFER, B., & SIMMONS, J. Q. Building social behavior in autistic children by the use of electric shock. *Journal of Experimental Research in Personality*, 1965, *1*, 99–109.
LOVAAS, O. I., & SIMMONS, J. Q. Manipulation of self-destruction in three retarded children. *Journal of Applied Behavior Analysis*, 1969, *2*, 143–157.
LUISELLI, J. K. The effects of multiple contingencies on the rocking behavior of a retarded child. *Psychological Record*, 1975, *25*, 559–565.
LUTZKER, J. R. Reducing self-injurious behavior by facial screening. *Mental Retardation*, 1978, *82*, 510–513.
MARTIN, J., WELLER, S., & MATSON, J. Eliminating object-transferring by a profoundly retarded female by overcorrection. *Psychological Reports*, 1977, *40*, 779–782.
MATSON, J. L., & STEPHEN, R. M. Overcorrection treatment of stereotyped behaviors of adult retardates. *Behavior Modification*, in press.
MATTOS, R. L. *Operant control of facial ticking and finger sucking in a severely retarded child.*

Paper presented at the annual convention of the American Association on Mental Deficiency, San Francisco, 1969.

Menzel, E. W. The effects of cumulative experience on responses to novel objects in young isolation-reared chimpanzees. *Behavior*, 1963, *21*, 1–12.

Menzel, E. W., Davenport, R. K., & Rogers, C. M. Effects of environmental restriction upon the chimpanzee's responsiveness in novel situations. *Journal of Comparative and Physiological Psychology*, 1963, *56*, 329–334.

Miron, N. B., & Rooney, J. R. *The accidental acquisition of stimulus control during the extinction of self-injurious behavior in severely retarded children.* Unpublished manuscript, Sonoma State Hospital (California), 1973.

Mulhern, T., & Baumeister, A. A. An experimental attempt to reduce stereotypy by reinforcement procedures. *American Journal of Mental Deficiency*, 1969, *74*, 69–74.

Nissen, H. W. Individuality in the behavior of chimpanzees. *American Anthropologist*, 1969, *58*, 407–413.

O'Brien, F., & Azrin, N. H. Symptom reduction by functional displacement in a token economy. *Journal of Behavior Therapy and Experimental Psychiatry*, 1972, *3*, 205–207.

O'Brien, F., Azrin, N. H., & Bugle, C. Training profoundly retarded children to stop crawling. *Journal of Applied Behavior Analysis*, 1972, *5*, 131-137.

O'Brien, F., Bugle, C., & Azrin, N. H. Training and maintaining a retarded child's proper eating. *Journal of Applied Behavior Analysis*, 1972, *5*, 67–72.

Ollendick, T. H., Matson, J. L., & Martin, J. E. Effectiveness of hand overcorrection for topographically similar and dissimilar self-stimulatory behavior. *Journal of Experimental Child Psychology*, 1978, *25*, 396–403.

Pendergrass, V. E. Time-out from positive reinforcement following persistent, high-rate behavior in retardates. *Journal of Applied Behavior Analysis*, 1972, *5*, 85–91.

Polvinale, R. A., & Lutzker, J. R. Elimination of assaultive and inappropriate sexual behavior by reinforcement and social-restitution. *Mental Retardation*, 1980, *18*, 27–30.

Provence, S., & Lipton, R. C. *Infants in Institutions.* New York: International Universities Press, 1962.

Repp, A. C., & Deitz, D. E. On the selective use of punishment: Suggested guidelines for administrators. *Mental Retardation*, 1978, *16*, 250–254.

Repp, A. C., Deitz, S. M., & Speir, N. C. Reducing stereotypic responding of retarded persons by the differential reinforcement of other behavior. *American Journal of Mental Deficiency*, 1974, *79*, 279–284.

Kimland, B. *Infantile autism*. New York: Appleton-Century-Crofts, 1964.

Rincover, A. Sensory extinction: A procedure for eliminating self-stimulatory behavior in psychotic children. *Journal of Abnormal Child Psychology*, 1978, *6*, 299–310.

Rincover, A., & Koegel, R. L. Research on the education of autistic children: Recent advances and future directions. In G. G. Lahey & A. E. Kazdin (Eds.) *Advances in clinical child psychology* (Vol. 1). New York: Plenum Press, 1977.

Rincover, A., Cook, R., Peoples, A., & Packard, D. Sensory extinction and sensory reinforcement principles for programming multiple adaptive behavior change. *Journal of Applied Behavior Analysis*, 1979, *12*, 221–233.

Risley, T. The effects and side effects of punishing the autistic behaviors of a deviant child. *Journal of Applied Behavior Analysis*, 1968, *1*, 21–34.

Roberts, P., Iwata, B. A., McSween, T. E., & Desmond, E. F. An analysis of overcorrection movements. *American Journal of Mental Deficiency*, 1979, *83*, 588–594.

Rollings, J. P. *The establishment of extroceptive stimulus control of stereotypic responding of retarded persons by the differential reinforcement of other behavior.* Unpublished doctoral dissertation, University of Alabama, 1975.

ROLLINGS, J. P., BAUMEISTER, A. A., & BAUMEISTER, A. A. The use overcorrection procedures to eliminate the stereotyped behaviors of retarded individuals: An analysis of collateral behaviors and generalization of suppressive effects. *Behavior Modification*. 1977, *1*, 29–46.

TIZARD, B. Observations of over-active imbecile children in controlled and uncontrolled environments. II: Experimental studies. *American Journal of Mental Deficiency*, 1968, *72*, 548–553.

WARREN, S. A., & BURNS, N. R. Crib confinement as a factor in repetitive and stereotyped behavior in retardates. *Mental Retardation*, 1970, *8*, 25–28.

WEHMAN, P., & MCLAUGHLIN, P. J. Teachers' perceptions of behavior problems with severely and profoundly handicapped students. *Mental Retardation*, 1979, *17*, 20–21.

WEISBERG, P. Operant procedures with the retardate: An overview of laboratory research. In Ellis, N. R. (Ed.), *International review of research in mental retardation (Vol. 5)*. New York: Academic Press, 1971.

WELLS, K. C., FOREHAND, R., HICKEY, K., & GREEN, K. D. Effects of a procedure derived from the overcorrection principle on manipulated and non-manipulated behaviors. *Journal of Applied Behavior Analysis*, 1977, *10*, 679–689.

WHITMAN, T. L., & SCIBAK, J. W. Behavior modification research with the severely and profoundly retarded. In Ellis, N. R. (Ed.), *Handbook of mental deficiency, psychological theory and research* (2nd ed.). Hillsdale, N. J.: Erlbaum, 1979.

WOLF, M. M., RISLEY, T., JOHNSTON, M., HARRIS, F., & ALLEN, E. Application of operant conditioning procedures to the behavior problems of an autistic child: A follow-up and extension. *Behavior Research and Therapy*, 1967, *5*, 103–111.

YARROW, L. J. Maternal deprivation: Toward an empirical and conceptual re-evaluation. *Psychological Bulletin*, 1961, *58*, 459–490.

5 Teaching Self-Help Skills to the Mentally Retarded

LUKE S. WATSON, JR., AND RANDY UZZELL

INTRODUCTION

The behavior modification (operant) approach to teaching independent living skills is a relatively new technology that has been in existence for approximately fifteen years. Antecedents to this technique can be found in the writings of Skinner (1953, 1958), Ellis (1974), Bijou (1966), Bijou and Orlando (1961), and Ferster (1961). Skinner (1953) speculated about ways the operant conditioning method could be used to develop social/educational systems. Shortly thereafter he published a paper on programmed instruction in which operant conditioning procedures were shown to have utility for teaching certain "cognitive" skills (Skinner, 1958). The implication of this paper was that the operant conditioning approach to programmed instruction could be used to train complex cognitive skills that might not be learned by more conventional educational methods. In 1958, Ellis presented a paper entitled "Behavioral Engineering in Development of Self-Help Skills" at the Southeastern American Association on Mental Deficiency Convention. At this presentation, he described a procedure for teaching toileting, dressing, and feeding skills to severely retarded persons living in residential institutions (Ellis, 1974). Shortly thereafter, Bijou and Orlando (1961) published a paper showing that mentally retarded persons were controlled behaviorally by schedules of reinforcement. Bijou (1966) later published a treatise on how the physical, biological, and social environments contribute to the condition known as mental retardation. It was a rather simple matter to conclude that if mental retardation could be caused, in part, by a person's psychological environment, then special psychoeducational techniques could reverse the condition, to some extent. Ferster (1961) put forth a similar argument about autistic children. He conducted studies showing that token reinforcement

LUKE S. WATSON, JR., AND RANDY UZELL • Partlow State School and Hospital, Tuscaloosa, Alabama 35401.

could serve as an incentive with autistic children, and that these children were responsive to the operant conditioning method. Thus, the conceptual framework for the development of behavior modification techniques for teaching independent living skills was laid.

The formal birth of the behavior modification approach to teaching independent living skills to the mentally retarded occurred around 1963. Ellis (1963), who was at Pinecrest State School at that time, published an operant analysis of how clients could be toilet trained. Dayan (1964), also at Pinecrest State School, demonstrated how Ellis's model could be used to toilet train severely and profoundly retarded persons. Then Bensberg, Colwell, and Cassell (1965), also at Pinecrest, published a paper that described how the same approach could be used to teach basic undressing and dressing skills as well as toileting. The method they used was labeled the *backward chaining* technique and consisted of teaching self-help skills in a backward sequence. This technique was based on the original concept of chaining (Keller & Schoenfeld, 1950), and was used in a number of training programs which came later (Minge & Ball, 1967; Patterson & Overbeck, 1968; Watson, 1973).

During the same period, Girardeau and Spradlin (1964), who were at Parsons State School, taught severely and moderately retarded girls self-grooming skills. This project was also noteworthy in that they introduced *token systems* as a reinforcement technique for training in practical living skills. Gorton and Hollis (1965), also at Parsons, published a paper on teaching utensil-feeding skills and self-help skills to the mentally retarded. They, too, used the backward chaining approach to train clients (Hollis, 1979).

One of the most sophisticated training programs for the mentally retarded that emerged during this earlier period was one developed by Lent and his associates at Parsons State School (Lent, LeBlanc, & Spradlin, 1970). They designed a program for teaching complex self-help and grooming skills, as well as social skills, to institutionalized moderately retarded teenage girls. An outgrowth of the program initially developed by Girardeau and Spradlin (1964), this program utilized a token reinforcement system and was specifically designed to return clients to the community. All these early programs were moderately successful, but a significant proportion of the clients did not respond to the training techniques, and teaching basic self-help skills often took several months (Azrin, Schaeffer, & Wesolowski, 1976). However, these early training attempts clearly demonstrated the potential of this approach for teaching practical living skills to the mentally retarded.

The next major milestone in self-help skill training occurred when Azrin and Foxx (1971) published their article on toilet training. One important component of their system was the *graduated guidance* approach. This method was basically a sophisticated application of the successive-approximation technique used to teach rats and pigeons to operate manipulanda in laboratory settings. Azrin and his colleagues later adapted this procedure for teaching the mentally retarded to eat with utensils (Azrin & Armstrong, 1973), and undressing and dressing skills (Azrin, Schaeffer, & Wesolowski, 1976). Clearly, the Azrin and Foxx method held great promise for teaching severely and profoundly retarded persons. The success rate of the approach was extremely high, and clients were taught rapidly.

A third behavior modification approach to teaching practical living skills to the mentally retarded emerged around 1974. Lent (1975) developed a training procedure that utilized a forward training sequence. A skill was task analyzed and was taught in the order in which it was usually carried out. The first step in the sequence was taught first, the second step taught second, etc. In contrast, when the backward chaining approach is used, the client is taught task-analyzed steps in reverse (i.e., the last step first, and the first step last).

These three approaches to behavior modification are the main techniques used to teach practical living skills. All three techniques are currently being utilized in residential facilities and special educational programs for the mentally retarded and in parent-training programs with varying degrees of success (Ayllon, Garber, & Pisor, 1976; Becker & Engelmann, 1974; Birnbrauer, Wolf, Kidder, & Tague, 1965; Heifetz, 1977; Lent, LeBlanc, & Spradlin 1970; Watson, 1967, 1978a; and Watson & Bassinger, 1974).

In the remainder of this chapter the three training procedures, backward chaining, graduated guidance, and forward sequencing, will be described and assessed. Finally, there will be a discussion of the factors which appear to be responsible for mentally retarded persons' failing to make progress in training programs for independent living skills.

Backward Chaining, Graduated Guidance, and Forward Sequencing

In this section, the three approaches to teaching utensil-feeding, self-help, and grooming skills will be reviewed. Each procedure will be described and compared with the other two procedures. Strengths and weaknesses of each approach will be considered. Programs selected for review were those which would be classified as complete programs, such as those developed by Azrin, Lent, and Watson. These training approaches typically present relatively well organized methods, which include reinforcement and fading techniques, and they often provide a number of client-training programs.

Backward Chaining

In backward chaining, clients are taught the last step in a training sequence first, and the first step last. For example, if a client is being taught to take off his or her pants, the steps in the sequence will be taught in the following order:

1. Removes pants from one foot
2. Removes pants from both feet
3. Pushes pants down from calves
4. Pushes pants down from thighs
5. Pushes pants down from groin
6. Pushes pants down from waist

Each task-analyzed step in this type of program constitutes a functional unit that is taught to clients, one unit at a time. The client is taught step 1 first, removing his or her pants from one foot, and always receiving the primary reinforcement when step 1 is completed, although social reinforcement (praise and pats) may be received as other steps or components in the program are completed as well. Thus, one of the identifying characteristics of this approach is that the last step in the training sequence is taught first, and the client always receives his or her primary reinforcement when he or she completes the last step in the program. Once the client completes step 1, he or she receives training on step 2, removing the pants from both feet. Now he or she practices step 2 followed by step 1, receiving primary reinforcement when step 1 is completed. The client takes his or her pants off one ankle and foot, followed by the other ankle and foot. After the client passes step 2, he or she begins to train on step 3, pushing the pants down from his or her calves, taking them off one ankle and foot, removing them from the other ankle and foot, and then being reinforced. This procedure continues until the client can independently push his or her pants down from the waist and remove them from both feet.

A second characteristic of the backward chaining approach is the type of reinforcement that is used, and the manner in which it is given. Three types of reinforcement are typically used: verbal reinforcement, a primary reinforcement (such as edibles, toys or tokens), and some kind of social-physical reinforcement (e.g., a hug). A sophisticated trainer may frequently give verbal reinforcement as the client completes each step or component in the training sequence, such as saying, "good." When the client completes the sequence, that is, the last step in the program, he or she usually is told that he or she did a good job, is given a primary reinforcement, and then is given a hug or a pat on the arm, shoulder, or leg.

A third characteristic of the procedure is the manner in which prompts are used. There are three types of prompts: verbal, gestural, and physical. When verbal prompts are used, the client is told what to do, for example, "Billy, take off your pants." In the case of gestural prompts, the trainer typically points or gestures. If the client is being taught to take off his or her pants, the trainer gestures downward with a sweeping motion of both hands, palms down, with arms extended outward to indicate that he wants the client to take off his or her pants. When a physical prompt is used, the trainer takes the client's hands in his, and if, for example, the client is being taught to take off his or her pants, the trainer hooks the client's hands in the waistband and pushes down, thus lowering the pants from the waist to the ankles.

Bensberg, Colwell, and Cassell (1965) developed the first backward chaining program. They also wrote a manual that described how to use the procedure (Bensberg, 1965). For teaching basic undressing, dressing, and feeding skills, programs were written in a step-by-step format. Specific instructions were given for the use of edible and social reinforcement. There also was some general reference to the use of prompts. Their training sessions typically ran from 15 to 30 min a day, and each client received an average of two training sessions a day.

The programs in this manual are fairly structured, and staff at Pinecrest who used this approach did receive inservice training prior to teaching clients. The only field testing that was reported was the paper by Bensberg, Colwell, and Cassell (1965). These programs were moderately successful with severely and profoundly retarded clients. The greatest importance of the Pinecrest program was that it was the first, and it stimulated tremendous interest throughout the United States in training self-help skills. Many of the procedures used in this prototype were the basis for later developments in the area.

A second backward chaining program, which is highly structured, is the one developed by Watson and his associates. Three manuals were written for staff training. There was an instructor's manual (Watson, 1974a), a student's text (Watson, 1973), a manual that contained a series of practical living-skill training programs (Watson, 1972), and an inservice training assessment checklist (Gardner, Brust, & Watson, 1970; Watson, 1974b). Staff attended an inservice training program before attempting to train clients. The instructor gave a series of lectures that used slide sequences to illustrate the major points made in the student's text and the lectures. Trainees were taught principles of reinforcement, shaping, and stimulus control, plus data collection techniques.

At the conclusion of the academic phase of training, trainees received practicum training. They learned how to determine reinforcement preferences, shape eye contact, obtain compliance, conduct baselines, and teach self-help skills. Practicum training began with trainees role-playing with one another. When they met criteria based on an assessment by the instructor using the Training Proficiency Scale Checklist, they began a four-month internship. During this internship, they taught utensil-feeding, self-help, and grooming skills to clients, and were assessed periodically with the Training Proficiency Scale (Watson, 1978a).

The training approach was quite similar to the Pinecrest program,[1] except that the prompting procedure was more structured. Staff were taught always to begin a training trial with a verbal prompt. If the client did not respond to the verbal prompt or did not respond to it correctly, the trainer repeated the verbal prompt and paired it with a gestural prompt. If the client still did not respond to the gestural prompt or did not respond correctly, the trainer repeated the verbal prompt again and paired it with a physical prompt. Each trial began with a verbal prompt (gestural prompts were used only if the verbal prompt failed, and physical prompts were used only if the client did not respond to the gestural prompt). This was followed by a crude type of fading procedure.

This program has received field testing in a parent-training, a classroom, (Watson, 1978a; Watson & Bassinger, 1974), and several residential settings (Watson, 1978a). Teachers, parents, and professional and paraprofessional staff were able to teach self-help skills and grooming skills to clients. During the past three years, staff at Partlow State School who attended this training program have taught dressing, grooming, and feeding skills. A summary of

[1] Pat Aycock, who was involved in staff training at Pinecrest, served as a consultant when we established our backward chaining prototype.

TABLE I
Summary of Self-Help and Social-Recreational Skills Taught to Severely and Profoundly Retarded Clients

Wiping with toilet tissue	Putting on a belt	Picking hair (afro)
Eating with a fork	Taking off a belt	Shaving face with safety razor
Using a napkin	Buckling belt	Shaving face with electric razor
Tying shoelaces	Snapping	Shaving armpits
Washing hands	Hooking	Unbuttoning
Washing face	Taking off a bra	Shaving legs
Brushing teeth	Sweeping	Taking off a skirt
Applying deodorant	Mopping	Putting on a skirt
Showering	Hanging clothes on a hanger	Unbuckling a belt
Cleaning fingernails	Folding clothes	Zipping
Shampooing	Buttoning	Putting on a bra
Noseblowing	Brushing hair	Making a bed
Untying shoelaces	Combing hair	

the programs that have been taught can be found in Table I. Approximately 90% of the severely and profoundly retarded residents who have been taught with this program have learned some dressing, grooming, and feeding skills. Less than 10% have been unable to learn these skills. There are clearly problems with this technique, and they will be reviewed in detail later in this chapter.

Other backward chaining programs have been developed. Patterson and Overbeck (1968) generated a program that was similar to that of Bensberg *et al.* (1965). They used a manual in which the basic principles of reinforcement and behavior shaping were presented. The manual had a section on compliance training. There was a series of undressing, dressing, and utensil-feeding programs, all of which were illustrated with drawings. The manual appeared to be well suited as a basic introduction for behavior shaping. Because there are no field test data, it is difficult to assess the program's effectiveness, however.

Baker, Brightman, Heifetz, and Murphy (1976) have published a series of self-help skill programs that employ the backward chaining technique and are designed specifically for parents. The manuals are designed to be either self-instructional or supplemented by an instructor. They are easy to read and liberally illustrated with drawings to make them more appealing. There are two manuals concerned with self-help skills. The first manual reviews basic readiness skills, selecting target behaviors and reinforcement. The three categories of reinforcement that are recommended are: (1) praise and attention, (2) snacks, and (3) games and toys. Verbal, gestural, and physical prompts are reviewed. The programs presented in the first manual are imitation; following simple instructions; basic motor activities; other motor activities, such as standing up or sitting down in a chair, walking, and ascending and descending stairs. Self-help-skill programs consist of drinking from a cup, eating with a spoon and a fork, taking off and putting on pants, putting on a pullover shirt, socks, and shoes. There also are programs for teaching clients to wash and dry their hands.

The second manual reviews the same basic shaping and reinforcement principles presented in the first self-help skill manual. The programs presented are buttoning, zipping, shoetying, hanging up clothes, cutting with a knife, bathing, shampooing hair, tablesetting, bedmaking, changing a bed, sweeping, and drying dishes and utensils.

Heifetz (1977) has assessed these program manuals under four different training conditions. He divided parents into five instructional groups: (1) no-treatment control, (2) manuals only, (3) manuals plus telephone consultation by a staff member, (4) manuals plus group training by two staff members, and (5) manuals, group training, and home visits by a staff member. Parents who had only manuals and no assistance from staff members did as well in training their children as the other three groups and were clearly superior to the control group. The dependent variables in this study were knowledge of behavior modification principles by the parents and self-help skill acquisition by the children. The implications of this study are that self-instruction using Heifetz's manuals saves the expense of professional consultation.

Another parent-training program that utilizes the backward chaining technique was developed by Elliott, Osteen, Falgione, Guthrie, and Skidmore (1978). The authors recommend that their manual be used to teach parents in a classroom setting by an instructor who is familiar with behavior modification. They also employed home visits following classroom instruction, to ensure that parents applied behavior modification principles properly. They consider these home visits to be a key part of parent instruction. In this program, parents are shown how to select target behaviors or training goals. The number of goals is based on a "developmental quotient." The self-help skills taught using this program are eating with a spoon and drinking from a cup, self-dressing and undressing. To date there are no empirical data available on these procedures.

DeVore (1977) has published a set of self-help skill programs which are designed for teachers and parents. A backward chaining approach is the primary procedure used, although some programs are written using forward sequencing. Programs are presented using a lesson plan format. Programs in the manual are eating with utensils, undressing and dressing, washing and drying hands, and noseblowing. As with the Elliott *et al.* (1978) program, no field test data were available.

The advantage of the backward chaining technique is that it is relatively easy to teach to paraprofessional staff with limited education, and a large number of independent living skills can be taught with this method. One of the major problems is that staff have a difficult time fading physical prompts with some severely and profoundly retarded clients. This is probably owing to the fact that a gradual fading procedure is not used (Watson, 1978b). The backward chaining approach lacks a procedure for gradually fading verbal prompts, and some verbal clients may become dependent on such prompts. Another shortcoming is that most persons who are trained to use backward chaining give only limited reinforcement and feedback, primarily at the completion of the last step in the training sequence (Azrin, Schaeffer, & Wesolowski, 1976). In addition, this approach lacks a procedure for preventing incorrect responses. Incorrect responses can add hours to the completion of a training program or prevent a severely or profoundly retarded client from completing it at all. Finally, many severely and profoundly retarded clients learn these programs relatively slowly, as compared with the graduated guidance approach (Azrin, Schaeffer, & Wesolowski, 1976).

Graduated Guidance

The graduated guidance approach is a highly sophisticated one that utilizes most of the principles that have come from operant learning theory, especially from programmed instruction. High-density reinforcement procedures are used to provide the client with frequent feedback. They are not permitted to make errors in training, and a fading procedure is used that should allow most clients to overcome their dependency on both physical and verbal prompts. This method appears to be ideally suited for both the severely and the profoundly retarded. Developed by Azrin and his associates, this procedure has been used successfully to carry out mealtime training programs (Azrin & Armstrong, 1973) and dressing-skills training (Azrin, Schaeffer, & Wesolowski, 1976). Clients learn the skills rapidly, and field tests have shown that all clients learn the skills on which they are trained, that is, Azrin's success rate for mealtime training and dressing-skill training has been 100%.

Putting on pants provides an excellent example of this training method.[2] A pair of shorts with an elastic waistband, about two sizes too large, would be used. The client probably would not have a shirt on, since the hem ("shirt-tail") could interfere with pulling the pants up. The trainer would seat the client in a chair, call his name to get his attention, and say, "Put on your pants." The trainer would use a physical prompt to hook the client's thumbs inside the waistband of the pants and make a pincer grip. Then he would get the client to place one of his legs into one pants "leghole," using a physical prompt if necessary, and get him to put the other leg into the other "leghole" while repeating the command to put on the pants. If the client did not begin to pull the pants up once he had them on both ankles, the trainer would say, "Pull them up." If the client did nothing, the trainer would use a physical prompt to start the client pulling up the pants. If he began to self-initiate after the physical prompt was given, the trainer would release the client's hands and *shadow* them, keeping his hands one to two inches from the client's hands. If the client paused while pulling up the pants, the trainer would repeat the command to pull them up and resume the physical prompt. He would grasp the client's hands again in a pincer grip, so as to hold onto the waistband of the pants and guide the hands upward.

If the waistband of the pants became "hung up" on the client's buttocks, the trainer would tap the waistband of the pants at the buttocks and say, "Pull them up here." If the client failed to reach in back and grasp the waistband of the pants at the buttocks, the trainer would use a physical prompt to insert the client's hand into the waistband of the pants at the buttocks, and say, "Pull them up," using physical guidance to get the pants up over the buttocks.

Any time the client self-initiated when physical guidance was being used, the trainer would release his hand and resume shadowing. This procedure would be continued until the pants were pulled up to the normal waist position, at which point the client would receive a primary, verbal, and physical reinforcement. Any time the client attempted to self-initiate, he would receive verbal reinforcement from the trainer, and all physical prompts were gradually faded out. Training sessions continued until the client could put on his pants independently after a single request to initiate the behavior.

As indicated in the above example, clients are taught using a "forward sequence" approach; the primary characteristic of this procedure is the manner in which prompts are used. The three types of prompts used are verbal,

[2] This example is taken from the movie *Teaching Independent Living Skills Using Graduated Guidance* (Watson, 1977). Richard Foxx. PhD., provided the demonstrations in this movie.

gestural, and physical, as in backward chaining. However, prompts are employed on an *intuitive* basis. The trainer uses prompts in any order he feels they should be used, but always gives the client the least amount of assistance needed for him to be successful. In early stages of training, physical prompts and verbal prompts are used primarily. The trainer tells the client what to do, and keeps his hands in a *shadowing* position. He follows the client's hands with his hands, keeping them one to two inches away from the client's hands. If the client does not perform a step correctly, the trainer immediately gives the necessary physical guidance to ensure that the client will carry out the step correctly. Then the trainer returns to the shadowing posture, in case the client will need additional physical guidance to complete another step. As the client achieves greater independence in training, the trainer uses fewer physical prompts and more gestural prompts.

The order in which prompts are faded in the graduated guidance approach is somewhat different from the manner in which they are faded in backward chaining. In backward chaining, the trainer typically fades physical prompts first, followed by fading gestural prompts and finally verbal prompts, in an effort to teach the client independence. In contrast, persons using the graduated guidance procedure usually would fade physical prompts first, followed by verbal prompts, with gestural prompts faded last (Foxx & Azrin, 1973; Watson, 1977). The advantage of this alternative is that it should work with clients who become dependent on either physical prompts or verbal prompts. By fading gestural prompts last, the client who is dependent on verbal prompts may achieve independence from these prompts. Another advantage of graduated guidance concerns preventing incorrect responses. Because trainers maintain a shadowing hand position as they train, their hands are close enough to the client's hands to allow them to prevent clients from making errors.

The high-density reinforcement procedure used is another characteristic of the graduated guidance approach. Clients receive verbal reinforcement and physical reinforcement almost continuously as they train, as long as they are successful (Azrin, Schaeffer, & Wesolowski, 1976). The trainer tells the client he is doing a good job for each small success or successful approximation, and also rubs the client's back or pats him on the arm or shoulder frequently throughout a training trial. Sometimes two trainers are used, such as in a dressing-skill program (Azrin, Schaeffer, & Wesolowski, 1976). This should provide the client with considerable verbal and physical reinforcement. In addition, the client receives primary reinforcement, additional praise, and pats or hugs when the trial is completed.

An additional feature of the graduated guidance approach is massed trials. In the meal program, Azrin and Armstrong (1973) used several small meals a day. In the dressing-skills program, they employed three-hour training sessions. Seven profoundly retarded clients required a median of 10 hours (range = 4-20 hours) to learn undressing and dressing skills when this approach was used with two trainers per client. Clients were taught to take off and put on their underpants, pants, shirts, socks, and shoes.

In conclusion, the graduated guidance approach seems to be highly effective with severely and profoundly retarded clients. Three major problems with the technique are evident. First, it appears to be more difficult to teach to staff than the backward chaining and forward sequencing methods. College graduates appear to learn to use it fairly well, but some paraprofessionals have difficulty learning this approach. Preliminary attempts to develop a staff-training program at our facility support this hypothesis. The second problem with graduated guidance is that it typically employs general principles and not structured, task-analyzed training programs. This unstructured approach will make it difficult for many people to apply the technique to teaching a variety of self-help skills. Also, work still needs to be done to demonstrate its application to programs more complex than utensil feeding and basic undressing and dressing. A final criticism is the two-person training approach used in dressing-skill training, and the lengthy training sessions. It may be extremely difficult to get administrators to deploy two staff to train one client, even though it may result in a dramatic saving of time. In addition, most staff will probably be highly resistive to carrying out lengthy training sessions with severely and profoundly retarded clients.

Forward Sequencing

The forward sequencing approach to teaching practical living skills is the third client-instructional technique. Clients are taught skills in the natural order in which they are performed, using four types of prompts. Since Lent's Project MORE program (1975) was the first formalized forward sequencing program, it will be used as an example of this training method. The Project MORE deodorant application program provides an excellent example of this approach (Lewis, Ferneti, & Keilitz, 1975). The steps in the application of roll-on deodorant are taught in the following sequence: (1) pick up the deodorant; (2) shake the deodorant container; (3) remove the cap; (4) hold the bottle up; (5) rub the deodorant onto the underarm; (6) put the deodorant in the other hand; (7) hold the bottle up; (8) rub the deodorant on the other underarm; (9) put the cap back on the deodorant.

Training begins with the instructor placing the deodorant in front of the client on a table. The instructor waits five sec for the client to carry out step 1, picking up the deodorant. If the client makes no attempt to pick up the deodorant after five sec, the trainer tells him what to do. "Pick up the deodorant," he says. If the client picks up the deodorant, the trainer reinforces him with praise, and then waits five sec for him to carry out step 2, shake the deodorant container. If the client fails to shake the deodorant, the trainer says, "Shake the deodorant." Many severely and profoundly retarded clients do not respond to such instructions, and if the client did not respond within 10 sec, the trainer would use either a gestural prompt or model the correct response for the client (in this case, modeling would seem more appropriate). If the client responds correctly to this cue, the trainer praises him and waits five sec to see whether he performs the third step without assistance, removing the cap from the deodorant. If not, the trainer uses a verbal prompt to cue him. If the client responds correctly at this point, he receives another social reinforcement. The trainer then waits five seconds for the client to carry out the fourth step in the sequence, holding up the bottle. If the client performs this step on his own, the trainer reinforces him and go to step five, rubbing the deodorant container onto the underarm. If he does not self-initiate, the trainer uses the first prompt, verbal instructions. If the client does not respond within 10 sec after the verbal prompt is given, the trainer uses either a gestural prompt or models the step for the client. If the client still fails to do this step correctly, the trainer uses a physical prompt. The remainder of the steps in this program are taught in this manner, and training continues until the client applies the deodorant independently, that is, without the instructor's assistance.

The prompting sequence used in the Project MORE approach is quite similar to the prompting sequence used by Watson in his backward chaining program. The trainer begins with a verbal prompt if the client needs assistance. If he fails to respond correctly, the trainer goes either to a gestural prompt of models for the client, whichever one seems most appropriate. If the client still fails to respond correctly, the trainer uses a physical prompt. This sequence of prompts is used with each step in the program. In this sense, a crude fading technique is used, just as in Watson's backward chaining program. Each trial begins without the trainer's providing any prompts.

In the Project MORE manuals, social reinforcement (smiles, praise, pats, and hugs) is recommended in preference to tangible reinforcement (things to eat or drink, games, or tokens), although the use of tangible reinforcement is not precluded. Our experience has been that some clients require tangible reinforcement.

These programs are published individually in manuals, with one program to the manual. All prompting and reinforcement techniques are presented in each manual, as well as a data-recording procedure. Each manual is well organized, and the training procedure is presented clearly, with each programmatic step illustrated. The manuals are designed to be self-instructional. The only manual needed for understanding the training procedure, other than the particular program manual of interest, is *How to Do More* (Bieberly, 1974). This manual reviews the prompting sequence and reinforcement procedure, and provides a rationale for their use. Each program manual is field-tested before it is published, and the field test data are presented in the manual. These programs appear to work well with the severely, moderately, and mildly retarded.

Watson (1978b) and his associates also have developed a practical living-skill training program that utilizes forward sequencing. It is similar to the Project MORE program, with certain exceptions. Trainers go through a formal staff-training program, whereas the Project MORE program is self-instructional. Staff are taught principles of reinforcement, shaping, stimulus control, and data collection in an academic phase. In practicum training they develop skills to motivate clients and obtain eye contact and compliance. Also, trainees learn how to take a baseline and how to teach self-help skills. In addition, there is a four-month internship.

The prompting sequence is similar to that of the Project MORE program, except that special fading programs are included for clients who become dependent on physical or verbal prompts. Basically, prompts are faded in the same manner as described in Foxx and Azrin (1973). Physical prompts are faded first, followed by verbal, then gestural prompts. Each type of prompt is gradually faded in four to five stages. A second alternative is available for clients who become dependent on verbal prompts. The trainer uses a modeling procedure exclusively, except for the initial command, "Do it like this." A procedure for preventing incorrect responses also has been developed. The trainer physically prevents the client from making the error, and then uses the necessary prompt to get the client to make a correct response.

The reinforcement procedure used by Watson also is somewhat different. If a client is being taught a program, such as deodorant application, he is given verbal reinforcement each time he completes a step in the program, and may receive a pat on the arm or shoulder as well. In addition, he receives

TABLE II
Summary of Self-Help Skills Taught to Moderately and Severely Retarded Clients

Clipping nails	Taking a coat off a hanger
Putting a coat on a hanger	Folding clothes
Vacuuming	Shining shoes
Putting on lipstick	Tablesetting
Applying base makeup	Ironing
Applying blush makeup	Telephoning for help
Applying eye makeup	Handwashing lingerie
Changing clothes regularly	Putting on pantyhose
Carrying on a conversation	Self-identification
Relating to facility staff	Crossing sidewalks and interesections
Operating a clothes washer	Matching clothes
Operating a clothes dryer	Taking care of personal possessions
Ordering meals in restaurants	Shopping
Wearing clothes appropriate to situation	

enthusiastic praise, a token, a pat on the arm or shoulder, or a hug when the entire sequence has been completed.

This program has been virtually 100% effective for teaching self-help skills to over 100 moderately and severely retarded clients (Watson, 1978a). However, this approach is designed for clients who can follow verbal instructions, and field tests have been limited to this population. A summary of skills taught using this approach can be found in Table II.

A third self-help skill training program that employs the forward sequencing approach is one by Bender and Valletutti (1976). They developed a manual that contains self-help skill, grooming-skill, and utensil-feeding programs. Programs are presented using a special-education curriculum guide format. No field tests to determine the effectiveness of this approach were found.

In conclusion, the forward sequencing approach appears to be an effective training technique that works well with severely, moderately, and mildly retarded clients. Clients readily learn self-help skills with this approach, and there appear to be a large number of practical living skills that can be taught to the mentally retarded using this training technique.

PROBLEMS WHICH INTERFERE WITH CLIENT TRAINING

There are a number of problems that cause client failure in skill-training programs, regardless of the training procedure used. Some of these problems are directly related to staff behavior, and others are related to difficulties encountered by clients during training. It seems appropriate to review these problems, since additional progress in the development of self-help skill programs will be dependent, to some extent, on resolving these difficulties.

Staff Problems

Two primary categories of staff problems that interfere with client progress in practical-living-skill training programs have been identified: staff training and staff management.

Staff Training

The observation has been made that the effectiveness of self-help skill training programs for the mentally retarded is a function of staff training (Kazdin, 1976; Watson, 1970). Staff who are not trained specifically to teach self-help skills to clients are not very effective (Watson & Bassinger, 1974). As a result, clients make little or no progress in programs of this kind. However, with proper training, most professional and paraprofessional staff can become effective trainers (Watson, 1978a; Watson & Bassinger, 1974.) The authors have conducted field test of backward chaining and forward sequencing programs with psychologists, teachers, nurses, psychiatric aides, and parents. It has been found that over 95% of these personnel could learn to teach self-help skills to mentally retarded clients. Staff training appears to be the first step that should be taken to ensure that a self-help skill training program is effective.

Staff Management

A second consideration in operating an effective self-help skill training program is the development of a staff management system. Observational studies have shown that psychiatric aides spend relatively little of their total work day training retarded residents (Bensberg & Barnett, 1966; Harmatz, 1973). It has been estimated that the staff in residential facilities for the mentally retarded train clients only about 40% of the time they are scheduled to train them (Watson, 1978a). Such a low rate of training by staff is probably partially responsible for the inordinate length of time often required for severely and profoundly retarded clients to learn even basic dressing skills (Azrin, Schaeffer, & Wesolowski, 1976). A solution to this problem is a staff management system (Watson, 1976).

Watson (1978a) has developed and field-tested a staff management system in several residential institutions in the United States. Staff are organized so that they can carry out routine resident management, for example, dressing, bathing, and feeding, and, in addition, recreational activities and self-help skill training. They contract with their supervisors to conduct resident training programs on a daily basis. Then they are monitored and reinforced with feedback by supervisors and administrators for meeting their resident training criteria each week. A field test of this program was carried out at Partlow State School, and staff met 100% of their resident training contracts (Watson, 1978a). A majority of staff required only recognition from supervisors and administrators to train consistently. However, others required feedback from their unit director about failure to meet their resident training responsibilities. Their basic problem appeared to be scheduling resident training at times when other duties did not interfere. Once the unit director assisted these staff members in resolving scheduling problems, they also trained on a consistent basis.

Client Problems

There are various problems related to client behavior which result in failure to acquire self-help skills. Generalization of independent living skills can be a problem (Stokes & Baer, 1977). Once a client has been taught a particular skill, he does not always exhibit this skill in the presence of staff, other than the original trainer, or in physical locations other than the original training area (Watson, 1978b). To deal with this problem, clients should receive generalization training after they are taught each independent living skill. Therefore, a generalization procedure that appeared to resolve the problem was developed (Watson, 1978a). After a client completed a particular self-help skill program, he then was trained to produce that skill in the presence of other staff who worked with him on his home unit. This was accomplished by having the original trainer ask the client to carry out the task in the presence of another staff member. Once the client completed the task for the original trainer, he was asked to do the task again by the other (novel) staff member, who was standing beside the original trainer. The client routinely complied. Generalization training was then repeated in the same manner with other staff until the client demonstrated the task in the presence of all relevant staff.

To obtain generalization of self-help skills to new or novel locations, such as other buildings, a similar procedure was used (Watson, 1978a). The original trainer escorted the client to the new location. As before, a novel staff member also was present with the original trainer. The original trainer asked the client to carry out the task in question, and when he completed it the novel trainer asked him to complete the task with the original trainer standing beside him. The client typically responded correctly. This procedure has been used successfully to carry out generalization training with a large number of moderately, severely, and profoundly retarded clients at Partlow State School (Watson, 1978a).

A second problem related to generalization training is maintenance of self-help skills after they are taught. Many clients do not use a certain self-help skill after they learn it. This is particularly true in residential facilities. Two procedures were used to ensure clients would maintain their skills after they were taught them (Watson, 1978a). First, staff carried out a maintenance procedure daily in which clients were required to use these skills at the appropriate times and places. They filled out a maintenance checklist each day, and were spotchecked by their supervisors. Second, clients were reinforced with natural reinforcement for using these skills (Ferster, 1967). However, as clients were taught numerous self-help skills it became increasingly difficult to maintain them because of the amount of time involved.

Several factors related to client failure in training programs were determined by tracking 124 severely and profoundly retarded residents for a two year period (Watson, 1978b). The definition used for a training problem was that the client failed to pass a step in a training program for a two-week period (Watson, 1978b). These problems and their incidences are summarized in Table III. As Table III indicates, uncooperativeness was the greatest factor that interfered with training, followed by attention problems, then fading prompts, and, finally, program difficulty. Uncooperativeness consisted of the client's simply refusing to respond, resisting physical prompts, having temper tantrums, engaging in self-destructive behavior, leaving the training area, and throwing training materials. There were two attention problems. The resident either would not look at the trainer when his name was called, or he would not look at the task at hand. Sometimes inattention was owing to the fact that residents spent their time engaged in self-stimulatory activity. Training problems related to prompts were almost exclusively due to problems concerned with the resident's dependency on physical prompts, although there was an occasional problem with dependency on verbal prompts. Program difficulty was always related to a resident's failure to pass a particular step in a program, that is, he could not perform the step to criterion.

TABLE III
Summary of Training Problems Encountered with Severely and Profoundly Retarded Residents

Problem	Incidence (%)
Uncooperativeness	35.2
Attention	21.9
Fading prompts	19.1
Program difficulty	13.9
Blindness, deafness, motor coordination	7.6
Extended illness	2.2
Aggressive toward trainer	0.2

Moderately retarded clients at Partlow State School and Hospital have presented far fewer training problems than the severely and profoundly retarded clients. However, there is one type of problem that occurs consistently. Some residents refuse to train, or fail to attend training sessions.

We have attempted to develop strategies to deal with these client-training problems over the past two years (Watson, 1978b). The greatest problem, uncooperativeness, has been dealt with by using a second trainer. Two trainers can maintain almost complete physical control over a client, and prevent self-destructive behavior, temper tantrums, etc. In addition, they can physically prompt the client more effectively. As he becomes cooperative, both trainers verbally and physically reinforce the client, and give him some type of primary reinforcement. When the client's negativistic behavior is eliminated, the second trainer is faded. This same two-trainer approach also is used to deal with attention problems and self-stimulation (Watson, Owen, & Uzzel, 1980).

Problems related to refusal to train among the moderately retarded have been dealt with by increasing the number of items available for purchase in a token store. Originally, exchange items were limited to snacks and various forms of tobacco. Now clients can purchase a variety of wearing apparel, cosmetics, jewelry, radios, or rent a bicycle and go on special outings (Watson, Owen, & Uzzel, 1980).

Problems related to fading physical and verbal prompts have been dealt with by developing special fading techniques, based on those used by Azrin and his associates (Watson, 1978b). Program difficulty problems have been attacked by using three procedures. If a client fails to make progress on a program, staff check to see whether he may lack certain prerequisite skills. For example, a client may not succeed in a deodorant application program because he does not know how to unscrew the deodorant top. If this is the case, the client is placed in a screwing program (involving a simple wooden nut and bolt), and when this is completed, he is returned to the deodorant program. Second, if a step in a program appears to be too large for a client, the trainer breaks it down into several smaller steps. The third approach to dealing with program difficulty involves sequencing the programs to be taught to a client from simplest to most difficult. Certain self-help skill programs appear to be easier to learn than others. For example, it seems to be easier to teach a client to take off clothing than to put it on. Further, learning to take off clothing items may provide a client with a behavioral repertory that facilitates teaching him to put on these same clothing items (Azrin, Schaeffer, & Wesolowski, 1976; Watson, 1972). One of the topics we cover in an advanced phase of our forward sequencing staff-training program is sequencing programs to be taught to clients in a manner that maximizes their chance to be successful (Watson, 1978b).

A final point related to client problems in training is what appears to be a plateau effect that occurs rather early with severely and profoundly retarded clients in self-help skill training programs. When a group, ward, or unit of severely and profoundly retarded residents are placed in a self-help skill training program, they start out as a group learning programs at a fairly reasonable rate. In five to eight months their group rate of program completion increases, and there is a period of six to eight months during which they make maximum progress. Then, 12 to 15 months after the program began, their performance slowly begins to drop off, and they complete fewer and fewer programs per month. This trend is illustrated in Figure 1, which summarizes the mean number of programmatic steps passed each month for a unit of severely and profoundly retarded ambulatory clients. Stage I refers to the initial stage in training, where residents are learning programs at a lower rate than in Stage II. In Stage II clients acquire programs at the maximum rate. During Stage III, clients pass increasingly fewer programmatic steps each month.

A possible explanation for this trend is that that residents assigned to a unit who make the greatest progress quickly learn all the self-help skills assigned to that unit within 12 to 18 months. There were clients (who are reflected in Figure 1) who learned 25 to 30 self-help skills during this interval. These clients were then transferred to the next unit in the progression system, and the ones who remained behind learned at a slower pace, as a group, than

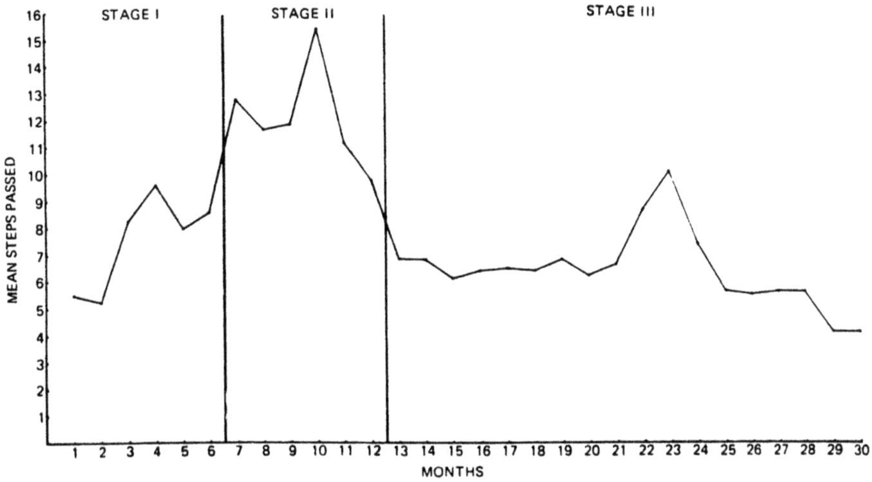

Figure 1. Summary of mean steps passed in self-help skill training programs each month by a group of 124 severely and profoundly retarded ambulatory adults.

the ones who "graduated" to the higher level unit. This factor accounted for part of the reduction in monthly progress, but the clients who remained behind also were increasingly placed in programs that were apparently extremely difficult for them, and they failed to make progress. As time went by, more and more of these clients encountered programs that presented training problems, or a greater number were placed in programs that were extremely difficult for them, and their progress was reduced. It may be that there are *learning plateaus* that occur fairly early with a large proportion of the severely and profoundly retarded who are receiving self-help-skill programming. The clients we tracked appeared to reach this plateau after they had received training on an average of 17.7 programs (range = 1 to 49). A partial solution to this problem is to increase the staff's training skills. In addition, more powerful reinforcement techniques need to be developed for the severely and profoundly retarded to make them more cooperative during training.

Conclusions

The three procedures used to teach self-help skills to the mentally retarded are backward chaining, graduated guidance, and forward sequencing. Backward chaining works well with the severely and profoundly retarded, and there are a large number of training program that can be adapted to this procedure. This technique is relatively easy to teach to paraprofessional staff. Its main disadvantage is that clients who become dependent on physical prompts do not seem to do well with this procedure. Graduated guidance is an extremely effective training procedure, and is ideally suited for the severely and profoundly retarded and/or clients who become dependent on physical prompts. Severely and profoundly retarded clients appear to learn skills faster with this approach than with backward chaining, and the success rate is greater. Its disadvantages are that some paraprofessional staff may find it to be difficult to learn. Also there are only a limited number of programs that have been adapted to this technique. The forward sequencing approach seems to work well with severely, moderately, and mildly retarded clients with receptive language skills who do not require extensive physical prompting. There is a large number of programs that can be taught using this technique. It appears to be ideally suited for training the moderately and mildly retarded.

Problems that interefere with clients' succeeding in training programs are both staff related and client related. Staff who do not receive relevant inservice training do not seem to train as well as those who receive inservice training. Staff who carry out self-help skill training under an effective management system train more than those who do not. The main client-related problems that interfere with clients making progress in training are uncooperativeness, inattention, dependence on prompts, and the application of programs with steps too difficult for the client to pass. Two possible solutions to client uncooperativeness are more powerful reinforcement procedures and two-trainer techniques. Solutions to the problem with prompts may be the use of more sophisticated fading procedures, such as those used in graduated guidance.

In conclusion, the technology of teaching practical living skills still needs further development in three areas: reinforcement techniques, fading of prompts, and simplification of program steps. In addition, more field test data are needed.

The next decade should prove to be an eventful one as the technology of teaching independent living skills to the mentally retarded continues to develop. With the advent of the deinstitutionalization movement, Public Law 94-142, and the general trend toward the education of all mentally retarded persons, there should be more support for the development of these kinds of psychoeducational techniques.

References

Ayllon, T., Garber, S., & Pisor, K. Reducing time limits: A means to increase behavior of retardates. *Journal of Applied Behavior Analysis*, 1976, *9*, 247–252.

Azrin, N. H., & Armstrong, P. M. "The Mini-meal": A method for teaching eating skills to the profoundly retarded. *Mental Retardation*, 1973, *11*, 9–11.

Azrin, N. H., & Foxx, R. M. A rapid method of toilet training the institutionalized retarded. *Journal of Applied Behavior Analysis*, 1971, *4*, 89–99.

Azrin, N. H., Schaeffer, R. M., & Wesolowski, M. D. A rapid method of teaching profoundly and retarded persons to dress. *Mental Retardation*, 1976, *14*, 29–33.

Baker, B. L., Brightman, A. J., Heifetz, L. J., & Murphy, D. N. *Steps to independence: A skills training series for children with special needs*. Champaign, Ill.: Research Press, 1976.

Becker, W. C., & Engelmann, S. *Achievement gains of disadvantaged children with IQ's under 80 in follow through*. Technical Report, 74-2 (Eugene: University of Oregon Follow Through Project, October, 1974).

Bender, M., & Valletutti, P. J. *Teaching the moderately and severely handicapped: Curriculum objectives, strategies and activities*. Baltimore: University Park Press, 1976.

Bensberg, G. J. (Ed.) *Teaching the mentally retarded: A handbook for ward personnel*. Atlanta: Southern Regional Educational Board, 1965.

Bensberg, G. J., Colwell, C. N., & Cassell, R. H. Teaching the profoundly retarded self-help activities by behavior shaping techniques. *American Journal of Mental Deficiency*, 1965, *69*, 674–679.

Bieberly, C. *How to do more: A manual of basic teaching strategy*. Parsons, Kansas: Project MORE, 1974.

Bijou, S. W. A functional analysis of retarded development. In Ellis, N. R. (Ed.), *International review of research in mental retardation*. New York: Academic Press, 1966.

Bijou, S. W., & Orlando, R. Rapid development of multiple-schedules performance with retarded children. *Journal of Experimental Analysis of Behavior*, 1961, *4*, 7–16.

Birnbrauer, J. S., Wolf, M. M., Kidder, J. D., & Tague, C. E. Classroom behavior of retarded pupils with token reinforcement. *Journal of Experimental Child Psychology*, 1965, *2*, 219–235.

Dayan, M. Toilet training retarded children in a state residential institution. *Mental Retardation*, 1964, *2*, 116–117.

DeVore, S. M. *Individualized learning program for the profoundly retarded*. Springfield, Ill.: Charles C Thomas, 1977.

Elliott, C. B., Osteen, K. D., Fagione, B. K., Guthrie, S. C., & Skidmore, L. J. *Happiness is. . . helping parents to help themselves: A guide for training parents to teach*. Gainesville, Fl.: Health and Rehabilitation Service, 1978.

Ellis, N. R. Toilet training the severely defective patient, an S–R reinforcement analysis. *American Journal of Mental Deficiency*, 1963, *68*, 98–103.

Ellis, N. R. Personal communication, 1974.

Ferster, C. B. Positive reinforcement and behavioral deficits of autistic children. *Child Development*, 1961, *32*, 437–456.

Ferster, C. B. Arbitrary and natural reinforcement. *Psychological Record*, 1967, *17*, 341–347.

Foxx, R. M., & Azrin, N. H. *Toilet training the retarded: A rapid program for day and night-time independent toileting*. Champaign, Ill.: Research Press, 1973.

Gardner, J. M., Brust, D. J., & Watson, L. S. A scale to measure skill in applying behavior modification techniques to the mentally retarded. *American Journal of Mental Deficiency*, 1970, *74*, 633–636.

GIRARDEAU, F. L., & SPRADLIN, J. E. Token rewards in a cottage program. *Mental Retardation*, 1964, *2*, 345–351.

GORTON, C. E., & HOLLIS, J. H. Redesigning a cottage unit for better programming and research for the severely retarded. *Mental Retardation*, 1965, *3*, 16–21.

HARMATZ, M. G. Observational study of ward staff behavior. *Exceptional Children*, 1973, *39*, 554–558.

HEIFETZ, L. J. Behavioral training for parents of retarded children: Alternative formats based on instructional manuals. *American Journal of Mental Deficiency*, 1977, *82*, 194–204.

HOLLIS, J. H. Personal communication, 1979.

KAZDIN, A. E. Implementing token programs: The use of staff and patients for maximizing change. In R. L. Patterson (Ed.), *Maintaining effective token economies.*, Springfield, Ill.: Charles C Thomas, 1976.

KELLER, F. S., & SCHOENFELD, W. N. *Principles of psychology*. New York: Appleton-Century-Crofts, 1950.

LENT, J. R. Teaching daily living skills. In J. M. Kaufman & J. S. Payne (Eds.), *Mental retardation: Introduction and personal perspectives*. Columbus, Ohio: Charles Merrill, 1975.

LENT, J. R., LEBLANC, J., & SPRADLIN, J. E. Designing a rehabilitation culture for moderately retarded adolescent girls. In R. Ulrich, T. Stachnik, J. Maybry (Eds.), *Control of human behavior: from cure to prevention.*, Glenview, Ill.: Scott, Foresman, 1970.

LEWIS, P. J., FERNETI, C. L., & KEILITZ, I. *Use of deodorant*. Parsons, Kansas: Project MORE, 1975.

MINGE, M. R., & BALL, T. S. Teaching of self-help skills to profoundly retarded patients. *American Journal of Mental Deficiency*, 1967, *71*, 864–868.

PATTERSON, G. E., & OBERBECK, D. B. *Behavior shaping: A handbook*. Austin, Texas: Austin State School, 1968.

SKINNER, B. F. *Science and human behavior*. New York: Macmillan, 1953.

SKINNER, B. F. Teaching machines. *Science*, 1958, *128*, 969–977.

STOKES, R. F., & BAER, D. M. An implicit technology of generalization. *Journal of Applied Behavior Analysis*, 1977, *10*, 349–367.

WATSON, L. S. Application of operant conditioning techniques to institutionalized severely and profoundly retarded children. *Mental Retardation Abstracts*, 1967, *4*, 1–18.

WATSON, L. S. Behavior modification of residents and personnel in institutions for the mentally retarded. In A. Baumeister & E. Butterfield (Eds.), *Residential facilities for the mentally retarded*. Chicago: Aldine, 1970.

WATSON, L. S. *How to use behavior modification with mentally retarded and autistic children: Programs for administrators, teachers, parents and nurses*. Columbus, Ohio: Behavior Modification Technology, 1972.

WATSON, L. S. *Child behavior modification: A manual for teachers, nurses and parents*. New York: Pergamon, 1973.

WATSON, L. S. *A manual for teaching behavior modification skills to staff: An inservice training program for parents, teachers, nurses and relevant direct care staff*. Libertyville, Ill.: Behavior Modification Technology, 1974. (a)

WATSON, L. S. *Training proficiency scale: An assessment instrument for evaluating behavior modification training proficiency of staff*. Libertyville, Ill.: Behavior Modification Technology, 1974. (b)

WATSON, L. S. Shaping and maintaining behavior modification skills in staff using contingent reinforcement techniques. In R. Patterson (Ed.), *Maintaining effective token economies.*, Springfield, Ill.: Charles C Thomas, 1976.

Watson, L. S. (Executive Producer) *Shaping independent living skills using graduated guidance.* Parsons, Kansas: Words and Pictures, 1977 (film).

Watson, L. S. *A management system approach to teaching independent living skills and managing disruptive behavior.* Tuscaloosa, Ala.: Behavior Modification Technology, 1978. (a)

Watson, L. S. *How to teach independent living skills and manage disruptive behavior.* Tuscaloosa, Ala.: Behavior Modification Technology, 1978. (b)

Watson, L. S., & Bassinger, J. F. Parent training technology: A potential service delivery system. *Mental Retardation,* 1974, *12,* 3–10.

Watson, L. S., Owen, J. R., & Uzzell, R. *A positive approach to managing disruptive behavior.* Tuscaloosa, Ala.: Behavior Modification Technology, 1980.

6 Reducing Aggressive Behavior of Mentally Retarded Persons

ALAN C. REPP AND ANDREW R. BRULLE

INTRODUCTION

Aggressive behavior by mentally retarded persons is a cause for concern for all helping professionals. One reason is that aggressive behavior may endanger the safety of the client himself, other mentally retarded clients, and/or the staff who deal directly with the clientele. Obviously, behavior such as attacking other clients or throwing furniture can cause serious safety hazards. A second reason is that this behavior can and does demand considerable staff attention, and thus subtracts from the total time that the staff can devote to more habilitative procedures (e.g., job training, self-care, etc.). It is precisely for these reasons that many techniques have been developed to help reduce aggressive responding in mentally retarded clients.

The purpose of this chapter is to address these techniques, and to do so in two ways. The first is to provide a brief review of several behavioral procedures shown to have been effective with mentally retarded persons; the second is to suggest some of the ways in which future research can be directed to show us how to implement or arrange these procedures more effectively. Neither of these is intended to be exhaustive; rather, they are intended to be illustrative, and to provide a point from which the serious practitioner can begin.

Because behavioral procedures are often combined in applied work, no review can offer studies only on single procedures. As such, before beginning the review, we shall list and define the procedures to be discussed, so that the reader unfamiliar with all the terms will have a reference as he or she progresses through the chapter. The procedures are classified into three groups,

ALAN C. REPP AND ANDREW R. BRULLE • Department of Learning and Development, Northern Illinois University, DeKalb, Illinois 60115.

which are described here as positive, neutral, or aversive techniques. The positive procedures involve the delivery of reinforcement; the neutral procedures involved the systematic absence of reinforcement or attention; and the negative procedures involve the use of aversive stimuli. The positive procedures discussed, and their definitions, are the following: (1) *differential reinforcement of other behavior* (DRO)—reinforcement is delivered if the client does not emit the target response for a specified interval; (2) *differential reinforcement of low rates of responding* (DRL)—reinforcement is delivered if the rate of responding is less than or equal to some criterion; (3) *differential reinforcement of incompatible responding* (DRI)—reinforcement is delivered if a response occurs that is topographically incompatible with the target response; (4) *differential reinforcement of alternative behavior* (DRA)—reinforcement is delivered if a particular alternative but not topographically incompatible response occurs. The neutral procedures discussed are often quite similar: (1) *extinction*—in which a previously reinforced response is no longer reinforced; (2) *ignoring*—in which a response being maintained for unidentified reasons is not consequated with attention. Finally, the aversive procedures are as follows: (1) *aversive conditioning*—in which an aversive stimulus is contingent upon responding; (2) *overcorrection*—in which the client excessively restores a disrupted environment to its prior state (called restitution) and/or practices over and over again acceptable forms of the disruptive behavior just exemplified (called positive practice); (3) *time-out*—in which access to reinforcement is removed contingent upon responding; and (4) *response cost*—in which previously accumulated reinforcement is removed.

POSITIVE PROCEDURES

These procedures are positive in two different ways. In one, they are positive in that some reinforcer is added to the environment. The term "added to" denotes a positive intervention. The positive techniques to be discussed generally include the introduction of some reinforcer whenever the target aggressive behaviors are absent or reduced. This definition of "positive" is extremely important, as will be seen later, when positive and negative punishment (both aversive techniques) are discussed. Two, these techniques are positive in the more generally accepted sense of the word—that is, the procedures are in no way aversive to the client. Furthermore, positive techniques, the client will not be subjected to any procedures that when using positive techniques, the client will not be subjected to any procedures that will substantially deprive him or her of any accepted reinforcers.

The use of positive techniques to reduce aggressive behavior is highly recommended on a legal, human, and logical basis. Martin (1975) has cautioned against the use of aversive techniques unless positive procedures have been tried first. Possible legal complications may arise if aversive techniques are used other than as a last resort. Secondly, it is logical to suggest that professionals concerned with helping mentally retarded individuals should naturally refer to positive techniques whenever possible. Ours is a profession filled with idealists, not sadists, and although aversive techniques can and should be used in a helping vein (Repp & Deitz, 1978), positive techniques should be the *prima facie* method. Finally, positive techniques are generally better accepted by the clientele because these techniques do not substantially interfere with the client's naturally occurring reinforcers (with the exception of extinction). Although there is no specific guarantee of a substantial behavior change, chances of such a change are realistic, and can be influenced by the utilization of less restrictive techniques that do not normally result in initial resistance by clients.

Differential Reinforcement of Other Behavior (DRO)

Representative Studies

The differential reinforcement of other behavior is a procedure in which reinforcement is delivered if the client does not emit the target response for a specified interval. Any *other* behavior within that interval will be reinforced. If the client does emit a response of the target behavior, however, he or she will not receive reinforcement for that interval.

Let us examine, for example, a hypothetical situation in which a client exhibits a high rate of attacking behavior (15 times/hour during baseline), and the researcher decides to use a DRO interval of three min. In this procedure, the client would receive reinforcement after every three-min interval in which he did not attack another client, *no matter what other behavior he exhibited during that interval.* After reinforcement, the interval is begun anew. If, however, the client does make an attacking response, no reinforcement is delivered, and the interval time is started again. Gradually the researcher will attempt to lengthen the interval until the client no longer needs reinforcement in order to refrain from attacking other clients.

Repp and Deitz (1974) used DRO in combination with a number of other techniques to reduce effectively a number of aggressive behaviors of mentally retarded clients. In experiment one, DRO (initial interval of five sec, rapidly increased to 15 min) combined with a 30-sec restraining time-out was exceptionally effective in eliminating the tantrums, self-mutilation, and attacking behaviors of a 12-year-old severely mentally retarded male client. Experiment two combined DRO (initial interval of 5 min, gradually increased to 15 min) and a minor verbal reprimand in an attempt to eliminate the aggressive and attacking behaviors of an 8-year-old severely mentally retarded male. Again, the procedure was effective. Experiment three combined a 15-min DRO, mild verbal reprimand, and a response-cost procedure to eliminate abusive language, physical abuse, and aggressive misuse of materials on the part of a 13-year-old moderately mentally retarded male; and experiment four utilized DRO (1-sec initial interval increased to 120 min) and a mild verbal reprimand to eliminate the self-aggressive responses of a severely mentally retarded 10-year-old female.

Bostow and Bailey (1969) used a combination of DRO procedures and time-out to reduce the number of loud verbalizations emitted by a 58-year-old severely mentally retarded female. The time-out procedure consisted of two min out of her wheelchair; the DRO interval began at 5 min, but increased rapidly to 30 min. This procedure was quite effective, as demonstrated by an ABAB design. Bostow and Bailey (1969) also combined time-out (2 min in a booth) and DRO (2-min intervals) to reduce severe aggressive behaviors of a 7-year-old severely mentally retarded boy. The authors commented that relatively short time-out procedures when used in conjunction with reinforcement procedures can be very effective in alleviating chronic aggressive responses.

Vukelitch and Hake (1971) also used DRO in combination with time-out in an attempt to reduce the choking responses of a severely mentally retarded resident. The researchers found that time-out, by itself, was not effective in reducing choking. However, when time-out was used in conjunction with noncontingent and continuous attention (DRO), the procedures then proved to be effective. At a later time, attention was made contingent upon differential reinforcement of incompatible responses (DRI). The researchers also noted that grabbing responses increased when choking responses decreased, but these too were reduced when time-out and DRO were combined.

Deitz, Repp, and Deitz (1976) explored the effectiveness of three different differential reinforcement procedures (DRO, DRL, DRI). In the DRO experiments, they were able effectively to use the procedure to reduce disruptive talking-out behaviors of four mildly mentally retarded students. The same researchers (Repp, Deitz, & Deitz, 1976) used DRO exclusively to reduce effectively the handbiting behavior of a severely mentally retarded male. The initial DRO interval was begun at 1 sec, but was extended to 5 min. This exceptionally short initial interval demonstrates how DRO can be used for high-rate responding (42.8 responses per min during baseline).

Repp (in press) has suggested that the initial DRO interval size be selected so that the client's chances of receiving reinforcement for not exhibiting the target behavior will be greater than that for exhibiting that target behavior during the initial interval. Recall, for example, the hypothetical situation discussed at the beginning of this section. In that case, the client was making an attacking response 15 times per hour, or once every 4 min. The researcher decided to use an initial DRO interval of 3 min, so that the client's chances of receiving reinforcement for *not* exhibiting that attacking behavior during the initial interval were greater than his chances of receiving reinforcement for exhibiting it.

As has been demonstrated above, differential reinforcement of other behaviors can be very effective, when used either exclusively or in conjunction with other procedures, in reducing aggressive responding by mentally retarded clients. However, some cautions here are appropriate. DRO can be a time-consuming procedure, as has been evidenced with some interval sizes being as short as one sec. In such cases as this, one would need a staff member whose sole responsibility was the administration of the DRO program. This technique can also be relatively weak in that the only consequences for an exhibition of the target behavior is a delay in the reinforcement. This problem may or may not manifest itself, depending of course on the individual preferences of each client. Finally, DRO may also result in what has been termed "behavioral contrast" (Reynolds, 1968). In this case, the decrease of some aggressive behavior in one situation (e.g., math class) may precipitate an increase in the same behavior in a different situation (e.g., social-studies class). In cases such as this, we should make plans to generalize the effectiveness of our DRO program across settings.

Some Areas for Future Research

The success of a DRO program depends on at least two factors: (1) the potency of the reinforcer relative to the potency of whatever is maintaining the behavior itself and (2) procedural elements inherent in the DRO schedule. The first factor seems relatively idiosyncratic to the individual and the situation in which he is responding, and the second seems more fruitful for other individuals with the same problem behaviors. Within the second factor, the need for research in three areas is immediately evident; these are (a) the definition of the DRO schedule, (b) the size of the DRO interval, and (c) the rule for increasing the DRO schedule so that larger and more manageable interval sizes are used.

Although we have defined DRO here in the same manner that Reynolds (1968) has (i.e., the scheduled delivery of reinforcement when responding has not occurred during a prescribed interval), others have offered an alternative definition. Sulzer-Azaroff and Mayer (1976) and Harris and Wolchik (1979) have conceptualized DRO as delivering reinforcement if responding is not occurring at the *end* of a prescribed interval. Harris and Wolchik (1979) compared this procedure with overcorrection and found it ineffective. However, when successful, it requires a practitioner to look for the target response only at the end, rather than during, an entire interval. Research with more subjects is needed to indicate: (a) whether this altered DRO procedure as described could ever be effective; and (b) whether there are arrangements that could be added to produce or enhance its effectiveness.

A second area of concern is the size of the initial DRO interval. Studies where DRO proved effective have typically begun with short intervals between reinforcement, generally based on the rate of responding during baseline, whereas studies which have shown DRO to be ineffective have generally begun with larger intervals between reinforcement. One study has shown that the initial interval size can have an enduring effect on the success of a DRO program. In this laboratory experiment with mentally retarded persons, Repp and Slack (1977) followed a DRL baseline period with a four-ply multiple schedule (DRO_A-DRO_B-DRO_C-DRL). The DRO schedule values varied in an ascending series through which the subjects progressed as they met criterion at each prior value. For DRO_A, those values were 1, 2, 6, 12, 20, 30, 42, 56, and 72 sec; for DRO_B, they were 12, 20, 30, 42, 56, and 72 sec; and DRO_C, they were 20, 30, 42, 56, and 72 sec. Eventually, all the DRO components shared the same DRO values (i.e., 20, 30, 42, 56, 72 sec). Results were as follows: (a) there were fewer total responses in the DRO_A series than in the DRO_B or DRO_C series, and, for two of three subjects, there were fewer responses in DRO_B than in DRO_C; (b) the order of efficiency in establishing schedule control was DRO_A-DRO_B-DRO_C; and (c) a prior history of DRO schedules with small values resulted in reduced responding under larger DRO schedules (for example, there was less responding on the 30-sec value in

DRO_A than in DRO_Bthan in DRO_C, despite the fact that responding had met criterion for the 20-sec value for all three components). This study suggests that the initial DRO size can have both immediate and lasting effects, and one reason why some studies may have failed to demonstrated the effectiveness of DRO schedules was suggested. Further research, however, is needed to determine whether this effect would exist outside the controlled laboratory environment.

A third area of concern is the formula by which DRO schedule values should be increased. Currently, there have been no applied studies addressing this issue. Alternatives would include: (a) some prestated arithmetic progression—for example, 10–20–40–80–160 secs, etc.; or 10–20–30–40–50 secs, etc., or 10–20–30–50–80–130 secs, etc.; or (b) some progression based on the current level of responding. We have used the latter to generate initial DRO values, but have not used it to determine successive values of the DRO schedule. Research is needed to determine the manner in which schedule control could be maintained while the DRO value is being increased.

Differential Reinforcement of Low Rates of Responding (DRL)

Representative Studies

The differential reinforcement of low rates of responding (DRL) is a procedure in which rates of responding less than or equal to a criterion are reinforced. For example, one may determine that it is not excessive for a child to "talk out" approximately 5% of the time during a classroom session. If this or a lesser rate were achieved, then reinforcement would occur. Repp (in press) has listed three different types of DRL schedules. One, *interresponse time* or *spaced responding*, is a procedure in which a response is reinforced if and only if it followed a similar response by a specified time period. As can readily be seen, in an applied study, this type of DRL schedule follows an inappropriate response with reinforcement. As such, it seems to be appropriate only in the experimental laboratory, where it has long been used to control low and steady rates of responding against which the effects of independent variables have been measured.

In *full-session DRL* scheduling, reinforcement is delivered only if the rate for a *full* session has been below a predetermined rate. For example, one may determine that out-of-seat behavior 3% of the time for a particular mildly mentally retarded boy is not excessive. If, during a class period, the boy exhibits 3% or less of this out-of-seat behavior, he will receive reinforcement at the end of the period. However, if the rate is greater than 3%, than no reinforcement will be delivered. Finally, in the *interval* method of scheduling DRL, the session is broken into a number of intervals, and reinforcement is delivered at the end of each of these intervals if the response rate has been below the predetermined level. In this procedure, good behavior that follows a brief early period of excessive responding may still be reinforced. As can be inferred, DRL scheduling often reinforces inappropriate behaviors. However, in most cases, the behavior is a problem only because of its excessive rate of occurrence. The therapeutic aspect of DRL is the fact that only *low rates* of these behaviors are reinforced. It is precisely for this reason that DRL has *not* been extensively used in dealing with dangerously aggressive behavior in mentally retarded clients. A procedure, such as DRO, which totally eliminates the aggressive responding is much more appropriate.

The initial rates for DRL scheduling can be determined in much the same way that the initial interval for DRO is determined. An added feature of DRL scheduling, though, is that as the client steadily progresses through the various steps until he reaches the predetermined final goal, the record of his progress provides the researcher with a changing criterion design, thus eliminating the need for reversals or extended baselines.

Deitz and Repp (1973) worked with a classroom of moderately mentally retarded children and, by using a DRL schedule, were able to reduce the talking-out behaviors of these children. The same researchers (Deitz, Repp, & Deitz, 1976) also used a DRL schedule to reduce disuptive responses by a 12-year-old mildly mentally retarded male. The behaviors (not dangerous) were: (1) talking when not called on by the teacher; (2) talking about a subject other than classwork; (3) leaving his seat; and (4) yelling at the other students in the class (p. 157). The student could go to the library for 10 min if he exhibited two or fewer responses during the class period. As was effectively demonstrated, the DRL schedule did lower the student's responses to an appropriate rate. In the same study, the researchers reported the effects of DRL on a classroom of 14 mildly mentally retarded students. Again, no extremely dangerous behaviors were exhibited, but the disruptive behaviors included: (1) talking aloud; (2) being out of one's assigned seat; (3) making loud noises; (4) hitting or shoving other students; and, (5) throwing objects (p. 159). Tokens were earned when the disruptive rate was less than 1.3 responses per minute, and again DRL proved effective.

Other variations of DRL include the "Good Behavior Game" (e.g., Barrish, Saunders, & Wolf, 1969; Harris & Sherman, 1973; Maloney & Hopkins, 1973; Medland & Stachnik, 1972) which essentially is a procedure in which two or more groups of students either (1) compete against each other to determine who could be the least inappropriate or (2) compete against a preset DRL limit to determine whether all "teams" could be below that limit. The variations within this paradigm are considerable, and allow a teacher creatively to plan ways for students to have fun while learning to "be good" (e.g., appropriate classroom behavior).

As mentioned earlier, on several occasions DRL is appriopriate only when the behavior selected for remediation is not dangerous. One could conceivably use DRL in attempting to reduce less severe forms of aggressive responding, and verbal aggression would be an example of such behavior.

Some Areas for Future Research

As with DRO schedules, the success of DRL schedules can be conceptualized as a function of the potency of the reinforcer being dispensed, and properties of the schedule itself. Unfortunately, applied studies of the properties of DRL schedules do not exist. Fruitful topics for research, however, are apparent, such as what value to establish as the initial DRL value, what method to use to determine values of ensuing DRL schedules, and the relative effectiveness of the three DRL methods discussed. The first two areas are quite similar to areas of investigation in DRO studies. In our research, we have determined the initial DRL value by summing the number of responses over the last (stable) sessions of baseline, and dividing that number into the cumulative length of these sessions. This quotient provides us with the mean interresponse time for those sessions. However, more rapid schedule control might occur if the value selected approximated the shortest interresponse time over the last several sessions. Using that value, one could ensure that a subject would earn a greater number of reinforcers for reduced responding than he could earn for excessive responding. If the cumulative value of the reinforcer for excessive responding did not exceed the value of the reinforcer for decreased responding, then behavior should decrease. An examination of these two procedures could show us whether the effort required by the practitioner to determine minimal interresponse times would be beneficial to schedule control.

The question of how to determine ensuing DRL values is essentially the same question asked when using DRO schedules. Basically, it is whether some preestablished mathematical formula shoul be followed, or whether the value of each phase should be based on responding during the last few sessions of the prior phase. Although the latter seems intuitively to be the better choice, and although it has been suggested for laboratory studies (Sidman, 1960), it has been curiously neglected in a *systematic*, applied sense. If studies showed the latter to be the better choice, one would still have the problem of determining the value within any phase. Should it be the mean of the last several sessions? Or 10% less than that mean? Or 20%? Or should it be equivalent to the lowest value of the last several sessions of the prior phrase?) The questions, of course, can become large, but through systematic replications, generality should emerge at least over the question of whether to base the decision on an average or on a low point in the last phase.

A third area for study would be which of these three reinforcement methods has been shown to be effective (and ineffective); the question remains whether the simple structure of the DRL schedule itself can lead to a more efficient reduction of responding. That question should be relatively easy to answer.

Differential Reinforcement of Incompatible Responding (DRI)

Representative Studies

The differential reinforcement of incompatible behavior (DRI) varies from the other two differential reinforcement procedures in that only behaviors which are *topographically incompatible* with the target behavior are reinforced. For example, if one wished to decrease the fighting responses of an educable mentally retarded (EMR) boy, one could reinforce this boy whenever he was *not* fighting. "Not fighting" is, of course, topographically incompatible with "fighting," and the reinforcement of this incompatible behavior could lead to a decrease in the aggression.

Reinforcement in DRI can be scheduled in different ways depending on which incompatible behavior is being reinforced. In the prior example, one would not be able to deliver reinforcement continually; therefore, some schedule must be determined based on data obtained during baseline. If, for example, the aggressive responding were occurring every 4 min, then a DRI schedule which presented reinforcement every 3 min initially would probably be more appropriate than one which presented reinforcement every 10 min.

In a study discussed earlier (Vulelich & Hake, 1971), DRI was used to help reduce choking and grabbing by a severely mentally retarded client. Initially, DRO was used, but as the client became more adept at controlling her behavior, DRI was instituted. This technique of using different reinforcement strategies suggests a logical flow of reinforcement. In some cases, reinforcement must occur almost continually in order to eliminate aggression. In the initial stages of a behavioral-change program, one could begin with a DRO schedule in order to quickly reduce this responding. As time progressed, however, one could gradually fade into a DRI schedule, in which more appropriate responses would be learned and other aggressive responses reduced.

In two studies with nonhandicapped children (Thomas, Becker, & Armstrong, 1968; Becker, Madsen, Arnold, & Thomas, 1967), a DRI schedule was used to help reduce disruptive classroom behaviors. By simply concentrating teacher attention on the students who were exhibiting appropriate behaviors, and by ignoring disruptive behaviors, a significant decrease in disruptive behaviors was effected. Deitz, Repp, and Deitz (1976) also used a DRI procedure to reduce talking-out and verbal-threatening behavior of a 14-year-old mildly mentally retarded male. Although this client's responses were not very frequent (approximately four per hour), they were severe and often disrupted the class for as long as 10 min. In this study, reinforcement was delivered on a variable-interval schedule of three min. In the postbaseline phase, the teacher reinforced the student for appropriate classroom behavior and ignored inappropriate behaviors. In the third phase of the study, reinforcement was withdrawn, but the teacher continued to ignore the disruptive behavior, and it quickly increased to baseline level. When DRI was reinstated in the fourth phase, an appreciable drop in the inappropriate behavior was evidenced.

Pinkston, Reese, LeBlanc, and Baer (1973) worked with a nonhandicapped preschool child who exhibited attacking behaviors. The first effective treatment had the teacher attending to the attacked child while ignoring the aggressive behavior of the subject. The second treatment included a DRI component where the child was reinforced for appropriate social interaction. This phase also proved to be effective.

Perline and Levinski (1968) used a combination of DRI, response cost, and time-out to reduce a number of aggressive behaviors by four severely mentally retarded preschoolers in a residential setting. The categories of behaviors were aggression toward peers, rising from chair, aggression toward teacher, throwing objects, and taking possessions. Clients were intermittently given tokens contingent upon behaviors incompatible with the behaviors selected for treatment. However, each time an inappropriate response occurred, one token was confiscated and the child was physically restrained for 5 to 15 min. Although the greatest decrease in behavior occurred in the category of aggression toward peers, a decrease in all the inappropriate behaviors was evidenced.

As with the other differential reinforcement procedures, DRI must be used cautiously. When attempting to eliminate a dangerous, aggressive behavior, one must be *certain* that the initial DRI schedule is designed to guarantee reinforcement for an incompatible behavior, or it is conceivable that DRI will fail because the client would receive no initial reinforcement. It is also conceivable that DRI will fail because either the reinforcement or the procedure is not strong enough to alter long-standing patterns of behavior. However, DRI is a positive and effective procedure and should be a part of the behavioral-change repertoire of all professionals who deal with the mentally retarded.

Some Areas for Future Research

Research on the differential reinforcement of incompatible responding shares some of the research questions germane to the DRO and DRL schedules. However, the question of the reinforcement schedule itself persists in a different fashion. In the DRO and DRL schedules, reinforcement is given for the absence or reduction of inappropriate responding. With DRI, an appropriate response is reinforced with the intent being to increase the rate of a specified behavior. The question then is whether a particular response, with its relationship to the inappropriate behavior, will be subject to the same schedule effects as other responses. Will the same effects be achieved by ratio and interval schedules? Could the topographically incompatible responses be considered to be two responses which could be treated as if in a conjunctive schedule? If so, it may be more efficient to deliver reinforcement only if the appropriate response occurred according to some schedule *and* the inappropriate response did not. Traditionally, practitioners seem either to schedule these consequences quite independently or to schedule no particular consequence for the inappropriate response. Perhaps considering these behaviors in a conjunctive sense would make the results more powerful.

Differential Reinforcement of Alternative Behaviors (DRA)

Representative Studies

The differential reinforcement of alternative behaviors (DRA) is a procedure similar to DRI. The major difference is that the behavior reinforced in DRA is not topographically incompatible with aggression. It is assumed, however, that while the client is engaged in the alternative behavior, he will not be engaged in aggression. The definition then of DRA is that reinforcement is delivered if a particular alternative but not topographically incompatible response occurs. For illustrative purposes, let us consider fighting. With DRI, we would reinforce the client for not fighting; however, with DRA, we would provide reinforcement for some alternative (e.g., seat work). It is obvious that while the client is concentrating on seat work she will not be fighting, and hence fighting will decrease. A very positive feature of DRA is the fact that only appropriate responses are reinforced and, therefore, that the client is able to learn a new response to substitute for the aggressive response.

Ayllon, Layman, and Burke (1972) used a DRA procedure to reduce disruptive behavior by four mildly mentally retarded students. Before the study began, the four were categorized as "the most unmotivated, undisciplined and troublesome children in the school" (p. 316). Rather than selecting DRI in which the students would be reinforced for not disrupting, the researchers chose to use a DRA procedure in which only appropriate academic responding would be reinforced. In the first few phases of the study, an extremely structured academic environment was provided, and disruptive responding decreased from 98% to 17%. Although the structured environment substantially reduced the disruptive behaviors, when DRA was also introduced (reinforcement via tokens for correct academic responses), the results were extraordinary. In addition to maintaining the disruptive responses at a low level, academic functioning increased tremendously, with improvements noted in reading of up to *three years*! This study underscores the twofold advantage of DRA: A decrease in inappropriate responding with a concomitant increase in appropriate responding.

As in all the other differential reinforcement procedures, one must be certain that, while programming DRA, the client is more likely to receive reinforcement for the alternative behavior than for a manifestation of the aggressive response. Although DRA can be exceptionally effective in two different aspects, it is also conceivable that (because the alternative behavior is not topographically incompatible with the target aggressive behavior) a client may continue to engage in the aggressive response while concurrently engaging in the alternative response, and thus receive reinforcement for inappropriate responding. For example, a client could be completing her macrame project while still verbally abusing the staff and other clients. If this becomes the case, one may simply increase the amount of work required by the alternative behavior or institute a DRO or DRL program until aggressive responding is either eliminated or reduced to an appropriate level.

Some Areas for Future Research

There have been only a few systematic DRA studies, although the procedure is inherent in any reduction program in which one is simultaneously trying to teach adaptive and reduce maladaptive responding. Nevertheless, the studies of Ayllon and his colleagues demonstrate the efficacy of such an approach. The major question with DRA is the same as that with DRI: can we presume that the alternative response will be subject to the same principles as most other adaptive responses, or does the maladaptive response exert more influence than one would otherwise find? One could reasonably presume that it would, because more than likely the events maintaining the aggressive behavior would not be the same as the consequences used to increase the adaptive alternative behavior. If this presumption is correct for some cases, then for those the issue could be more complex than it first seems.

NEUTRAL PROCEDURES: EXTINCTION AND IGNORING

The term "extinction" denotes a procedure in which a previously reinforced response is no longer reinforced, and the term "ignoring" simply means that attention will not be delivered when a certain response occurs. Unfortunately, many people presume that these two procedures are always the same, and they operate in that fashion. As a result, many procedures that have been categorized as extinction may instead have been examples of ignoring, since it was assumed that the *removal of attention* (which establishes that attention was a reinforcer in the first place) will result in a decrease in behavior. This difference in terminology may seem trite, but it is actually quite important from a therapeutic standpoint. If we were to ignore aggressive behavior on the assumption that our attention had been reinforcing that behavior, whereas in actuality it had not, then our "treatment" would be totally ineffectual. While believing that we were instituting a behavioral-change program, actually by this approach we would be denying our client treatment. Only when attention had been maintaining behavior would extinction and ignoring be the same. This source of confusion may be the reason that so many practitioners believe that extinction does not work.

In the previously discussed study with a nonhandicapped preschool child, Pinkston, Reese, LeBlanc, and Baer (1973) used an extinction process to eliminate the attacking of others. Prior to the onset of treatment, the teachers had verbally responded to the child's attacking behaviors. The reinforcing properties of this responding were clearly demonstrated when the teachers ceased responding to the attacking child and instead turned their attention to the attacked children. When baseline conditions were reinstituted, the child's aggressive behavior showed an abrupt increase.

Becker, Madsen, Arnold, and Thomas (1967) used an extinction and DRI program to reduce disruptive classroom behaviors. When teacher attention was directed toward appropriate behaviors and removed from the disruptive behaviors, a marked decrease in disruption resulted. Forehand (1973) also used an extinction program with a six-year-old mildly mentally retarded male. The boy manifested a behavior categorized as spitting where each response had been attended to by the teacher. However, when the teacher learned to ignore the behavior (an extinction process), spitting disappeared.

Martin and Foxx (1973) worked with a 22-year-old institutionalized female in three behavioral categories: (1) physical aggression toward victims, (2) self-aggression, and (3) physical aggression toward objects. As would be expected, each of these episodes had resulted in significant staff attention. However, when an extinction program was instituted, and these aggressive episodes were ignored, they decreased.

Although extinction in this last study was effective, one must be exceedingly cautious when attempting to use either extinction or ignoring with aggression, because both procedures frequently require considerable time, in comparison to other methods, before they are effective. If a rapid decrease in behavior is necessary (as would be the case when dealing with a dangerous aggressive behavior), then some other procedure must be instituted. Repp (in press), along with many others, has noted a number of other characteristics of extinction which must be considered before instituting a program. One, extinction may trigger an initial increase in the number of responses. It is only natural to expect that a client who has become accustomed to receiving reinforcement for various behaviors will "try harder" (increase behavior) to regain that lost reinforcement, hence an initial increase in the number of responses. This same client may also become frustrated when the accustomed reinforcement is no longer delivered, and this frustration may lead to an outburst of aggression. This aggression is a frequent phenomenon which must be considered before extinction programs are instituted. Third, the response, many months after successful extinction, may spontaneously recover at a high rate. This "last ditch effort" at regaining the lost reinforcement may not occur if alternative means of earning reinforcement are provided, but it too warrants consideration. Finally, we must be very careful not to reinforce inappropriate responses accidentally. For example, if attention were a reinforcer for a child and we ignored the first 29 episodes of an inappropriate response but "gave in" to the 30th, then we might be producing a variable-ratio 30 reinforcement schedule, and behavior would probably increase rather than decrease.

The effectiveness of extinction and ignoring has been clearly demonstrated, but their use, particularly with aggressive behavior, demands careful thought and planning. Some behaviors cannot be safely ignored, and this safety factor will necessarily preclude the use of either extinction or ignoring as the sole behavioral-change procedure. The dangers of such a program have been clearly demonstrated by Lovaas and Simmons (1969), who used extinction with the self-destructive behaviors of two boys. One required ten, 90-min sessions to stop hitting himself in the room in which the sessions were held; during this period, he hit himself more than 9,000 times. A second boy was under extinction for 17 sessions, the last of which found him exhibiting more than 500 self-destructive behaviors. The inappropriateness of this procedure when used alone was well summarized by these authors:

> We have replicated the extinction operations on other institutionalized children. . . . In each instance, the self-destructive behavior showed a very gradual drop over time, being particularly vicious in the early stages of extinction. . . . In summary, we can conclude that although extinction seemingly works, it is not an ideal form of treatment because the large amount of behavior during the early stages of extinction subjects the child to much apparent discomfort. (pp. 146–147)

When used in conjuction with other reinforcement procedures (DRL, DRO, etc.), or in conjunction with some punishment techniques, however, extinction or ignoring can be an effective and integral part of any reductive process.

Aversive Procedures

The aversive techniques to be described in this section include both positive and negative punishment. Positive punishment is defined as a procedure in which responding results in the *addition* of something aversive to the client's environment, with a concomitant reduction in responding. Conversely, in negative punishment, responding results in the *subtraction* of a reinforcer, with a concomitant reduction in responding. This definition of positive and negative is the only meaning that will be used in this section, and in no way denotes whether one procedure is better than another.

Before implementing any behavioral-change technique (much less any punishment technique), one must consider whether or not there are sufficient objective data to demonstrate the need for intervention. In this era of Civil Rights, any intervention that is based solely on the whim of a well-meaning, but naive, practitioner would (and should!) be open to question. Legally (P.L. 94-142; Federal Regulations 45CFR249.13, 1977), and ethically, one must always be certain that objective data are available that *clearly* demonstrate the need for an intervention.

Second, one must question whether or not the behavior to be changed is a legitimate interest of the state. Personnel in state institutions and in public schools have recently been defined as agents of the state (Martin, 1979), and, as such, any intervention in which they participate must be designed to change behavior that is in the interest of the state. This is a rather gray area, open to judicial interpretation; however, one may logically surmise that only severe behaviors should be subject to aversive techniques.

A third consideration in the use of aversive techniques is whether or not nonaversive techniques have been tried first. As illustrated in the prior sections of this chapter, many effective nonaversive techniques exist for intervention in the aggressive behaviors of mentally retarded clients. A documented record demonstrating that nonaversive techniques have been professionally and correctly implemented, but to no avail, is necessary before any aversive technique should be considered.

If these three prerequisites have been met, however, and the client is still exhibiting aggressive responding, then one has no choice (considering the welfare of the client, the other clients, and the staff) but to institute a punitive behavioral-intervention technique. Careful planning must precede any application of this technique, however, and must include such aspects and answer such questions as:

1. Will the application of this technique be injurious to either the client, the staff or the other clients?
2. Is the treatment a proven accepted one, or is it experimental in nature?
3. Has notice been served and has consent been given by both the client (where appropriate) and/or his parents?
4. Have the proper committees (e.g., Human Rights Committees) given their approval?

When these questions have been satisfactorily answered, one will have met some of the legal and ethical prerequisites of instituting punishment procedures.

During the administration of this technique, many other components must also be satisfied. Adequate records of all administrations of the punitive procedure must be kept, and staff who administer this procedure should be thoroughly trained and well-versed in the procedure itself. Additionally, the punitive procedure should be witnessed as often as possible, and end goals must have been established. Finally, one must also determine how long the procedure will continue if it is ineffective and, in this case, have alternative procedures developed for immediate implementation.

Gardner (1969) has stated that "Punishment, as frequently used in institutions for the mentally retarded, is likely to produce negative reactions to authority figures" (p. 100). This statement is logical, since most people do not like to be punished, hence the term *aversive techniques*. However, with careful planning and thoughtful implementation, punishment can play a useful role in the alleviation of aggressive behaviors in mentally retarded clients.

Aversive Conditioning

Representative Studies

Aversive conditioning is a procedure which reduces inappropriate responding by introducing an aversive stimulus contingent upon an inappropriate response. Aversive conditioning is an example of positive punishment, in that an aversive stimulus is *added to* the subject's environment.

When one hears the term "aversive conditioning," one may conjure up images of mad, sadistic doctors shocking innocent victims. Although electric shock can prove to be an effective aversive stimulus, all aversive conditioning need not be this severe, and it may take the form of a simple verbal reprimand (e.g., "No!"). The term "aversive conditioning" should not evoke avoidance responses on the part of professionals. Rather, skilled behaviorists will recognize that aversive conditioning has and will continue to be important in the alleviation of aggressive response in mentally retarded clients.

Wallace, Burger, Neal, VanBrero, and Davis (1976) surveyed 207 institutions concerning their use of aversive conditioning. Of the 115 that responded, only 45% indicated that they used aversive conditioning; 100% of those using aversive conditioning and 74% of those not using it felt that aversive conditioning is legitimate and acceptable when used to alleviate certain behaviors; 88% indicated that they felt that aversive conditioning would be a treatment of last resort, and 87% recommended a multidisiplinary decision before any aversive-conditioning techniques were used. This study illustrated that the behaviorists who staff the institutions understand the legitimate uses of aversive conditioning, and that the aforementioned guidelines may formally or informally be followed.

Tanner (1973) discussed four major issues concerning the use of aversive shock. He found that, physically, it was no more dangerous than many other accepted modes of treatment, and that, emotionally, there was no evidence to support that it adversely affected the subject's emotional adjustment. The effectiveness of aversive shock was unsurpassed in modifying homosexual behavior, and there was considerable evidence of its effectiveness in eliminating aggressive and self-aggressive behaviors. Finally, he stated that the argument of "dehumanization" was purely semantic, and that no real evidence had been put forth in this area.

Aversive shock has been used effectively to control violent behaviors of a schizophrenic female (Ludwig, Marx, Hill, & Browning, 1969) and of a mentally retarded female adult (Brandema & Stein, 1973). In the latter study, a 24-year-old client exhibited physically assaultive behavior. The punishment for this assaultive behavior was an electric shock, and although the shock drastically reduced the behavior, it did not totally eliminate it. This result was similar to one advanced by Birnbrauer (1968), who found that the effects of shock were highly discriminated, and did not transfer to other behaviors. Risley (1968) worked with a 6-year-old child who had been labeled at various times mentally retarded, autistic, and brain damaged. The two major target behaviors were physical assaults on her younger brother and climbing and rocking in high places. Risley attempted many procedures, including time-out, extinction, and DRI, all of which proved to be unsuccessful. The introduction of electric shock, though, proved to be a successful alternative. This procedure was effective in the clinic, but did not transfer to the home; hence, the mother had to administer the shock in the home in order to alleviate the behaviors in that situation.

In a milder application of aversive conditioning, Paluck and Esser (1971) studied the territorial behaviors of severely mentally retarded boys. When placed in a large room together, 21 boys (ages 5 through 10, IQ $\leq$ 50) quickly demonstrated the phenomenon known as "territorial behavior" by claiming certain areas of the room as their own, and by protecting their areas by physically aggressive acts. The territorial behavior was not affected any more by punishment than by ignoring, but verbal punishment succeeded in reducing the physical aggression of these boys. Doleys, Wells, Hobbs, Roberts, and Cartelli (1976) compared the effects of a mild form of aversive conditioning with time-out and positive practice. Four children (8-year-old male, mildly mentally retarded; 10-year-old female, mildly mentally retarded; 10-year-old male, mildly mentally retarded and autistic; and 10-year-old male, moderately mentally retarded) were evaluated on their compliance to commands. The three techniques included (1) time-out (40 sec in the corner), (2) positive practice (see the next section of this chapter), and (3) social punishment (scolding and glaring). They demonstrated that the procedure of social punishment (a mild form of aversive conditioning) was more effective than either time-out or positive practice.

Another alternative that has recently become a popular aversive stimulus for stereotypic and aggressive behaviors is an aversive taste solution (usually concentrated lemon juice). Sajwaj, Libet, and Agras (1974) used it to decrease life-threatening ruminating behavior, and Mayhew and Harris (1979) used it to decrease both tantrumlike screaming and self-injurious behavior. In each case, the concentrated lemon juice was effective.

As has been demonstrated by the aforementioned studies, aversive conditioning can be an effective technique, and one need not shy away from it if all the prerequisites have been met. Indeed, when severe aggressive or self-aggressive responses are present, one owes it to the clients to attempt any procedure which might alleviate the problem.

Some Areas for Future Research

The area of aversive conditioning probably has less need of systematic applied research into the factors controlling effectiveness than any other area. The reason is that, far more than in any other area, there was an excellent base from laboratory research that guided the workers in the applied area. That base, of course, was the work by Azrin, Hake, Holz, Hutchinson, and others (cf. Azrin & Holz, 1966), and it was an extraordinary contribution to our field. Since that time, there have been some applied studies that were concerned with generalization, whether the punishing agent would be avoided, and so forth. But today, with the realistic and appropriate restraint on the use of aversive procedures, a primary need is the development of aversive stimuli that are functionally aversive but do not evoke such strong emotional reactions from observers. Two such attempts have been made and replicated. One is the procedure labeled "overcorrection"; it, however, has come under considerable criticism recently and may become, at least in some cases, as objectionable as electric shock. Another is the use of aversive taste solutions, such as concentrated lemon juice, which most of us have tasted and find objectionable, but generally do not consider cruel for treating aggressive behaviors. The demonstrated effectiveness of such alternatives, found in the natural environments of us all, seems to be a prime research goal in this area.

Overcorrection

Representative Studies

Overcorrection is a positive punishment procedure in which the individual is required to: (1) excessively restore the disrupted environment to its condition prior to the disruption (reinstitutional overcorrection) and/or (2) practice over and over again the acceptable forms of the disruptive behavior just exhibited (positive-practice overcorrection). For example, a student who has turned a wastepaper can over in class may be required to put everything back, to straighten the entire room, and to wash the blackboards (restitutional overcorrection). Or a client who has just verbally abused another client may be required to apologize to the offended client, and compliment him on some other aspect (restitutional overcorrection), *and* approach every other client in that setting and compliment them (positive-practice overcorrection). It may not always be possible to institute both forms of overcorrection for every behavior, and in such cases one form will suffice. Overcorrection is a relatively new positive-punishment technique, yet its popularity has rapidly increased in the 1970s as many found it useful when other procedures had failed. It has been used to decrease toileting accidents (Azrin & Foxx, 1971), to reduce stereotypic responding of severely mentally retarded persons (Azrin, Kaplan, & Foxx, 1973), and to eliminate vomiting responses (Duker & Seys, 1977).

Foxx and Azrin (1972) used overcorrection in conjunction with aversive conditioning to eliminate successfully a variety of aggressive behaviors by mentally retarded clients. The first experiment involved a 50-year-old profoundly mentally retarded female who successfully disrupted the institutional environment by throwing and overturning furniture. The client was verbally chastised, and required to correct the damage she had wrought and to practice her correction procedure over and over. For example, if the client had overturned one table, she was required to straighten that table, and to straighten all the other tables in the room. The researchers used physical guidance to facilitate learning the corrective tasks. The second experiment involved a 22-year-old profoundly mentally retarded female who attacked and bit other residents and employees. The researchers had previously used a 15-minute time-out procedure in an attempt to eliminate this behavior, but to no avail. In the overcorrection procedure, after her biting another person, the client's mouth was first cleansed with an oral antiseptic. She was then required to assist the staff in the medical treatment of the attacked person. This twofold overcorrection technique resulted in a drastic lowering of the attacking behaviors. The client in the third experiment was a 56-year-old brain-damaged female who exhibited screaming and throwing behaviors. The overcorrection procedure consisted of 15 min of "Quiet Training" (required to lie in bed and stay quiet), "Social Reassurance Training" (required to apologize to the staff and patients), and "Household Orderliness Training" (required to straighten magazines, chairs, etc.). Again, the results demonstrated the effectiveness of the procedure.

Webster and Azrin (1973) used required relaxation as an overcorrection procedure to reduce the disruptive behavior of mentally retarded clients. Eight severely mentally retarded adults were required to spend two hours relaxing in bed for each disruptive behavior. The agitated resident was required to remove his clothes and don a hospital gown, and told "You are disturbed and upset and need to relax. You need to lie down for awhile. I will tell you when you've relaxed enough and may get up" (p. 72). If there were any disruptions during the last 15 min of a relaxation period, the period was extended for another 15 min, or until the resident had had at least 15 min of relaxation. There were no special considerations made for the residents in bed—they were simply ignored. None of their beds was moved to a special area, nor was traffic in and out of the area restricted. This procedure of required relaxation proved to be very effective in eliminating the disruptive behaviors, and a survey of the staff showed that this procedure was preferred three to one over time-out or other procedures.

Finally, Azrin and Wesoloski (1974) used an overcorrection procedure to eliminate the stealing responses of 34 mentally retarded clients. In the restitutional phase of the procedure, the thief was required to return the stolen item to the victim. In the positive practice phase, the thief had also to present the victim with an item identical to the stolen one. This procedure eliminated thefts by the fourth day.

Foxx and Azrin (1972) have recommended that overcorrection and restitution be (1) directly related to the misbehavior, (2) required immediately after the behavior, (3) extended in duration, (4) performed actively by the offender without pausing, and (5) free from positive reinforcement. Some aspects of overcorrection may take the form of aversive conditioning (in which the client intensely dislikes the overcorrective procedure and, therefore, refrains from manifesting the target response) or negative punishment (in which some positive reinforcer, such as free time, is removed from the client's environment by the overcorrection procedure). Although the exact classification of the procedure may be difficult, overcorrection has become a popular positive punishment procedure and can be arranged to provide both therapeutic and learning components.

Some Areas for Future Research

Overcorrection is a relatively new procedure, and, as such, may produce criticism not found in the publications of its originators. For example, Rollings, Baumeister, and Baumeister (1977) questioned the validity of Foxx and Azrin's (1973) conclusions about the effectiveness of overcorrection, finding that

> (a) overcorrection may produce decelerations, but that the magnitude of the effect varies considerably between subjects; (b) punishment and non-punishment conditions are well discriminated by the subject, partly on the basis of trainer proximity; (c) increased collateral stereotypic and emotional responding may accompany deceleration of target behaviors; (d) no spontaneous generalization of suppression is observed from training to living areas; and (e) suppression effects obtained under the procedures used here are not durable. In general, we conclude that the overcorrection procedure is actually a very complex package of contingencies and that the effects on behavior may also be complex. (p. 43)

These criticisms suggest a number of research questions that are quite obvious. More important, however, they demonstrate that the seemingly free and abundant use of this procedure today may be premature. From the comments of Rollings *et al.*, and from the unpublished comments of practitioners having used overcorrection for aggressive clients, the choice of this procedure should be made cautiously and should be under the auspices of appropriate committees (e.g., Human Rights Committees, Behavior Modification Committees).

Time-Out

Representative Studies

Time-out is a negative punishment procedure in which an inappropriate response results in the client's access to reinforcement being removed for a specified period of time. It is assumed that the removal of this accessibility to reinforcement will result in a decrease in the inappropriate response. It is in this sense that time-out is a negative-punishment procedure—accessibility to reinforcement is removed from the environment (negative), and this removal results in a subsequent reduction in behavior (punishment). Obviously, if the procedure does not result in a decrease in behavior, then the procedure cannot be deemed punishment. There have been a few studies in which this has been the case. For example, Vukelich and Hake (1971) found that time-out was not effective in reducing the choking responses of a severely mentally retarded client. When a DRO procedure was added to the time-out procedure, a decrease in the responses was noted. Plummer, Baer, and LeBlanc (1977) also found that time-out was ineffective even when a reinforcer was operating in the environment. When a total-reinforcement procedure was substituted, however, positive results were seen. The researchers suggested that time-out from instructions was actually reinforcing in this case. Solnick, Rincover, and Peterson (1977) noted similar results in a six-year-old autistic girl where time-out procedures instituted from tantrums actually resulted in an increase in the number of tantrums, because the time-out provided time for the girl to engage in self-stimulatory behavior. In the same study, though, with a 16-year-old mentally retarded male who exhibited spitting and self-injurious behavior, a 90-sec time-out procedure was found to be very effective. The authors concluded that "there can be no standard time-out procedure that will reliably reduce problem behaviors" (p. 423). The authors also noted that "Often we find that dreary institutional dayrooms or highly demanding learning tasks constitute the 'time-in' setting while escape from these situations is time-out" (p. 423). In response to this problem, the authors suggested that, in order for time-out to be effective, the "time-in" situation must be enriched. In spite of the difficulties experienced with time-out and the fact that time-out is not always an effective technique, many other studies have demonstrated the significant effects that a time-out program can have in reducing aggressive behaviors.

Repp (in press) has discussed five different types of time-out procedures: (1) ignoring, (2) isolation, (3) removal of materials, (4) withdrawal, and (5) contingent observation. *Ignoring* is a procedure in which attention to responding is removed for a period of time, the assumption being that attention had previously been reinforcing. In *isolation time-out*, the client is physically removed from the environment for a set period. This procedure is by far the most common, and reports of its use abound in the literature. As an example, Hamilton, Stephens, and Allen (1967) used confinement in a time-out area to reduce unaccaptable behaviors in severely mentally retarded female adults. Using either a 30-min or a two-hour confinement period, they found time-out to be a very effective (yet severe) procedure. In *removal-of-materials time-out*, reinforcing materials which had been available to the client are removed. Barton, Guess, Garcia, and Baer (1970) used this procedure to help train mentally retarded persons in appropriate eating habits. When these behaviors were displayed by an individual client, this client's food tray was removed. In *wtthdrawal-of-the environment time-out*, the client is left in place, yet everyone around him moves to a different environment. The premise for this procedure is that the removal of the client to an isolation area may result in physical attention which, in turn, may result in further complications. An interesting application of this procedure was developed by Foxx and Shapiro (1978), who applied it to the disruptive behaviors of five severely mentally retarded children in an institution's classroom. While in class, these children wore a ribbon which signified that they were eligible for positive reinforcement (attention, edibles, etc.) every few minutes. During the baseline phase of the study, disruptive behaviors occurred in 32% of the intervals. When the time-out phase was introduced, this ribbon was removed for three minutes whenever a misbehavior occurred, and teacher attention and participation in activities ceased for the child who was not wearing the ribbon. This procedure was effective, as evidenced by the 6% misbehavior rate during treatment. A similar procedure is *contingent-observation time-out* in which the client is present, but does not participate in any of the activities. The major difference is that all the other clients and staff remain in place, while the offending client is removed to the periphery of the activities. This procedure assumes that the client, by observing the activities of the other clients and staff, will want to return to the activities being offered, and will thus cease his misbehaviors.

Time-out procedures have also been used in conjunction with other reinforcement procedures to reduce successfully a variety of aggressive responses. Bostow and Bailey (1969) combined time-out with DRO to reduce the number of loud verbalizations emitted by a 58-year-old severely mentally retarded female and to reduce the attacking behaviors of a seven-year-old severely mentally retarded male. In the first case, the time-out consisted of the client's being removed from her wheelchair for a 2-min period (a type of contingent observation time-out) and in the second case, time-out was defined as two min in a time-out booth (isolation time-out). In both cases, time-out was combined with DRO procedures, and this combination proved to be very effective. Repp and Deitz (1974) also used DRO in conjunction with a time-out procedure to eliminate severe tantrums, self-mutilating, and attacking behaviors of a severely mentally retarded 12-year-old male. In this case, the time-out was a 30-sec restraint. Perline and Levinsky (1968) used a combination of time-out, response cost, and DRI to reduce aggressive behaviors in four severely mentally retarded preschoolers. The children were given tokens intermittently contingent upon behaviors that were incompatible with the misbehaviors. However, for each misbehavior that occurred, the child lost one token and was physically restrained for 5–15 min. This particular combination of procedures was effective, as evidenced by an abrupt decrease in all misbehaviors.

One of the most important considerations in the utilization of time-out procedures is the determination of the length of the time-out period. Time-out has been shown to be effective when it has been as long as two hours (Hamilton, Stephen, & Allen, 1967), or as short as 90 sec (Solnick, Rincover, & Peterson, 1977). In assessing this problem, Burchard and Barrera (1972) utilized a combination of response cost (token loss) and time-out to reduce antisocial behavior in mildly mentally retarded adolescents. They found that higher values (30 tokens or 30 minutes) were much more effective than were lower values (5 tokens or 5 minutes). Contrarily, White, Nielsen, and Johnson (1972) found that although 15- and 30-min time-out periods were more effective than a 1-min time-out period, there was no difference between a 15-min period and a 30-min period. They also noted that the one-min time-out period was most effective when it was presented first, which suggests that, if time-out has not been previously used, then relatively short time-out periods may be as effective as longer ones. Finally, Clark, Rowbury, Baer, and Baer (1973) worked with an 8-year-old Down's Syndrome female in a preschool setting. The three target behaviors were (1) chokes and armwraps, (2) attacking people, and (3) attacking materials. In a multiple-baseline study, the researchers were able effectively to decrease all the behaviors by use of a 3-min time-out period in a booth. More interestingly, in the second part of the study, the researchers compared different schedules of intermittent time-outs. By using schedules in which time-out occurred on the average after every 1, 3, 4, or 8 responses, or in which high rates were temporarily punished (i.e., where the time-out was contingent on the occurrence of a disruptive behavior within 10 min of the last behavior), the authors were able to demonstrate a nonlinear relationship between the different schedules of time-out. Occurring after every one to three responses, time-out was equally effective. Time-out occurring after about every three responses, however, was more effective than when it occurred after about every four responses, which in turn was more effective than when it occurred after about every eight responses. The temporal time-out schedule was as effective as the most effective of the other schedules. This interesting relationship suggests that some schedules of intermittent time-out may be nearly as effective as a continuous schedule.

Although time-out procedures can be effective, and should be an integral part of any behaviorist's treatment inventory, one must be certain that the institution of a time-out procedure does not deny the client's constitutional right to treatment by separating him for long periods from the regular school program. Similarly, as with any other punishment procedure, documentation demonstrating which positive techniques have first been attempted and proving that all due process procedures have been precisely followed are necessary before any time-out procedure can be instituted.

Some Areas for Future Research

Time-out has long been in use, both systematically and unsystematically, for aggressive and nonaggressive behaviors. But its persistent use with aggressive behaviors is questionable, because of a trap that often develops: (a) student is aggressive, (b) staff attends verbally and/or physically to calm student, (c) student is placed in time-out area, and (d) student often aggresses in time-out and requires staff intervention. Time-out is certainly one of the most ubiquitous procedures today, but perhaps its high use betokens not its effectiveness, but rather its ineffectiveness, and hence its repeated use in situations in which staff know of no alternative.

The crux of the ineffective use of time-out is that it is often treated only as a procedure in which someone is removed from his environment. Too often its users ignore the requisite that this environment must be a rich, stimulating, reinforcing environment. The work of Solnick, Rincover, and Peterson (1977) points out what may be the most fruitful area of research that would enhance the punishing properties of time-out—how to make the present environment maximally reinforcing for the individual. Then the functional aspects of the time-out procedure would be met. With this objective, many research questions become obvious. One is how do we determine naturally and efficiently that the individual's environment is reinforcing? Presently, we usually presume that it is reinforcing; occasionally, we demonstrate that at specific times some reinforcers are effective for increasing some behaviors. An intriguing fact is that one of the best ways to evaluate the reinforcing properties of the environment is to consequate a particular response with time-out—if that behavior is decreased, then the environment is reinforcing. However, if that behavior is the aggressive one, then we do not have the critical information needed before we even begin the time-out program. If, on the other hand, we choose an innocuous behavior by which to test the environment, we are probably countervailing current legal and ethical standards by using a punishment procedure with a response too innocuous to be punished. Without information on the reinforcing nature of the environment from which the student is removed, our use of time-out is presumptuous. It may be analogous to (1) presuming that all students like chocolate, (2) using chocolate to reinforce some behavior, and (3) never bothering to find out that this student does not like chocolate.

The second research area then becomes that of discovering those factors that make the environment reinforcing. The questions are numerous: (1) Are there particular rates or densities of reinforcement that would make the environment more reinforcing? (2) Are environments of tangible reinforcers (e.g., tokens) more reinforcing than environments of nontangible reinforcers (e.g., praise)? (3) Are environmental effects related to the functioning level of the individual (e.g., profoundly vs. mildly retarded)? (4) Would group rather than individual contingencies make the total environment more reinforcing? Questions such as these, directed toward the variables enriching the present environment, rather than questions directed toward the parameters of the removal procedure itself, may well be the more valuable in the long run. For with answers to questions about what makes an environment more reinforcing in the first place, we are likely to reduce some aggressive responding, not through consequences, but through preventive engineering.

Response Cost

Representative Studies

The final procedure to be discussed has been termed *response cost*, and refers to that procedure which involves the loss of previously earned reinforcement. Response cost, like time-out is a negative form of punishment, because a reinforcer is removed from the environment. The difference is, of course, the fact that time-out involves a set period of *time* during which the client can no longer earn reinforcement, whereas in response cost the client loses some reinforcer already earned prior to the manifestation of the undesired behavior. Response cost is not a new form of behavioral management. Indeed, its effects are well known by anyone who has ever been guilty of a minor traffic violation and has had to pay a fine. The scientific study of its effects on mentally retarded populations, though, is a relatively new endeavor, and one which merits serious consideration.

Sulzbacher and House (1968) used response cost in a group-contingency plan to eliminate obscene gestures in a classroom of mildly mentally retarded children. In this procedure, a free-time period was set aside at the end of each day for the class. However, any gesture or reference to it, or tattling, or comments about it, resulted in a loss of one minute of free time for the entire class. This procedure was extremely effective in reducing the average level of behavior from 16 to 2 per day. Greene and Pratt (1972) used an almost identical procedure to reduce the misbehaviors of institutionalized mentally retarded adolescents. In this procedure, a half-hour reward period was set aside each day for the clients to use as they pleased. Again, any misbehavior resulted in the loss of one minute of this free time. The categories of misbehaviors included (a) rudeness, (b) insulting others, (c) "uncalled for" obscenity, (d) refusal to follow directions, and (e) creating a disturbance. The categories were relatively broad and allowed interpretation on the part of the teacher. Again, this procedure was very effective, and significant declines were shown for all misbehaviors.

Iwata and Bailey (1974) compared the effects of a reward program and a response cost program with 15 elementary mildly mentally retarded students by modifying their off-task and disruptive behaviors. During the first intervention phase, each child in one group received tokens (up to a maximum of 10 per session) for following the rules. Each child in the other group was given 10 tokens at the beginning of the period. They were allowed to keep these tokens; however, any misbehavior resulted in the loss of one token. Students who met a set criterion (six tokens at the beginning of the intervention phase raised to eight tokens toward the end of the phase) were then served a snack at the end of the period. During the second intervention phase, the identical procedures were followed except that the groups were reversed. The researchers found that there was no significant difference between the response cost or the reward system. They also found that there was no difference in student preference. However, they did note that the frequency of teacher-approving comments increased under the reward system, whereas no change was noted when the response cost system was in effect.

In programming response cost, Repp (in press) has suggested that an assessment be made of the client's economy in order to maximize the effect of the response cost program. One would need to determine how much reinforcement the client is currently earning and how often inappropriate responding is occurring. By dividing the former by the latter, one could determine the maximum fine for each response that would still generally leave the client with some reinforcement. The use of a maximum fine has been recommended by Burchard and Barrera (1972), who used a response cost and time-out procedure to reduce antisocial behavior in mildly mentally retarded adolescents. The higher values of the fines (30 tokens or 30-min time-out) were much more effective than were the lower values (5 tokens or 5-min time-out). This concept of a maximum fine while still leaving some reinforcement is a very logical, yet an often overlooked, premise. In order to reduce aggressive behaviors quickly through the use of a response cost program, however, this determination should be made.

Some Areas for Future Research

Because response cost is so directly related to positive punishment, it probably shares many of the common principles of punishment (e.g., increased density is more effective, increased intensity is more effective) and does not have such obvious areas of need in terms of research. One of the most obvious, however, is the extent to which it can control aggressive behaviors. Most of the research has not gone beyond mild and often verbal aggression; its effectiveness with more serious behaviors has not often been demonstrated. Second, its use with persons who function at different levels of mental retardation should be more carefully studied. Because response cost generally relies on token programs, it may not be meaningful for mentally retarded persons at lower functioning levels. Yet, "counting" devices could be studied to determine whether they could provide a functional definition of significant loss. Third, and perhaps most important, response cost can be studied in a manner similar to time-out (e.g., not in terms of the parameters of the cost procedure itself, but rather in terms of what makes the accumulated reinforcer more reinforcing, and hence its loss more punishing).

CONCLUDING REMARKS

The purpose of this chapter has been to discuss in two ways some behavioral procedures that have been shown to have been effective in reducing aggression. The first has been to present definitions and brief reviews of these procedures. The second has been to suggest that in many areas we have been rather limited and that a great deal of research remains to be done.

The behavioral study of aggressive behavior has been to this date primarily a study of how to consequate behavior so that it will be rapidly reduced. Such a development is natural, because the behavioral researcher is often the person who is also responsible for ensuring that change occurs, not from a research perspective, but rather from a treatment perspective. He or she has quite often also been the teacher, supervisor, in-house psychologist, etc., whose primary responsibility has been to expedite treatment.

Since we now have some effective procedures in our arsenal, perhaps we could move into what might be a more fruitful area in the long run—that of preventative engineering. Beyond developing effective consequences, behaviorists have (to us) more importantly developed effective means of studying behavior. We have considerable technical skill at collecting data and at analyzing data on a single-subject basis. With these technologies, we can pursue two directions that may produce more success than has accrued to this point in dealing with aggressive behaviors. The first is a complex and careful analysis of antecedents and of setting events that control aggressive behaviors. Many researchers have shown that we can quite easily observe 20 or 30 events at one time, and that through computer operations we can determine their effect on behavior. When efforts in this direction are systematic, we should be able to isolate many events, with scientific assuredness, that lead to aggressive behaviors. When this has been done, we will have a far more significant contribution than the identification of procedures of consequation.

Second, with these technologies it should be possible to divorce ourselves from our insistent study of behavioral procedures. Much of our applied work is still grounded in the laboratory work of Ferseter and Skinner (1957) and of Skinner's students. Although that has certainly been a monumentally effective approach, and an appropriate one, it really is not one which we need follow so carefully anymore. We could and should be analyzing procedures, theories, etc., of nonoperant people. We do not, and should not, follow or even attend to the intervening-variable complex from which Skinner has led us. Nevertheless, there is little problem in translating the writings of cognitive theorists, hypnotists, acupuncturists, and Zen Buddhists into operational procedures. In this manner, we can break from the "behavioral-procedure" mold, and examine the much larger world; in this way, we may discover much more effective means of dealing with aggressive behaviors.

References

Ayllon, T., Layman, S., & Burke, S. Disruptive behavior and reinforcement of academic performance. *The Psychological Record*, 1972, *22*, 315–323.

Azrin, N. H., & Foxx, R. M. A rapid method of toilet training the institutionalized retarded. *Journal of Applied Behavior Analysis*, 1971, *4*, 89–99.

Azrin, N. H., & Holz, W. C. Punishment. In W. K. Honig (Ed.), *Operant behavior*. New York: Appleton-Century-Crofts, 1966.

Azrin, N. H., & Wesolowski, M. D. Theft reversal: An overcorrection procedure for eliminating stealing by retarded persons. *Journal of Applied Behavior Analysis*, 1974, *7*, 577–582.

Azrin, N. H., Kaplan, S. J., & Foxx, R. M. Autism reversal: Eliminating stereotyped self-stimulation. *American Journal of Mental Deficiency*, 1973, *78*, 241–248.

Barrish, H. H., Saunders, M., & Wolf, M. M. Good behavior game: Effects of individual contingencies for group consequences on disruptive behavior in a classroom. *Journal of Applied Behavior Analysis*, 1969, *2*, 119–124.

BARTON, E.S., GUESS, D., GARCIA, E., & BAER, D. M. Improvement of retardates mealtime behaviors by time-out procedures using multiple-baseline techniques. *Journal of Applied Behavior Analysis*, 1970, *3*, 77–84.

BECKER, W.L., MADSEN, C.H., ARNOLD, C.R., & THOMAS, D.R. The contingent use of teacher attention and praise in reducing classroom behavior problems. *Journal of Special Education*, 1967, *1*, 287-307.

BIRNBRAUER, J. S. Generalization of punishment effects. *Journal of Applied Behavior Analysis*, 1968, *1*, 201-211.

BOSTOW, D. E., & BAILEY, J. B. Modification of severe disruptive and aggressive behavior using brief time-out procedures. *Journal of Applied Behavior Analysis*, 1969, *2*, 31–37.

BRANDEMA, J. M., & STEIN, L. I. The use of punishment as a treatment modality: A case report. *Journal of Nervous and Mental Disease*, 1973, *156*, 30–37.

BURCHARD, J. D., & BARRERA, F. An analysis of time-out and response cost in a programmed environment. *Journal of Applied Behavior Analysis*, 1972, *5*, 271–282.

CLARK, H. B., ROWBURY, T., BAER, A. M., & BAER, D. M. Time-out as a punishing stimulus in continuous and intermittent schedules. *Journal of Applied Behavior Analysis*, 1973, *6*, 443–455.

DEITZ, S. M., & REPP, A. C. Decreasing classroom behavior through the use of DRL schedules of reinforcement. *Journal of Applied Behavior Analysis*, 1973, *6*, 457–463.

DEITZ, S. M., REPP, A. C., & DEITZ, D. E. D. Reducing inappropriate classroom behavior of retarded students through three procedures of differential reinforcement. *Journal of Mental Deficiency Research*, 1976, *20*, 155–170.

DOLEYS, D. M., WELLS, K. C., HOBBS, S. A., ROBERTS, M. W., & CARTELLI, L. M. The effects of social punishment upon non-compliance: A comparison of time-out and positive practice. *Journal of Applied Behavior Analysis*, 1976, *9*, 471–482.

DUKER, P. C., & SEYS, D. M. Elimination of vomiting in a retarded female using restitutional overcorrection. *Behavior Therapy*, 1977, *8*, 255–257.

FERSTER, C., & SKINNER, B. F. *Schedules of reinforcement*. New York: Appleton-Century-Crofts, 1957.

FOREHAND, R. Teacher recording of deviant behavior: A stimulus for behavior change. *Journal of Behavior Therapy and Experimental Psychiatry*, 1973, *4*, 39–40.

FOXX, R. M., & AZRIN, N. H. Restitution: A method of eliminating aggressive-disruptive behavior of retarded and brain damaged patients. *Behaviour Research and Therapy*, 1972, *10*, 15–27.

FOXX, R. M., & AZRIN, N. H. The elimination of self-stimulatory behavior by overcorrection. *Journal of Applied Behavior Analysis*, 1973, *6*, 1–14.

FOXX, R. M., & SHAPIRO, S. T. The time-out ribbon: A non-exclbsionary time-out procedure. *Journal of Applied Behavior Analysis*, 1978, *11*, 125–136.

GARDNER, W. I. Use of punishment procedures with the severely retarded: A review. *American Journal of Mental Deficiency*, 1969, *74*, 86–103.

GREENE, R. J., & PRATT, J. J. A group contingency for individual misbehaviors in the classroom. *Mental Retardation*, 1972, *10*, 33–35.

HAMILTON, J., STEPHENS, L., & ALLEN, P. Controlling aggressive and destructive behavior in severely retarded institutionalized residents. *American Journal of Mental Deficiency*, 1967, *72*, 852–856.

HARRIS, S. L., & WOLCHIK, S. A. Suppression of self-stimulation: Three alternative strategies. *Journal of Applied Behavior Analysis*, 1979, *12*, 185–198.

HARRIS, V. W., & SHERMAN, J. A. Use and analysis of the "Good Behavior Game" to reduce disruptive classroom behavior. *Journal of Applied Behavior Analysis*, 1973, *6*, 405–417.

IWATA, B. A., & BAILEY, J. S. Reward vs. cost token systems: An analysis of the effects upon students and teacher. *Journal of Applied Behavior Analysis*, 1974, *7*, 567–576.

Lovaas, O. I., & Simmons, J. Q. Manipulation of self-destruction in three retarded children. *Journal of Applied Behavior Analysis*, 1969, *2*, 143–157.

Ludwig, A. M., Marx, A. J., Hill, P. A., & Browning, R. M. The control of violent behavior through faradic shock. *Journal of Nervous and Mental Disease*, 1969, *148*, 624–637.

Maloney, K. B., & Hopkins, B. L. The modification of sentence structure and its relationship to subjective judgements of creativity in writing. *Journal of Applied Behavior Analysis*, 1973, *6*, 425–433.

Martin, G. Brief time-outs as consequences for errors during training programs with autistic and retarded children: A questionable procedure. *The Psychological Record*, 1975, *25*, 71–89.

Martin, P. L., & Foxx, R. M. Victim control of the aggression of an institutionalized retardate. *Journal of Behavior Therapy and Experimental Psychiatry*, 1973, *4*, 161–165.

Martin, R. *Legal challenges in regulating behavior change: Workshop materials*. Champaign, Ill.: Research Press, 1979.

Mayhew, G., & Harris, F. Decreasing self-injurious behavior. *Behavior Modification*, 1979, *3*, 322–336.

Medland, M. B., & Stachnik, T. J. Good behavior game: A replication and systematic analysis. *Journal of Applied Behavior Analysis*, 1972, *5*, 45–51.

Paluck, R. J., & Esser, A. H. Controlled experimental modification of aggressive behavior in territories of severely retarded boys. *American Journal of Mental Deficiency*, 1971, *76*, 23–29.

Perline, I. H., & Levinsky, D. Controlling maladaptive classroom behavior in the severely retarded. *American Journal of Mental Deficiency*, 1968, *73*, 74–78.

Pinkston, E. M., Reese, N. M., LeBlanc, J. M., & Baer, D. M. Independent control of a preschool child's aggression and peer interaction by contingent teacher attention. *Journal of Applied Behavior Analysis*, 1973, *6*, 115–124.

Plummer, S., Baer, D. M., & LeBlanc, J. M. Functional considerations in the use of procedural time-out and an effective alternative. *Journal of Applied Behavior Analysis*, 1977, *10*, 689–706.

Repp, A. C. *Mental retardation: A behavioral approach*. New York: Prentice-Hall (in press).

Repp, A. C., & Deitz, S. M. Reducing aggressive and self-injurious behavior of institutionalized retarded children through reinforcement of other behaviors. *Journal of Applied Behavior Analysis*, 1974, *7*, 313–325.

Repp, A. C., & Deitz, D. E. D. Ethical issues in reducing responding of institutionalized mentally retarded persons. *Mental Retardation*, 1978, *16*, 45–46.

Repp, A. C., & Slack, D. J. Reducing responding of retarded persons by DRO schedules following a history of low-rate responding: A comparison of ascending interval size. *The Psychological Record*, 1977, *27*, 581–588.

Repp, A. C., Deitz, S. M., & Deitz, D. E. D. Reducing inappropriate classroom and prescriptive behaviors through DRO schedules of reinforcement. *Mental Retardation*, 1976, *14*, 11–15.

Reynolds, G. S. *A primer of operant conditioning*. Glenview, Ill.: Scott, Foresman, 1968.

Risley, T. R. The effects and side effects of punishing the autistic behaviors of a deviant child. *Journal of Applied Behavior Analysis*, 1968, *1*, 21–34.

Rollings, J. P., Baumeister, A. A., & Baumeister, A. A. The use of overcorrection procedures to eliminate the stereotyped behaviors of retarded individuals. *Behavior Modification*, 1977, *1*, 29–46.

Sajwaj, T., Libet, J., & Agras, S. Lemon-juice therapy: The control of life-threatening ruminating in a six-month-old infant. *Journal of Applied Behavior Analysis*, 1974, *7*, 557–563.

SIDMAN, M. *Tactics of scientific research.* New York: Basic Books, 1960.

SOLNICK, J. V., RINCOVER, A., & PETERSON, C. R. Some determinants of the reinforcing and the punishing effects of time-out. *Journal of Applied Behavior Analysis,* 1977, *10,* 415–424.

Standards for intermediate care facility services in institutions for the mentally retarded or people with retarded conditions. 45CFR 249.13. U. S. Department of Health Education and Welfare.

SULZBACHER, S. I., & HOUSE, J. E. A tactic to eliminate disruptive behaviors in the classroom: Group contingent consequences. *American Journal of Mental Deficiency,* 1968, *73,* 88–90.

SULZER-AZAROFF, B., & MAYER, R. G. *Applying behavior analysis procedures with children and youth.* New York: Holt, Rinehart & Winston, 1976.

TANNER, B. A. Aversive shock issues: Physical danger, emotional harm, effectiveness and "dehumanization." *Journal of Behavior Therapy and Experimental Psychiatry,* 1973, *4,* 113–115.

THOMAS, P. R., BECKER, W. C., & ARMSTRONG, M. Production and elimination of disruptive classroom behavior by systematically varying teacher's behavior. *Journal of Applied Behavior Analysis,* 1968, *1,* 35–45.

Vukelich, R., & Hake, D. F. Reduction of dangerously aggressive behavior in a severely retarded person through a combination of positive reinforcement procedures. *Journal of Applied Behavior Analysis,* 1971, *4,* 215–225.

WALLACE, J., BURGER, D., NEAL, H. C., VANBRERO, M., & DAVIS, D. E. Aversive conditioning use in public facilities for the mentally retarded. *Mental Retardation,* 1976, *14,* 17–19.

WEBSTER, D. R., & AZRIN, N. H. Required relaxation: A method of inhibiting agitative-disruptive behavior of retardates. *Behaviour Research and Therapy,* 1973, *11,* 67–78.

WHITE, G. P., NIELSEN, G., & JOHNSON, S. M. Time-out duration and the suppression of deviant behavior in children. *Journal of Applied Behavior Analysis,* 1972, *5,* 111–120.

7 Training Skills for Community Adjustment

Allen Marchetti and Johnny L. Matson

Introduction

The move toward community placement of the mentally retarded has gained considerable momentum within the past few years. The push has come primarily from those who espouse a philosophical approach to treatment called "normalization." This concept originated in Europe and has been accepted in the United States primarily through the efforts of Wolfensberger (1972). The normalization movement in the United States has been accelerated by numerous legal decisions. For example, before 1971 no court action had been filed on the legal rights of the mentally retarded. Between October, 1971, and July, 1973, at least 41 proceedings were initiated in the federal and state courts (Freedman, 1974). The pace of such court-related attempts to gain rights for the mentally retarded has continued to accelerate since that time. These actions have been significant in that most of them either directly or indirectly support normalization.

The two legal decisions that have probably spurred on the normalization movement most were the 1972 Wyatt-Stikney decision and Public Law 94-142 (Kindred, 1976). In the former case, the institutionalized mentally retarded were guaranteed the right to treatment. Since no such right was guaranteed to those living in the community, and since sufficient funds have typically not been available in most states to provide optimum treatment, all but the most difficult residents were placed in group homes or independent living arrangements. The second major new development was Public Law 94-142, which mandated that all persons, regardless of their handicap, have the right to a publicly supported educational program designed to assist in

Allen Marchetti • Partlow State School and Hospital, Tuscaloosa, Alabama 35401. Johnny L. Matson • Department of Psychiatry, University of Pittsburgh, School of Medicine, Pittsburgh, Pennsylvania 15261.

remediating their deficits and/or providing a normalized living experience (Wolfensberger, 1972). Public Law 94-142 focuses on community action for children during the school day. However, what occurs outside the school day, and the development of any provisions for mentally retarded adults, has yet to be addressed. Such legal decisions are most likely on the horizon and emphasize the need for the development of effective treatment approaches.

Despite the prevalence of numerous deficits in skills necessary for proper community adaptation among the mentally retarded, many professionals working with this group assume that behavior modification approaches are less applicable for those who display the highest cognitive functioning (mild and moderate) versus the more severely mentally handicapped persons (Aanes & Haagenson, 1978; Zaharia, 1975). For higher functioning mentally retarded individuals, placement in a normalized environment is advocated as a treatment approach. As Aanes and Haagenson (1978) note, normalization as treatment is based on the assumption that associating with people who act normally is sufficient to induce normal behavior in the mentally retarded.

The minimal amount of experimental data that is available does not support the applicability of nonspecific treatments such as normalization, which basically consists of community placement with a deemphasis on formalized training. Furthermore, the literature describing treatment procedures with traditional unstructured educational and psychotherapeutic techniques has tended to be of little benefit (Ginzberg, 1979). One exception has been the application of behavior modification approaches. For the past 15 years, considerable effort has been placed on the development of successful methods for teaching more independent functioning skills, including toileting, grooming, and eating. Research with behavior modification procedures targeting other, complex behaviors (e.g., pedestrian and shopping skills) needed for semi-independent or independent living has also been successful. However, there has been limited research in this area. Given the legal and philosophical emphasis on more normalized living conditions, skill training in this latter area will undoubtedly expand much more rapidly in the next few years.

The present chapter will be a review of the accomplishments achieved to date in training community living skills to the mentally retarded and will also examine areas in need of further research. In this chapter, the literature on training programs aimed specifically at skills deemed necessary for the most "normal" adaptation possible in the community is reviewed. These programs have been organized into four subcategories, which are: practical living, physical care, leisure, and social skills. Methodological flaws and areas for future research are discussed.

PRACTICAL LIVING SKILLS

One of the areas that have received attention recently is the development of practical living skills. This area consists of self-help behaviors that enhance the integration and independent functioning of the mentally retarded person in the community. Unlike appropriate interpersonal behavior, these skills are helpful in ensuring proper maintenance of the home and mobility within the community. Skills that have been researched to date include telephone usage, sewing and mending clothes, and acquiring desirable pedestrian behavior. A review of each of these areas follows.

Telephone Usage

The rationale for treatment in this area is that community adjustment of the mentally retarded can be greatly enhanced by the acquiring of telephone-usage skills. Acquisition of this set of behaviors affords the individual a means of obtaining assistance in emergency situations, insures contact with others, and can save an individual the time and expense involved in travel (Risley & Cuvo, 1980).

In the first of these published studies, Leff (1974) described a method of teaching telephone dialing to the mentally retarded. A device was developed by the author and later patented (Leff, 1975) for teaching dialing. The study was designed to compare the relative efficacy of a standard number system and a color-coded system in training telephone usage with the mentally retarded, called "Dial-a-Phone." This method consisted of pairing colors with numbers to make discriminations of phone numbers more simple. In addition to this training method, the relation of dialing ability to chronological and mental age was also examined.

A pretest was administered to 124 mildly and moderately retarded children ranging from 6 to 21 years of age. Mental ages ranged from 2½ to 8 years. Each subject was asked to dial a given number without assistance. There were 24 subjects who correctly completed the task, and were dropped from the study, leaving 100 persons. Unfortunately, the instructional procedures employed in this study were not clearly specified. The results were that 47 subjects learned to dial with numbered discs, 44 required colored discs, and 9 were unable to learn the dialing procedure. A follow-up was conducted 2 weeks after the posttest with 25 randomly selected subjects. However, since assistance was provided to the subjects during this follow-up measure, the extent to which independent performance was maintained is unclear.

Additionally, methodological control was markedly absent, thus limiting what could be said about the effectiveness of treatment.

In a second study, Leff (1975) gave 117 mildly and moderately retarded children a pretest of phone dialing; 67 subjects were then excluded from the study owing to their ability to dial a telephone or their absences from the pretest session. The 50 remaining individuals were matched, based on initial skill level in phone dialing, and then placed in either the "Dial-a-Phone" (Leff, 1974) or the control condition which received treatment based on the best unsystematized efforts of the staff employed at the facility to teach telephone usage. Of the 25 subjects in the "Dial-a-Phone" condition, 24 (96%) learned the requisite skill, and 9 of 25 control subjects learned to dial a telephone (36%). All but two subjects who did not reach criterion in the control condition ($N=16$) were later taught dialing, using the "Dial-a-Phone Technique." Training the control subjects markedly strengthened the reliability of the results. In addition, follow-up data taken 10 days after the conclusion of treatment showed continued ability with the dialing skills.

Methodological problems exist in Leff's 1975 study. The methods of treatment used with subjects in the control groups were not standardized, and therefore cannot be replicated, nor was a no-treatment condition used so that the effects of the two treatment conditions could be more accurately evaluated. Also, follow-up was not based on empirical information, but rather on staff impressions.

In a third study by Leff (1975), 60 moderately mentally retarded children enrolled at a sheltered workshop were field-tested with the "Dial-a-Phone" procedure. Of these, 54 subjects (90%) learned to dial within 1–12 sessions. These findings are certainly impressive. However, the same shortcomings in methodology found in Leff's two earlier studies are also applicable here. Primarily, these problems are a lack of independent observers who could insure the reliability of data, and an insufficient description of target behaviors.

In a study that proved to be methodologically more rigorous, Risley and Cuvo (1980) screened 61 mentally retarded adolescents and adults who attended a community sheltered workshop for participation in a study aimed at teaching phone-usage skills. The three persons with the greatest skill deficits were included in the study. The goal of making emergency telephone calls was divided into four subgoals: (1) decision of whom to call (i.e., police, fire, doctor); (2) searching the telephone directory for the phone number; (3) dialing the number without error; (4) providing the service person with identifying information. Criteria for passing the program consisted of dialing the proper emergency number after being given a visual and verbal description of an event. (e.g.,the house is on fire). Subjects were given 5 seconds to perform each step of the task. If the response was not performed correctly, prompts were given in the following order: (a) verbal instruction, (b) verbal instruction and modeling, and (c) verbal instruction and physical guidance. Feedback to subjects was provided at various predetermined response stages and at the end of the training session by visually illustrating to the subject the number of steps he performed with no prompts.

The percentage of critical responses that each subject was required to perform was analyzed for the 61-step task. All subjects met 100% criteria in 6–29 practice trials. At the brief follow-up, which varied from one to two weeks, there was 100% maintenance of the trained skill for two subjects, and 85% for the third. Reliability data for percentage of scorer agreement during both training and testing ranged from 97% to 100%, with a mean of 99%. Although the authors did a thorough job of describing target behaviors and treatment procedures, there were several methodological shortcomings similar to those of the Leff studies. Paramount among these were an incomplete description of the training methods used and a small subject population.

Given that only one methodologically rigorous study was present among this group of papers (Risley & Cuvo, 1980), much more work is needed to establish empirically validated procedures for teaching telephone use.

Sewing and Mending

Sanders (1978) has defined physical presentability as a major goal for mentally retarded persons. Since this factor is important for the integration of the mentally retarded in the community, teaching sewing skills should increase the mentally retarded person's ability to care for him- or herself, and may promote awareness of personal appearance. Additionally, mending clothes is a potential money-saving activity; it increases garment life and reduces the need to purchase new clothing.

Some persons have seen the advantages of providing training in this important area. In one study, Nettlebeck and Kirby (1976) taught 36 mentally retarded females ranging in age from 16 to 38 years ($\overline{X}$ =23 years) to sew. Subjects whose full-scale I.Q. on the WAIS placed them in the mild to moderate range of retardation were trained at a rehabilitation center. The training program incorporated six components: (1) training was carried out in task-analyzed component steps; (2) subjects actively participated by carrying out all the work under guidance of staff; (3) supervision in the form of instructions and performance feedback was aimed at ensuring that errors were minimized; (4) feedback was given in the format of frequent verbal instructions; (5) work output was graphed, based on short periods during which a number of sewing tasks were practiced; and (6) the component steps were combined after the subject had become proficient in each. It was found that the 26 trainees without previous sewing experience were able to perform 53% of the standard tasks within 23 to 94 days of training ($\overline{X}$ = 51 days). For the 10 trainees with previous sewing experience, average achievement was 60%. However, because of major methodological flaws, such as failure to define adequately the target behaviors, the data were uninterpretable.

Cronin and Cuvo (1979) trained five moderately retarded adults with deficiencies in mending skills (17 to 20 years old) while they were attending public school. Inclusion in their study was based on a screening test that was designed to measure three prerequisite skills: (1) identification of sewing materials; (2) needlethreading, knot-tying, pinning; and (3) button and thread selection. Each step of the three sewing skills was scored as correctly or incorrectly performed. The test was administered prior to training, immediately after achieving criteria for the three tasks, and at one- and two-week follow-up intervals.

At the start of training, subjects were asked to identify what mending tasks were needed for a particular garment before being instructed to complete it. Prompts were utilized in the following sequence: (a) no help, (b) verbal instruction, (c) verbal instruction and modeling, (d) verbal instruction and physical guidance, and (e) verbal instruction and visual cues (e.g., marking on the garment, measuring stitch length, etc.). Verbal praise and information feedback by way of a graph were used as a response consequence. If performance on a previously trained task fell below criteria, maintenance training was implemented during the next training session with the addition of two prompts: (a) confirmation—participant verbalized the step they were on; (b) non-specific prompt—where subjects were asked after 5 sec, "What do you do next?" The authors utilized a multiple-baseline design across subjects and responses. Similarly, target behaviors were operationally defined and reliability data which proved to be adequate were taken in an appropriate fashion.

It was found that, prior to instruction, all tasks were performed at 35% accuracy or below. All five participants maintained their skills at 100% criteria with no prompting at the 2-week follow-up. Additionally, the need for prompts decreased as a function of trials for each task.

This study was an initial demonstration of the applicability of a well-specified treatment procedure for teaching mending skills. For this reason, it was not possible to state which element (e.g., task analysis, graduated sequence of prompts, and response consequences) was primarily responsible for skill acquisition. However, because of the well-controlled nature of the study, a good data base exists for further work. Hopefully, researchers interested in this area will replicate and extend the work of Cronin and Cuvo (1979), providing similar experimental rigor.

Money Management

An increasing trend is the belief that the mentally retarded should participate in all aspects of community living, such as recreational and social activities. Funding sources from both state and federal agencies as well as sheltered work facilities have also been instrumental in establishing income for the mentally retarded. With these sources, the mentally retarded, not unlike other members of society, have the added responsibility of managing these funds if they are to become more independent. Therefore, they must learn to spend these funds conscientiously in order to purchase the requisite goods and services needed to live in society. Although mentally retarded persons should acquire money-management skills in order to be successfully placed in the community (Edgerton, 1967; McCarver & Craig, 1974), a search of the literature indicates that there has been limited research examining procedures for teaching monetary usage. Additionally, the focus of most research has been on identifying and counting coins, to the exclusion of more complex monetary management skills.

In the first empirical study reviewed, Wunderlick (1972) explored the possibility of teaching children who ranged from 9 to 13 years of age coin values and currency-exchange equivalencies. IQ ranged from 49 to 70, with a mean of 59. Subjects were selected based on inability to distinguish among coin values and to make change. They first touched a slide containing a specific coin denomination, then selected the equivalent coin. A correct choice led to immediate reinforcement and advancement in the program. Wunderlick emphasized the importance of this method of training, since it required subjects to touch a stimulus before making a choice response. This method directed attention to the stimulus properties, a strategy which was assumed to be useful to increase the probability that the subject would attend to the relevant discriminative cues. Wunderlick indicated that error rate using this procedure was low. Pretest, posttest and follow-up data were not available, however. In addition, a method of determining whether the subject lacked these skills at pretest was not described. Another weakness of the study was the failure to mention the number or length of training sessions.

Monetary counting skills have also been taught to mentally retarded adolescents by Bellamy and Buttars (1975). Subjects were five moderately retarded adolescents whose mean age was 16.1 years. The training program was broken down into three phases, consisting of baseline, training academic skills, and teaching skills associated with counting money. The teaching phase utilized modeling procedures and physical guidance. If a subject made a correct response, verbal reinforcement and feedback using a point card were given. The training program required 206 trials and 100 hours of instruction. Treatment was carried out over a 6-month period, and resulted in the development of the students' ability to count money. Unfortunately, a general lack of detail was the case in this present study, which would make replication of the procedures difficult.

Lowe and Cuvo (1976) developed a program to sum various combinations of coins with two male and two female moderately retarded children ($\overline{X}$ age = 14.8 years and $\overline{X}$ I.Q. of 57). All the subjects were able to count to 100 by ones and fives, name the values of five basic coins, and sum combinations of coin values up to \$1.00.

A multiple-baseline design was utilized, with the primary dependent measure being summation of 51 coin combinations. Coins were presented in vertical piles, which subjects were required to count. Training sessions lasted approximately 30 min, and were carried out four times a week. Subjects were trained first in counting coins one at a time, and then in combination. In counting single coins, subjects were asked to use one finger to indicate the number of fives in the coin's value. The training sequence consisted of having the experimenter model the above-mentioned procedure, having the subject initiate the procedure concurrently with the experimenter, and requiring the subject to perform the task alone. The proportion of correct responses on the coin summation test was .29 at pretest and .92 at posttest. At the four-week follow-up the group mean was .79, an average decrement of .13 from the posttest scores, which suggests that the subjects maintained these skills. A positive aspect of the study was the fact that procedures were clearly identifiable and could easily be replicated.

Borakove and Cuvo (1976) used a pretest/posttest matched-group design to assess the teaching of coin summation in a more efficient manner, since it had been demonstrated that this skill could be taught to the mentally retarded (Bellamy & Buttars, 1975; Lowe & Cuvo, 1976). Despite these important initial results, some researchers had suggested that the counting technique described in the previous studies could be improved by placing the coin aside after it was counted. This procedure, they asserted, would facilitate increased attention on the next coin to be counted. To further enhance training, Borakove and Cuvo (1976) incorporated previous research in which Spradlin, Cotter, Stevens, and Friedman (1974) found that it was easier for groups to count moveable objects than those in a fixed order.

Fourteen subjects with a mean chronological age of 15 years and a mean IQ of 46.20 on the Stanford-Binet Intelligence test were included in the study. Two training procedures were tested. One method was a replication of the Lowe and Cuvo (1976) procedure, and the other utilized the same features, with the inclusion of an additional coin-displacement procedure in an attempt to improve on the latter technique. The inclusion of the displacement procedure enhanced the efficacy of treatment. Subjects in the displacement group acquired skills selected for treatment more rapidly, acquired significantly greater summing proficiency, and maintained proficiency in summation of coins better than subjects who did not receive treatment. The findings of this study further support earlier research in which displacement of objects minimized the reliance on memory skills and facilitated the effects of teaching coin summation (Spradlin *et al.*, 1974).

Using a pretest/posttest matched-group design, Trace, Cuvo, and Criswell (1977) taught coin equivalence. Seven male and seven female institutionalized residents in the mild-to-severe range of mental retardation were tested. The major dependent measure was a coin equivalence assessment which required subjects to select correct coin combinations. Training was accomplished through development of a response chain by moving coins, selection and counting, and depositing various monetary values in a coin machine. Modeling procedures and verbal instruction were utilized if subjects performed the task incorrectly, and correct responses were rewarded with social praise and M & M candy. The experimental group's mean performance increased significantly from pretest to posttest whereas subjects in the no-treatment control condition showed no significant gains. Improvements of experimental subjects were maintained at follow-up.

Procedures were specified in sufficient detail to make replication possible. The inclusion of a no-treatment control group as well as a treatment group was an additional strength of the study, since such a design feature provides better experimental control. As the authors indicated, a control condition which eliminated the use of the coin machine and compared the relative effectiveness of the instructional program without the machine could further demonstrate the efficacy of this training package.

In an extension of the research on coin summation, Miller, Cuvo, and Borakove (1977) tested whether it would be more efficient to teach verbal production of coin values directly or to teach auditory comprehension first. Subjects in the verbal-production condition were first instructed to point to the target coin when the experimenter named the value. This phase of training was followed by a production phase, in which the subject was asked to verbalize the value of identified coins.

Fourteen moderately retarded subjects participated in the study, which used a matched-group pretest/posttest design in a multiple-baseline format. Modeling and prompting were utilized to elicit correct responses. No significant differences in pretest data were noted between experimental conditions. Subjects in both experimental conditions improved significantly from pretest to posttest. Additionally, these gains were maintained at a four-week follow-up. Teaching production alone was found to be a more efficient training strategy than teaching production combined with comprehension.

In still another study, change-making skills were trained by Cuvo and his colleagues (Cuvo, Veitch, Trace, & Konke, 1978). Subject participation was contingent on the ability to identify the value of all American coins, sum combinations of coins, form equivalent combinations of coins, and state monetary values of price signs. A multiple baseline design across subjects and behaviors was used. In addition, a change computation test was administered at pretest, posttest, and a two-week follow-up. Four training sessions of 45–60 min each were held weekly. Three adolescent mentally retarded subjects were given a fixed amount of money and a picture of an item with a price tag attached, and then asked to purchase the item as well as state the amount of change they should receive. The training procedure, which included modeling as well as verbal and tangible reinforcers, resulted in rapid gains which were maintained at follow-up.

Smeets (1978), in a more recent study, investigated the use of a calculator to enable subjects with few numerical skills to demonstrate the ability to make independent purchases. The three moderately retarded subjects in the study ranged from 20 to 29 years of age. In 4–5 sessions per week averaging 30–60 min each, subjects were trained to enter numbers on the calculator as well as a letter key, and the price of one or more items. Other tasks included paying coins and banknotes to match the purchase price of an item, and checking their change. All subjects acquired the target behavior in 8-10 hours of training. Although the efficacy of the procedure was shown with Dutch currency, its replications with American coins and currency should be tested. The authors indicate that Dutch currency consists of more coins of different denominations than American money. In addition, the Dutch paper money's color differed across denominations, making discrimination between values easier than with American dollars, which is one reason why generalization of these findings to American money may not occur.

A considerable amount of study on training money management skills has been conducted with the mentally retarded. Certainly additional work is needed, particularly with respect to how money should be budgeted. However, relative to the other areas of training reported in this chapter, the work in teaching coin summation and related money-management skills is substantial, both from the standpoint of the number of studies conducted, and the methodological rigor employed.

Mobility Skills

The mobility to participate in all aspects of community living is without question a requisite skill for independent living in which many mentally retarded persons are deficient. This problem is of additional concern since the health and safety of the mentally retarded in the community is at issue (Nihira & Nihira, 1975a, b). Undeniably, dangerous situations exist which can be dealt with only by teaching the person how to handle these potentially hazardous situations. Additionally, the loss of freedom resulting from deficiencies in this area can greatly curtail the employability and independence of the mentally retarded.

In a 1971 census, O'Brien (1972) found that 18% of all traffic deaths involved pedestrians, with 64% of these involving street crossing. One-third of these accidents occurred at intersections, and 45% occurred in areas deemed unsafe for crossing. These statistics involve nonretarded populations. The frequency of accidents may be even greater with the mentally retarded, because of their frequent lack of such skills.

In the first study employing behavior modification procedures to teach pedestrian skills to the mentally retarded, Page, Iwata, and Neef (1976) treated five ambulatory, mildly retarded adults. Training was conducted in a classroom setting, using a model simulating four square city blocks. Subjects were taught specific skills utilized in a street crossing sequence: (1) intersection recognition; (2) pedestrian-light skills; (3) traffic-light skills; (4) responding appropriately to a stop sign facing cars traveling in the same direction as the pedestrian. Progression through the task-analyzed steps of the skills was trained, utilizing the model, and then tested *in vivo*. Verbal praise was given for correct responses, and incorrect responses were followed with instruction and modeling on how to perform behaviors appropriately. Skills generalized to the natural environment and were maintained at appropriate levels at a 2- to 6-week follow-up.

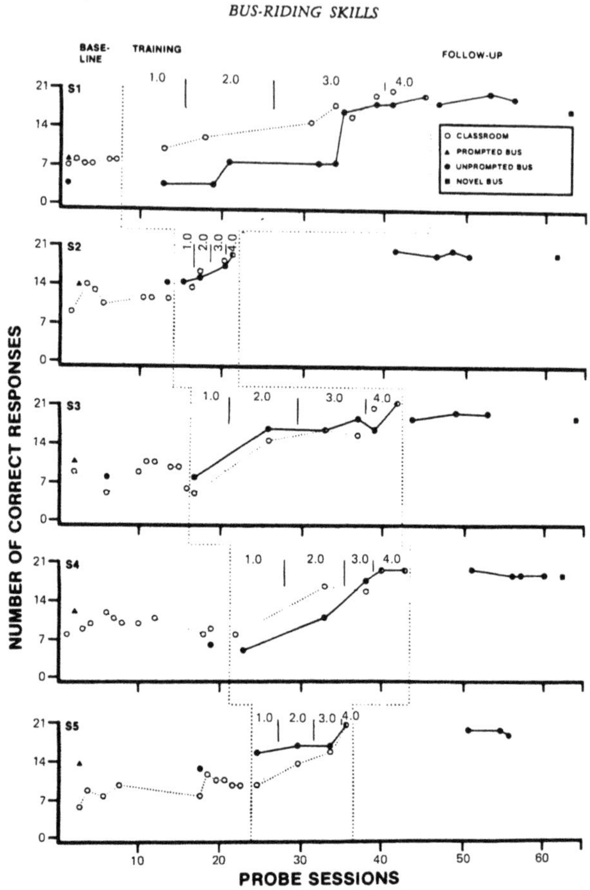

FIGURE 1. Number of correct responses on classroom and bus probes for the five classroom-trained subjects during baseline, training, and follow-up conditions.

The authors demonstrated that pedestrian skills could be taught to the mentally retarded in a classroom setting, and that such training would generalize to the natural environment (see Figure 1). Such a training approach can be seen as advantageous, since inclement weather and the dangers of training in the natural environment were avoided.

The positive results of Page *et al.* (1976) related to training pedestrian skills were supported in a study by Matson (1980). Thirty adult inpatients in the moderate-to-severe range of mental retardation served as subjects, with 10 persons being assigned to each of three experimental conditions. One condition received no treatment, a second condition received treatment similar to the classroom procedures described by Page and his colleagues, and the third condition was comprised of a package of techniques referred to as "independence training," a training program developed by Matson and his colleagues for treating the mentally retarded. This latter condition consisted of self-evaluation, social reinforcement, and participant modeling at a mock up of an intersection on the hospital grounds, with subjects physically practicing pedestrian skills. Independence training proved to be significantly more effective than the other treatment conditions, and classroom training proved to be more effective than no treatment. From these data it seems that an active treatment, closely approximating the target skill, is more efficient than classroom training.

Neef, Iwata, and Page (1978) later extended their research to the training of public transportation usage with five mild to moderately retarded adults. Subjects possessed basic pedestrian skills, but none could independently ride a bus. A multiple-baseline design was employed across subjects to evaluate training effects. The "city model" employed in their previous study was used in a manner similar to that described above. Two additional students were trained, utilizing an *in vivo* procedure, on a bus while riding in the community. The purpose of the *in vivo* condition was to test the efficiency of this procedure versus the classroom technique. Contrary to Matson's (1980) findings, classroom training proved to be highly effective for generalizing effects to the natural environment. These differences may be accounted for by the nature of the problem studied, differences in subjects, and the way *in vivo* training was carried out. A further consideration is the size of the groups used by Neef and his colleagues; $N = 5$ and $N = 2$. Certainly a between-group comparison with small numbers of subjects should be interpreted cautiously with respect to applicability to mentally retarded persons as a whole.

These three initial studies demonstrate the efficacy of teaching pedestrian skills to persons who are mildly to severely mentally retarded, on both an inpatient and an outpatient basis. This area deserves additional attention, however, given the potential ramifications of an error in pedestrian behavior. More comparisons of different treatment modalities and assessments of long-term follow-up are needed. Despite these shortcomings, the fact that the studies conducted were generally sound, from a methodological perspective, suggests that such training can indeed be beneficial.

PHYSICAL CARE

Recent studies have been aimed at developing skills which will enhance the physical well-being of the mentally retarded. Behavior modification procedures have been increasingly used for self-regulation of various types of behaviors. Brickey's (1978) contention that mentally retarded persons are sometimes overprotected and denied the opportunity to assume responsibility for self-management of their daily activities is well taken. As a result of such staff attitudes and patient care, these persons tend to become increasingly dependent on others to help them attend to their daily needs. Programs for reversing this situation are needed.

Self-Administration of Medication

Staff dispensing of medication is one example of possible overprotection, at least for some mentally retarded persons. Brickey (1978), in an attempt to increase independent use of medications, conducted a study in which he taught self-administration of drugs to 20 men and women (enrolled at a sheltered workshop) with moderate to borderline mental retardation. Subjects were informed of the type of medication they were currently taking and were instructed to come to the secretary at medication time (12 noon) to pick up their pills, with staff providing prompts as necessary to elicit correct responses. After two weeks of choosing the correct drug and dosage, subjects were required to carry and dispense their own medication. Spot checks were completed to ensure that dosages were taken properly. The final step of the program was for subjects to purchase their own medication, which required transportation and money-handling skills. Subjects successfully completed all but the last step of the program.

In the only other study on self-administered medication reported to date, McFarlane and Hames (1973) taught diabetic children in a summer camp. They utilized various techniques, such as counseling, films, and modeling. Unfortunately, there were a number of methodological flaws, such as the failure to specify behaviors to be treated and methods of adequately assessing them, which obscured the results. Despite these problems, the importance of such training and research seems evident.

Oral Hygiene

A number of studies have been designed for teaching oral-hygiene skills to the mentally retarded. Cheney, Kluft, and Levicki (1974) point out that, historically, dental diagnosis and treatment for the mentally retarded have been overlooked despite statistical evidence of overwhelming need. Fortunately, several studies specifically designed to treat such problems have recently appeared.

Saunders (1976) described in a nonexperimental report a method of teaching the mentally retarded to brush their teeth. Information was provided on how to select the proper toothbrush (i.e., considering the bristles, size of brush handle, and grips). Additionally, information was provided on how to adapt this equipment for the handicapped. Since data was not obtained using appropriate experimental methodology, nothing can be said about Saunders' training procedures.

Abramson and Wunderlick (1972) trained dental-hygiene techniques to the mentally retarded. In their study, the authors broke the training skills down into three stages: (1) being able to choose one's own toothbrush; (2) reinforcing successive approximations of toothbrushing; and, (3) modeling and reinforcing correct tooth-brushing behavior. Subjects were severely retarded institutionalized children between 9 and 14 years of age ($N=9$). Subjects completed the discrimination-training phase of the experiment in a mean of 88.7 trials, although one subject did not reach the criterion. Analysis of pretest data showed that subjects brushed the left, middle, and right side of the mouth only 10% of the time before training and 81% of the time while posttest measures were taken. Once again, a lack of operational definitions and ambiguous description of treatment procedures minimized the utility of the results.

Horner and Keilitz (1975) evaluated a comprehensive toothbrushing program which included a detailed task analysis and description of training. Eight severely to mildly retarded subjects (ranging in age from 9 to 17 years) who lived in a large institution were treated. Subjects were divided into two groups of four. The first group received tokens plus social reinforcement and were trained in a large experimental room containing a single sink with a mirror directly over it. The second group received only social reinforcement and was trained in the bathroom of the living unit of their residence. Baseline data was taken by providing subjects with a toothbrush, toothpaste, dispensable cup, and a box of facial tissues located near the sink. A progression of training procedures was utilized during training and included (1) no help, (2) verbal instruction, (3) demonstration and verbal instruction, and (4) physical guidance and instruction. A 5-sec delay occurred after a training procedure was used before proceeding to the next training procedure in the sequence.

All the subjects showed improvement in performance of tooth brushing compared to baseline. Limitations of the study include a failure to provide follow-up data and generalization of trained skills to other situations. However, the utilization of task analysis with operational definitions and the detailed description of training procedures was a marked improvement over previous research in this area. Similarly, the methodology used to test the experimental hypothesis was sound.

In another study, Dicks (1975) evaluated the effects of different communication techniques in the cooperation of mentally retarded children during the performance of dental procedures. Forty-eight mentally retarded subjects were placed in one of three experimental conditions: (1) verbal instruction, (2) verbal instruction and visual demonstration of dental equipment, and (3) verbal instruction along with visual demonstration of the equipment (demonstrated on a plastic model). It was found that the greater the degree of mental retardation, the less cooperation. Another finding was that no significant relationship could be found between the length of institutionalization, number of previous visits to a dental clinic, age or sex of the child, and subject cooperation. Verbal instructions along with visual demonstration of equipment proved to be the most effective treatment.

Weight Control Procedures

Another form of health care that has been studied is the development of procedures for weight control. One of the primary treatment methods has been self-monitoring. In one such study, Joachim and Korboot (1975) treated 32 mildly retarded residents from a residential training center, using a variety of procedures. Subjects were randomly assigned to one of four conditions: (1) weight and record with instruction, (2) weight and record, (3) instruction, and (4) an unspecified control group. These four groups were further divided, half of each receiving weekly experimenter contact and the remainder no contact. The treatment period was 8 weeks. Subjects in group one and two were required to weigh themselves before breakfast and before evening meal and to record their weight on a 12.5 cm by 7.5 cm card. Additional instructions for group one consisted of telling subjects that the experimenter wanted them to reduce their weight any way they could. Subjects in group three received these instructions before breakfast and the evening meal for an 8-week period. Subjects in group four (control) received no instruction and were not weighed. Additional activities of control subjects were not described. Self-monitoring of weight produced some weight loss, although it did not prove to be significant. Experimenter contact resulted in significant weight loss at the return to baseline and at 8-week follow-up periods.

In a follow-up to the Joachim and Korboot (1975) study, Joachim (1977) instituted a self-monitoring program for treatment of obesity in a 32-year-old mildly retarded institutionalized female. The program was based on three elements: (1) monitoring weight four times per day, (2) monitoring all food and drink intake, and (3) weekly contact with the therapist. Results were more significant than in the previous study, because after 38 weeks of treatment the subject had lost 38 pounds. Weight loss was greatest when the subject was required to record both her weight and her food intake. However, when there were variations in these procedures, no appreciable weight loss occurred. At a follow-up of 46 weeks the subject had regained 31 of the 38 pounds.

As with many of the procedures discussed in the present review, the results were mixed. Only one subject was employed in the second study. Therefore, comparing the effectiveness of the different treatment procedures is difficult. Perhaps the most surprising fact, however, was that few studies in this area have been conducted, given that weight control is a frequent problem with the mentally retarded.

Emergency Skills

A final area of physical care, examined in only one study, is how to handle appropriately an emergency situation. This is another area in need of study with the mentally retarded. National statistics on acute illnesses and injuries during 1975 were estimated at 443.1 million among America's civilian noninstitutionalized population, a figure that breaks down to 212 acute conditions per 100 persons. Although such data are not available for the mentally retarded, injury rates in this country are probably as high for them as for persons of normal intelligence.

To provide some initial information on the feasibility of training such skills to the mentally retarded, Matson (1980) using a multiple-baseline format, trained five moderately retarded adults how to escape from a fire, how to handle a seizure, and what steps to take in case of a minor cut. Training involved classroom instruction, participant modeling, and social reinforcement. The subjects who had been institutionalized most of their lives were able to acquire the requisite skills within 3 weeks of daily training, and maintained them at follow-up, which varied from 2 to 7 months, depending on the target behavior being measured.

Leisure Time Skills

Rationale for Treatment

The present trend in mental-retardation programming is to emphasize the utilization of community resources and services. With community placement, a major problem is how to use leisure time productively. Luckey and Shapiro (1974) emphasize the importance of recreation in the habilitation of the mentally retarded. They acknowledge that few provisions for leisure time with this group are available. Prior to the mid 1940s, recreation for mentally retarded persons was restricted primarily to residential institutions (Witt, 1971); leisure time was viewed primarily as a means to preserve order, maintain morale, and prevent boredom. Only after World War II was recreation viewed as beneficial for the mentally retarded. The widespread emphasis on recreation as a primary programmatic concern can be attributed to the direction provided by the National Association for Retarded Citizens (Sengstock & Stein, 1967). In 1964, the association adopted a list of provisions to insure a direction for recreational programming. This resolution emphasized equal access for the mentally retarded to publicly supported recreational agencies by making their facilities adaptable to the needs of these persons. Trends of this nature should further stimulate programmatic research in this area, since, as can be seen below, few studies have been conducted.

Play Behavior

In one of the studies that have been reported on play behavior, Katz and Yekutiel (1974) interviewed parents of graduates from two sheltered workshops for the mentally retarded concerning leisure time and social problems of their children. Parents indicated that the most significant problem facing their children was a lack of suitable companions, as evinced by the fact that 78 % of these children had no friends and had very little social interaction with others. The next most serious problem was insufficient facilities for leisure time activities, followed by a lack of interest in such activities. Parents of institutionalized individuals felt that this was a more pervasive problem for their children than did parents of mentally retarded persons living in the community. Most parents indicated that the greater part of leisure time activity was spent watching television or listening to the radio. The accuracy of these impressions has yet to be validated by correlation with direct behavioral measures. Despite this, these data, do give some idea of leisure time priorities for training with the mentally retarded. It can be seen in the following studies that priorities established in this study have not been followed in the treatment research that is available.

There has been a limited number of empirical studies on teaching the mentally retarded specific leisure skills. One such project was conducted by Bundschuh, Williams, Hollingsworth, Gooch, and Shirer (1972), who attempted to teach swimming. Participants were 14 moderately and 26 mildly retarded children, ranging in age from 5 to 19 years. It was found that 90% of the participants learned to swim, with 10% progressing from nonswimmer to swimming 75 feet or more. All of the mildly retarded children swam 6 feet or more at the conclusion of the 20-day instructional program. Conversely, the moderately retarded children made a successful adjustment to the water, although results were not so striking as those observed in the former group.

A major difficulty with the Bundschuh *et al.* (1972) study was the failure to describe clearly the training procedures and the therapist's role in implementing them. Also, pretest and posttest measures were not described, making it difficult to assess the efficiency of the training.

In another study of play behavior, Wehman and Rettie (1975) attempted to increase the use of play materials during a one-hour leisure time period. Participants were three severely retarded women who resided in a state institution. The main dependent variable was physical action on the play materials, such as touching, exploring, or manipulating toys. A multiple-baseline design was used across individuals. Following a baseline period, one subject began to receive social reinforcement and experimenter attention for playing with the designated materials. In addition, physical and verbal prompts and modeling were utilized as teaching methods. Initially, one subject received training to increase play actions; then a second subject was included in training, and then another, until everyone was involved. Play behavior was markedly increased with all the subjects treated.

A limitation of the present study was that follow-up measures were not used. Also, generalization of the learned responses, that is, increased social interaction and play interaction, were not attempted with novel subjects and/or materials. However, the most critical problem may have been the behaviors trained to these adults. Such skills are not age appropriate and thus may not constitute the most suitable type of leisure skills for this group. Certainly a focus on other forms of leisure activities for adults should be considered. Such alternatives are addressed in the following section.

Adult Leisure Skills

In one study aimed at teaching age-appropriate leisure skills to adults, Matson and Marchetti (1980) trained use of a stereo to 55 severely to moderately retarded adults. Subjects were matched on proficiency in stereo operation skills, and then one member of each matched group was assigned to one of the five treatment conditions: a no-treatment control group, placebo treatment, independence training, traditional classroom training, or independence training plus traditional classroom training. Independence training, which incorporated social reinforcement, *in vivo* modeling, instructions, and feedback proved to be the most effective method, followed by traditional classroom training, the combined-treatment package, and the two control groups.

Although there has been increased emphasis on the need for recreational activities for the mentally retarded (Luckey & Shapiro, 1974), and evidence has suggested that mentally retarded persons do not utilize their leisure time effectively (Katz & Yekutiel, 1974), research has been limited. Future research must be conducted to explore and identify what recreational and leisure activities are available to the mentally retarded in the institiution and in the community, and must begin to explore the most efficient training procedures to teach these skills. Additionally, a wide range of training strategies must be compared to determine the efficacy of various training components, and more studies such as Katz and Yekutiel's (1974) should be made so that some idea about treatment priorities can be established.

Given the trend in availability of recreational activities for the mentally retarded, increased development of techniques for assisting these persons to acquire requisite leisure skills seems probable. Research verifying the utility of appropriate treatment procedures is limited, but seems promising. A greater emphasis has been placed on play behavior, but the recreational needs of adults is beginning to be realized as well.

SOCIAL SKILLS

An area which has received perhaps more attention than any other, with respect to successful community functioning, is social or interpersonal skills. Capacity to make appropriate requests, eye contact, and related verbal and motoric responses that constitute social skills is generally lacking in the mentally retarded. There is such deficiency in this area, in fact, it has become a defining characteristic of mental retardation (Grossman, 1977). This problem is further exacerbated by long-term hospitalizatons, where the individual does not know and is not reinforced for displaying appropriate social behavior. Since many of these individuals are now, or will soon be, living in the community, an environment in which demand characteristics for appropriate social responding are much higher than in the institution, the need for social skills training is gaining in importance.

Initial Research

The first published study aimed at teaching social skills to the mentally retarded was conducted by Ross (1969). He attempted to increase knowledge of social responses to educable mentally retarded children, based on the assumption that educable retarded children exhibit antisocial behavior because they do not know the appropriate social responses and norms. Participants in the study were 32 mildly retarded children ranging from 3 to 10 years of age. These subjects were randomly assigned to a treatment or placebo-control condition. A third group consisted of 16 normal children (matched on age), who were assigned to a no-treatment condition.

Prior to the training phase of the experiment, subjects were assessed on social behavior. The training phase, which consisted of role playing and live modeling by the therapist, was then started for the treatment. Subjects were presented with social situations aimed at teaching appropriate play skills, (e.g., A asks B whether A may borrow a crayon to paint a sign. B says A may borrow the crayon, and A starts the sign. A presses too hard, breaking the crayon. B says, "Oh, you broke my crayon." A says, "I'm sorry I broke it. I'll buy you a new crayon." B says, "That's fine. You said you were sorry and you offered to buy me a new crayon, so you can still use my crayons.") The mentally retarded children in the placebo treatment group received equal time with the experimenter; however, they did not receive training. The children of normal intelligence had no therapist contact. It was found that the mentally retarded children in the active-treatment group improved significantly more than persons in the placebo or control groups in social responsiveness, and these gains were maintained at follow-up.

The procedures utilized by Ross (1969) incorporated primary and secondary reinforcers as well as modeling. The study was important, since the efficacy of employing these procedures for improving social skills was demonstrated. However, implementing the program as described on a routine basis might be difficult, owing to the utilization of live modeling, puppet play, and film slides. A second, more serious shortcoming of the study was the lack of reliability data collected by independent observers. Because of the shortcomings of the methodology, a more rigorous replication of these procedures would be valuable.

In another early attempt to train social skills, Whitman, Mercurio, and Caponigri (1970) utilized operant reinforcment procedures for developing social skills in two severely retarded children. Targeted behaviors were rudimentary social interaction in the form of mutual participation in ballrolling and blockpassing. Subjects were 6- and 10-year-old children who could not verbalize words or phrases. Ratings were made on the number, length, and type of social responses exhibited during 10 days of baseline. Training was then provided for 30 consecutive school days, in 30-min sessions. Treatment consisted primarily of contingent reinforcement and manual guidance. Subject 1 did not engage in social interaction during the baseline period, but he spent an average of 1.8 min per 15-min rating session exhibiting appropriate play during the reinforcement phase of the experiment. This behavior was maintained at follow-up. Subject 2 averaged one min in appropriate play during the baseline period, 4.3 minutes during the reinforcement phase, and 1.8 min during follow-up. These results support the contention that operant techniques can be effective in increasing social responsiveness. Additionally, the social skills learned were found to generalize to other situations including different stimuli and different children.

Modeling techniques have been utilized to teach a wide range of novel behaviors (Bandura, 1969). Ross (1969) demonstrated the effectiveness of these procedures in teaching social responses. However, the contribution of this component alone in the acquisition of social skills was not clear, because of the simultaneous use of edible and social reinforcers.

Nelson, Gibson, and Cutting (1973) employed modeling to teach a mildly retarded boy to use grammatically correct questions and to smile and speak appropriately. Training consisted of having the child watch two normal 7-year-old boys who were used as models and presented on videotape. For each target behavior, three consecutive training procedures were utilized: modeling, instructions plus social reinforcement, and modeling plus instructions and social reinforcement. The target behaviors significantly increased during training, and were maintained at the 3½-month follow-up.

The experimental design utilized in the Nelson *et al.* (1973) study does not permit a component analysis of the three training procedures. Also, investigation of the efficacy of individual components versus the combined use of modeling, instructions, and reinforcement should more clearly demonstrate the efficiency of these procedures. Although significant improvement on target behaviors was found, the results must be viewed cautiously, considering that the experiment involved a single subject.

Gibson, Lawrence, and Nelson (1976) extended the research of Nelson *et al.* (1973) by comparing the relative effectiveness of (1) modeling, (2) instructions and feedback, and (3) modeling, instructions, and feedback in improving peer interaction skills of three mentally retarded adults. Target responses were (a) verbalization between a subject and his peers, (b) recreation activities such as playing cards, etc. with peers, and (c) cooperation, which involved responses such as sweeping, or washing clothes with peers. Following baseline, each subject received nine training sessions utilizing one of three methods. Sequential effects were counterbalanced by utilizing a different order of treatment presentation for each subject. (Videotapes of nonretarded adults were employed with modeling.) Regardless of the response class trained, modeling, instruction, and feedback produced significantly greater increases than instructions and feedback or modeling alone. The former procedures were effective in improving the target responses, although gains were not maintained at follow-up. This lack of maintenance is a significant problem that deserves more attention, and it has been addressed in studies described later in this review.

Other rudimentary social skills have been taught to the mentally retarded, utilizing behavioral techniques. The modification and generalization of a 15-year-old girl's loud voice was demonstrated by Jackson and Wallace (1974). This goal was accomplished using token reinforcement for incompatible behavior. In a study using related techniques, Stokes, Baer, and Jackson (1974) employed a multiple-baseline design to evaluate the training of handwaving as a greeting response to four profoundly retarded children. Reinforcement along with prompting and shaping were effective in teaching the targeted behaviors. Similarly, Twardosz and Baer (1973) taught two mentally retarded children to ask questions about novel stimuli through imitation and reinforcement techniques, which transferred effectively to untrained stimuli—an impressive demonstration of generalization.

In a well-designed control-group study aimed at improving social skills, Lee (1977) investigated the effectiveness of a 10-week structured-group counseling program designed to enhance the social-adjustment skills of mentally retarded adults. Subjects were 48 institutionalized residents in the moderate-to-mild range who were randomly assigned to the treatment ($N =$ 24) or control group ($N = 24$). Group counseling sessions were carried out with groups of seven to eight residents in which social interaction, personal appearance, physical mannerisms, awareness of feelings, making friends, and social responsibility were trained. Social behaviors were taught through peer and counselor interactions, verbal instruction, discrimination training, role playing, and discussion. Improvement was assessed with the American Association on Mental Deficiency Adaptive Behavior Scale, the Peabody Picture Vocabulary Test, peer nominations (i.e., residents chose who they would prefer to work and play with), and ward staff nominations (i.e., staff rank ordered the residents to determine prevalance of socially inappropriate behaviors). The treatment group showed a significantly greater improvement than the control group at posttest on the Peabody Picture Vocabulary, Adaptive Behavior Scale, and peer nomination. Unfortunately, more sensitive measures of behavior change, such as direct behavioral observation or rating of the trained behaviors, were not made. Fortunately, such measures were used in later studies.

Complex Social Skills Package

A more complex social skills training package has become widespread for treating a number of populations, including the mentally retarded. In the first study using these procedures, Matson and Stephens (1978) treated four long-term chronic psychiatric patients whose diagnoses indicated psychosis and mental retardation. The subjects were referred because of high rates of arguing and fighting, and were trained in a number of discrete, operationally defined behaviors. Training was done using scenes developed from real-life situations in which these women typically started a fight and/or an argument. Social skills training sessions ranged from 10 to 40 min. Six role-played scenes were presented, then the subject responded. Feedback was given by the therapist concerning the adequacy of the response, along with instructions on more appropriate ways to respond. Appropriate responses for each scene were then modeled by the trainer. For example, if improvement was evident, the trainer might say, "That's better, Sue, you looked right at him when you spoke." Depending on the quality of the response, the therapist might (1) present the same scene, (2) instruct the role model to demonstrate appropriate responding, or (3) present and narrate the next scene in the sequence. All target behaviors were reviewed at least once for each scene, and social praise was provided for appropriate behaviors. When an inappropriate response occurred, the patient would be required to repeat a socially appropriate statement which was modeled by the trainer. Feedback and instruction was then provided until all target behaviors were handled correctly or until the subject had attempted to answer a scene three times.

The social skills training procedures employed in this study were found to be effective in controlling argumentative and physically combative behaviors with chronic patients. It can be concluded from the follow-up data that results were maintained up to three months, although there was evidence of deterioration of trained skills beyond this period. The efficacy of the social skills training procedures suggests that such training may be applicable with the mentally retarded, although results should be viewed cautiously, in light of the subject characteristics (e.g., chronic psychiatric female inpatients) and the small sample size ($N = 4$).

Using a similar methodology and experimental design, in a group format, Matson and Zeiss (1978) trained 12 patients (from a unit described in the previous experiment) assigned to one of four treatment groups ($N = 3$). Two groups received instructions, modeling, and performance feedback, and the other two groups received role playing in addition to these techniques. Moderate improvement in the performance of social behaviors was observed on the ward, along with a decrease in fighting and arguing. To ensure maintenance of learned social responses, a procedure was employed which utilized group sessions on a less frequent basis. This procedure resulted in maintenance of improvement over a 10-week period.

Turner, Hersen, and Bellack (1978) employed an intensive training program to teach prosocial behaviors to a 19-year-old mentally retarded adult. The social skills training package consisted of behavioral rehearsal, modeling, instruction, feedback, and verbal reinforcement. Target behaviors were seven behavioral components of social skills: eye contact, response latency, loudness of speech, number of words spoken, smiles, physical gestures, and overall assertiveness. Six months following the conclusion of the initial treatment, booster sessions were used to bolster the effects of the initial treatment. Training procedures identical to the initial training sessions were implemented in the booster and initial training sessions.

Overall assertiveness improved, although it was not specifically treated (see Figure 2). A slight decrement in gains was noted at follow-up for all dependent measures except eye contact. As the authors point out, booster sessions such as those employed here are infrequently used to augment treatment gains, but they seem important for training complex interpersonal skills.

Another method that enhances generalization and maintenance of gains on social behaviors was reported by Matson, Zeiss, Zeiss, and Bowman (1980).

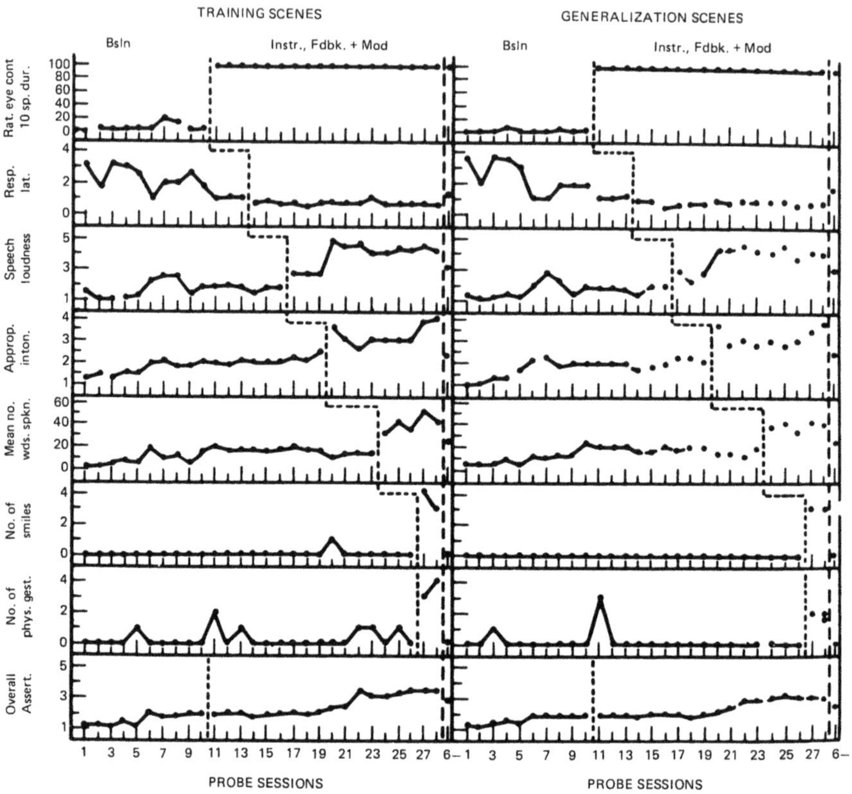

FIGURE 2. Initial training and six-month follow-up.

They utilized an assessment procedure for rating resident—staff interactions on a number of appropriate and inappropriate behaviors (e.g., reply to questions, helping on the unit, making positive statements, speaking with self). The 15 behaviors that staff were most likely to reinforce were selected for treatment, since these behaviors would be likely to generalize to the natural environment (Matson & Stephens, 1978).

Twelve male chronic institutionalized patients, six of whom were diagnosed as mentally retarded, served as subjects in one of four treatment groups. Two groups received contingent reinforcement for appropriate behavior, and the other two groups received the "standard social skills package" (e.g., scene presentation with instruction, feedback, modeling, and role-playing). The later condition proved to be the more effective mode of training, with treatment effects generalizing to the ward for those subjects who were mentally retarded as well as those who were not.

As in the Matson and Stephens (1978) and Matson and Zeiss (1978) studies, chronic psychiatric patients, with mixed diagnoses of schizophrenia and mental retardation, were treated. Results of these investigations should be viewed cautiously with respect to their applicability to mentally retarded persons as a whole.

As noted, one of the primary difficulties with the training of social skills is the ability to produce generalization and maintenance of gains. In an attempt to remedy this deficiency while training social skills, Matson (1978) trained six moderately mentally retarded adults with undesirable behaviors such as noncompliance and physical aggression. The training package included daily feedback (seven times per day) in the form of a check on a report card (indicating to the subject whether the undesirable behaviors occurred during the reporting time), instructions, and praise for appropriate behaviors. Short periods of social isolation in the form of restriction to one's bed area were used after daily training when a minus was reported for a check period that day. Of 22 inappropriate behaviors, 21 were decreased, and improvements were maintained at a 7-month follow-up.

Matson (1979) also treated a 28-year-old moderately retarded female who made negative statements about others. The subject met with a trainer in a therapy room, followed by a one-hour treatment period on the ward. Emphasis in the training room was on how to recognize and record negative comments in the living area via examples of appropriate recording procedures using events that had occurred in the subject's life. Staff modeling of appropriate behavior was employed to demonstrate how positive comments could be made instead of negative ones. Finally the subject demonstrated the alternative behavior, and the trainer provided feedback when a positive statement was made correctly. The second phase of training, which was conducted on the ward, required self-monitoring for one hour, followed by the trainer's asking the subject what had been done wrong (making negative statements) and how this could be modified. Then the trainer provided feedback to correct mistakes and gave praise when the subject told the truth and/or verbalized how the situation could be handled appropriately. Negative statements were decreased during the training period; however, gains deteriorated rapidly once training was discontinued. On a more positive note, the subject was able to learn how to record accurately (84%) and self-monitor her negative comments.

Matson and Earnhart (1981) extended the finding of Matson (1979) by treating four moderately to severely retarded adults who evidenced social skill deficits. The purpose of the study was to make a comparison of self-monitoring procedures. On-the-ward training proved to be necessary for establishing accurate performance of target behaviors in that setting. Once inappropriate behaviors had been decelerated, the intensity of training was faded to include only verbal prompts by staff.

In another test of the social skills training package, Matson and Zeiss (1979) varied the standard procedure (e.g., instruction, modeling, role-playing and feedback) in an attempt further to enhance generalization and maintenance. Two moderately mentally retarded adult females who were inpatients on a chronic ward of a psychiatric hospital were treated. Instructions, modeling, role-playing, and feedback were provided during daily problems situations, rather than using preselected scenes as in previous research (Matson & Stephens, 1978). Second, the two subject served as partners, monitoring behavior of others and their own (e.g., socially inappropriate statements, arguing, tantrum behaviors, or interruptions). Training was effective for teaching appropriate social behaviors on the ward and in therapy sessions. These improved skills were maintained at the 6-week follow-up.

The amount of research on social skills training is certainly more extensive and thorough than what is available with the other community adjustment skills reviewed. Despite this fact, considerably research on social skills training with the mentally retarded is still needed. Issues deserving further study are: what components of training are most critical, how can generalization be achieved most readily, and how effective is the standard social skills training package, relative to other forms of treatment, for remediating these deficits. Additionally, methods of establishing priorities for treatment and developing assessment instruments for these behaviors would be useful.

Overview of Methodology

In general, the programmatic research to date on training community adjustment skills has, with only a few exceptions, evidenced a lack of methodological control. Throughout this chapter, violations of common experimental control variables have been noted. For example, operational definitions of behaviors and adequate explanations of training procedures which would allow for replication are few, the use of AB rather than multiple-baseline or reversal subject designs is common, and the failure to include adequate control conditions in many of the group designs are frequent flaws in methodology. Thus, many of the studies proved to be incomplete descriptions of programs, rather than well-controlled experimental studies. Papers of the latter type are sorely needed if research in this area is to make a substantial contribution.

A few well-designed studies which have resulted in major contributions did appear in the literature. Examples of well-executed research include the papers by Garcia (1974) on conversational speech, Gibson, Lawrence, and Nelson (1976) on conversational speech, Horner and Keilitz (1975) on tooth brushing, Johnson and Bailey's (1977) study on leisure behaviors, and Neff, Iwata, and Page's (1978) paper on teaching public transportation skills. In thise papers, important research questions were evaluated in systematic ways that were thoroughly explained. These studies and the other research papers reviewed are evaluated and summarized in light of pertinent design features in Table I. Studies are summarized for each by the topic areas used in the preceeding sections of this chapter.

An analysis of the four subsets (practical living, physical care, leisure time, and social skills) under each of these general categories gives a better idea of the areas in which some research of a methodologically sophisticated nature has occurred. Areas in which such research has been conducted include money management (under practical living skills), oral hygiene, emergency skills (under physical care), play behavior, and adult leisure skills (under leisure time), and both the social skills subsets.

All four major areas of programming certainly deserve further systematic research, from our point of view. The area perhaps most in need of research is practical living skills, since few well-designed studies have been conducted in this area and since these skills are similar to many self-help behaviors that have been successfully trained in institutional settings (e.g.,dressing, toileting). This latter point is important because considerable effort has been made to work out a technology for less complex practical living skills and, therefore, it seems likely that this technology might be adopted in the practical living-skill areas for community living. Whichever area or areas are targeted for treatment, a concerted effort to apply sound methodological principles should be adapted if training techniques are to be accurately evaluated.

CONCLUDING REMARKS

The bulk of the studies reported in this chapter describe the potential utility of behavior modification procedures for training mentally retarded individuals in requisite skills that lead to more appropriate community adaptation. Two major weaknesses in the existing literature are particularly

TABLE I
Methodological Characteristics of Reviewed Community Living Skills Studies

	Design	Follow-up	Reliability
Practical living skills			
Telephone usage			
Leff, 1974	Pre/post, single condition, no control group, $N = 100$	2 weeks	No
Leff, 1975	a. Pre/post, two conditions, experimental and control group, $N = 50$	10 days	No
Leff, 1975	b. Pre/post, single condition (comparisons to groups in Leff, 1975a), no control group, $N = 60$	2-8 weeks	No
Risley & Cuvo, 1980	Multiple baseline, single condition, no control group, $N = 3$	1-2 weeks	Yes
Sewing/mending			
Nettleback & Kirby, 1976	Pre/post, single condition, no control, $N = 36$	None	No
Cronin & Cuvo, 1979	Multiple baseline, single condition, no control group, $N = 5$	1-2 weeks	Yes
Money management			
Wunderlick, 1972	Pre/post, single condition, no control group, $N = 5$	None	No
Bellamy & Buttars, 1975	Multiple baseline, single condition, no control group, $N = 5$	None	No
Lowe & Cuvo, 1976	Multiple baseline, single condition, no control group, $N = 4$	4 weeks	No
Borakove & Cuvo, 1976	Pre/post, multiple baseline, 2 experimental conditions, no control group, $N = 14$, $n = 7$	4 weeks	No
Trace, Cuvo, & Criswell, 1977	Pre/post matched groups and multiple baseline, 1 experimental condition, no treatment control group, $N = 14$, $n = 7$	1 week & 1 month	No
Miller, Cuvo, & Borakove, 1977	Pre/post matched groups & multiple baseline, 2 experimental conditions, no control group, $N = 14$, $n = 7$	1 week & 4 weeks	No
Cuvo, Veitch, Trace, & Konke, 1978	Multiple baseline, single condition, no control group, $N = 3$	2 weeks	Yes
Smeets, 1978	Multiple baseline, single condition, no control group, $N = 3$	None	No
Mobility skills			
Page, Iwata, & Neef, 1976	Multiple baseline, single condition, no control group, $N = 3$	2-6 weeks	Yes
Matson, 1980	Pre/post, 2 experimental conditions, no treatment control group, $N = 30$, $n = 10$		
Neef, Iwata, & Page, 1978	Multiple baseline, 2 experimental conditions, no control group, $N = 7$, $N = 2$, $N = 5$, respectively	1-12 months	Yes

TABLE I (*Continued*)

	Design	Follow-up	Reliability
Physical care			
Self-administration of medication			
Brickey, 1978	Design unclear, 1 experimental condition, $N = 20$	Unclear	No
Oral hygiene			
Abramson & Wunderlick, 1972	Pre/post, single condition, no control group, $N = 9$	None	Tested on instruments prior to experiment
Horner & Keilitz, 1975	Multiple baseline, 2 experimental conditions, no control group, $N = 8$, $n = 4$	None	Yes
Dicks, 1975	Pre/post, 3 experimental conditions, no control group, $N = 48$	None	No
Weight control			
Joachim & Korbott, 1975	4×2 factorial design, $N = 32$	8 weeks	No
Joachim, 1977	Multiple baseline, single condition, no control group, $N = 1$	46 weeks	No
Emergency skills			
Matson, 1980	Multiple baseline, single condition, no control group, $N = 5$	2-7 months	Yes
Leisure time skills			
Play behavior			
Katz & Yekutiel, 1974	Nonexperimental parents questioned on leisure time and social problems of their children	NA	NA
Bundschuh, Williams, Hollingsworth, Gooch, & Shirer, 1972	Pre/post, single condition, no control group, $N = 40$	None	No
Wehman & Rettie, 1975	Multiple baseline, single condition, no control group, $N = 3$	None	No
Adult leisure skills			
Matson & Marchetti, 1980	Multiple baseline, 3 experimental conditions, 2 control groups, $N = 55$	2 months	Yes
Social skills			
Ross, 1969	Multiple baseline, experimental condition, 2 control groups, $N = 48$	Varied, 14-94 days	No

(*continued*)

TABLE I (*Continued*)

	Design	Follow-up	Reliability
Whitman, Mercurio, Caponigri, 1970	Multiple baseline, single condition, no control group, $N = 2$	2 weeks	Yes
Nelson, Gibson, & Cutting, 1973	Modified multiple baseline, single condition, $N = 1$	3½ months	Yes
Gibson, Lawrence, & Nelson, 1976	Multiple baseline, single condition, no control group, $N = 3$	Yes	Yes
Jackson & Wallace, 1974	Multiple baseline, single condition, no control group, $N = 1$	Yes	Yes
Stokes, Baer, & Jackson, 1974	Multiple baseline, single condition, no control group, $N = 4$	1-6 months	Yes
Twardosz & Baer, 1973	Multiple baseline, single condition, no control group, $N = 2$	None	Yes
Lee, 1977	Pre/post test, 1 experimental condition, 1 no treatment control group, $N = 46$	None	Yes
Matson & Stephens, 1978	Multiple baseline, single condition, no control group, $N = 4$	3 months	Yes
Matson & Zeiss, 1978	Multiple baseline design, 2 experimental conditions, no control group, $N = 12$	5-10 weeks	Yes
Turner, Hersen, & Bellack, 1978	Multiple baseline, single condition, no control group, $N = 1$	6 months	Yes
Matson, Zeiss, Zeiss, & Bowman, 1980	Multiple baseline, 2 experimental conditions, no control group, $N = 12$	Yes	Yes
Matson, 1978	Multiple baseline, single condition, no control group, $N = 6$	7 months	Yes
Matson & Earnhart, 1981	Multiple baseline, single condition, no control group, $N = 4$	1 month and 4 months	Yes
Matson, 1980	Multiple baseline, single condition, no control group, $N = 1$	None	Yes
Matson & Zeiss, 1979	Multiple baseline, single condition, no control group, $N = 2$	6 weeks	Yes

evident when comparing these studies to those performed with more established problem behavior areas such as self-injury and self-help skills; many of the experiments have been loosely controlled from a methodological point of view, and few group studies have been conducted. These are points which the authors have attempted to emphasize in the preceding methodology section.

Another problem with the available literature is the emphasis on developing treatment techniques to the exclusion of improving service delivery systems, enlightening the general public and professionals about the mentally retarded, and parent and staff training and supervision in the community. These latter three areas have tended to be continuing problems with all behavior modification programs, and are major contributors to the implementation of such methods on a broad scale. However, these concerns are particularly troublesome for mentally retarded persons living in the community, since therapists, equipment, and related variables important for providing successful training tend to be spread over a much greater geographical area than for institutionalized persons, or school children.

Another major problem is that some community living skills have received a disproportionate amount of attention. For example, the number of studies on socially appropriate play skills is sparse, whereas coin summation has been studied in an extensive fashion. Establishing priorities for future treatment research and conducting studies designed to assess which skills are most necessary for community adjustment should be emphasized by future researchers. Hopefully, with the increased emphasis on promoting community placement of the mentally retarded, the development of behavior modification procedures necessary to improve community adjustment skills will attract greater attention from behavioral researchers.

REFERENCES

AANES, D., & HAAGENSON, L. Normalization: Attention to a conceptual disaster. *Mental Retardation*, 1978, *16*, 55–56.

ABRAMSON, E. E., & WUNDERLICK, R. A. Dental hygiene training for retardates: An application of behavioral techniques. *Mental Retardation*, 1972, *10*, 6–8.

BANDURA, A. Principles of behavior modification. New York: Holt, Rinehart, & Winston, 1969.

BELLAMY, T., & BUTTARS, K. L. Teaching trainable level retarded students to count money: Toward personal independence through academic instructions. *Education and Training of the Mentally Retarded*, 1975, *10*, 18–26.

BORAKOVE, L. S., & CUVO, A. J. Facilitative effects of coin displacement on teaching coin summation to mentally retarded adolescents. *American Journal of Mental Deficiency*, 1976, *81*, 350–356.

BRICKEY, M. A behavioral procedure for teaching self-medication. *Mental Retardation*, 1978, *16*, 29–32.

BUNDSCHUH, E. L., WILLIAMS, C. W., HOLLINGSWORTH, J. D., GOOCH, S., & SHIRER, C. Teaching the retarded to swin. *Mental Retardation*, 1972, *10*, 14–17.

CHENEY, H. G., KLUFT, G., & LEVICKI, G. A. Dental students' educational program for mentally handicapped children. *Mental Retardation*, 1974, *12*, 54–55.

CRONIN, K., & CUVO, A. J. Teaching mending skills to mentally retarded adolescents. *Journal of Applied Behavior Analysis*, 1979, *12*, 401-406.

CUVO, A. J., VEITCH, V. D., TRACE, M. W., & KONKE, J. L. Teaching change computation to the mentally retarded. *Behavior Modification*, 1978, *2*, 531–548.

DICKS, J. L. Cooperation of the mentally retarded child during dental procedures with some associated variables. *Mental Retardation*, 1975, *13*, 78.

EDGERTON, R. B. *The look of competence: Stigma in the lives of the mentally retarded*. Berkeley: University of California Press, 1967.

FREEDMAN, D. The retarded citizen and the law. In C. Cherington & G. Dybwad (Eds.). *The retarded citizen in quest of a home*, Washington, D. C.: Department of Health, Education, and Welfare, Publication No. (OHD) 74-21004, 1974.

GARCIA, E. The training and generalization of a conversational speech form in nonverbal retardates. *Journal of Applied Behavior Analysis*, 1974, *7*, 137–149.

GIBSON, F. W., LAWRENCE, P. S., & NELSON, R. O. Comparison of three training procedures for teaching social responses to developmentally disabled adults. *American Journal of Mental Deficiency*, 1976, *81*, 379–387.

GINZBURG, H. C. Editorial. *The British Journal of Mental Subnormality*, 1979, *25*, 1–4.

GROSSMAN, H. J. *Manual on terminology and classification in mental retardation*. Washington, D. C.: American Association on Mental Deficiency, 1977.

HORNER, D. R., & KEILITZ, I. Training mentally retarded adolescents to brush their teeth. *Journal of Applied Behavior Analysis*, 1975, *8*, 301–309.

JACKSON, D. A., & WALLACE, F. R. The modification and generalization of voice loudness in a fifteen-year-old retarded girl. *Journal of Applied Behavior Analysis*, 1974, *7*, 461–471.

JOACHIM, R. The use of self-monitoring to effect weight loss in a mildly retarded female. *Journal of Behavior Therapy and Experimental Psychiatry*, 1977, *8*, 213–215.

JOACHIM, R., & KORBOOT, P. Experimenter contact and self-monitoring of weight with the mentally retarded. *Australian Journal of Mental Retardation*, 1975, *3*, 222–225.

JOHNSON, M. M., & BAILEY, J. S. Modification of leisure behavior in a halfway house for retarded women. *Journal of Applied Behavioral Analysis*, 1977, *10*, 273–282.

KATZ, S., & YEKUTIEL, E. Leisure time problems of mentally retarded graduates of training programs. *Mental Retardation*, 1974, *12*, 54–57.

KINDRED, M. *The mentally retarded citizen and the law*. Washington, D. C.: The President's Committee on Mental Retardation, 1976.

LEE, D. Y. Evaluation of a group counseling program designed to enhance social adjustment of mentally retarded adults. *Journal of Counseling Psychology*, 1977, *24*, 318–323.

LEFF, R. B. Teaching the TMR to dial the telephone. *Mental Retardation*, 1974, *12*, 12–13.

LEFF, R. B. Teaching TMR children and adults to dial the telephone. *Mental Retardation*, 1975, *13*, 9–11.

LOWE, M. L., & CUVO, A. J. Teaching coin summation to the mentally retarded. *Journal of Applied Behavior Analysis*, 1976, *9*, 81–87.

LUCKEY, R. E., & SHAPIRO, I. G. Recreation: An essential aspect of habilitative programming. *Mental Retardation*, 1974, *12*, 33–35.

MATSON, J. L. Training socially appropriate behaviors to moderately retarded adults with contingent praise, instructions, feedback and a modified self-recording procedure. *Scandinavian Journal of Behavior Therapy*, 1978, *7*, 167–175.

MATSON, J. L. Decreasing inappropriate verbalizations of a moderately retarded adult by a staff assisted self-control program. *Australian Journal of Mental Retardation*, 1979, *5*, 242–245.

MATSON, J. L. A controlled group study of pedestrian skill training for the mentally retarded. *Behavior Research and Therapy*, 1980, *18*, 99–106.
MATSON, J. L. Preventing home accidents: A training program for the retarded. *Behavior Modification*, 1980, *4*, 397–410.
MATSON, J. L., & EARNHART, T. An analysis of the effects of self-monitoring on institutionalized retarded adults. *Behavior Modification*, 1981, *5*,27–38.
MATSON, J. L., & MARCHETTI, A. A comparison of leisure skills training procedures for the mentally retarded. *Applied Research in Mental Retardation*, 1980, *1*, 113–122.
MATSON, J. L., & STEPHENS, R. M. Increasing appropriate behavior of explosive chronic psychiatric patients with a social skills training package. *Behavior Modification*, 1978, *2*, 61–65.
MATSON, J. L., & ZEISS, R. A. Group training of social skills in chronically explosive, severely disturbed psychiatric patients. *Behavior Engineering*, 1978, *5*, 41–51.
MATSON, J. L., & ZEISS, R. A. The buddy system: A method of generalized reduction of inappropriate interpersonal behaviors of retarded-psychiatric patients. *British Journal of Social and Clinical Psychology*, 1979, *18*, 401–405.
MATSON, J. L., ZEISS, R. A., ZEISS, T., & BOWMAN, W. A. A comparison of social skills training and contingent attention to improve behavioral deficits of chronic psychiatric patients. *British Journal of Social and Clinical Psychology*, 1980, *19*, 57–64.
MCCARVER, R. B., & CRAIG, E. M. Placement of the retarded in the community: Prognosis and outcome. In N. R. Ellis (Ed.), *International review of research in mental retardation* (Vol. 7). New York: Academic, 1974.
MCFARLANE, J., & HAMES, C. Children with diabetes: Learning self-care in camp. *American Journal of Nursing*, 1973, *73*, 1362–1365.
MILLER, M. A., CUVO, A. J., & BORAKOVE, L. S. Teaching naming of coin values: Comprehension before production vs. production alone. *Journal of Applied Behavior Analysis*, 1977, *10*, 735–736.
NEEF, N. A., IWATA, B., & PAGE, T. Public transportation training: In vivo versus classroom instruction. *Journal of Applied Behavior Analysis*, 1978, *11*, 331–344.
NELSON, R. O., GIBSON, F., & CUTTING, D. S. Video taped modeling: The development of three appropriate social responses in a mildly retarded child. *Mental Retardation*, 1973, *11*, 24–28.
NETTLEBECK, T., & KIRBY, N. H. Training the mentally handicapped to sew. *Education and Training of the Mentally Retarded*, 1976, *11*, 31–36.
NIHIRA, L., & NIHIRA, K. Normalized behavior in community placement. *Mental Retardation*, 1975, *13*, 9–13. (a)
NIHIRA, L., & NIHIRA, K. Jeopardy in community placement. *American Journal of Mental Deficiency*, 1975, *79*, 538–544. (b)
O'BRIEN, J. G. *Death by ounces*. Hartford, Conn.: Travelers Insurance Company (Voices in Society Series), 1972.
PAGE, T. J., IWATA, B. A., & NEEF, N. A. Teaching pedestrian skills to retarded persons: Generalization from the classroom to the natural environment. *Journal of Applied Behavior Analysis*, 1976, *9*, 433–444.
RISLEY, R., & CUVO, A. J. Training mentally retarded adults to make emergency telephone calls. *Behavior Modification*, 1980, *4*, 513–526.
ROSS, S. A. Effects of intentional training in social behavior on retarded children. *American Journal of Mental Deficiency*, 1969, *73*, 912–919.
SAUNDERS, R. H. Take a giant step to independent living: Adaptive toothbrushing. *Teaching Exceptional Children*, 1976, *9*, 7.
SAUNDERS, R. M. Presentability as a goal for work activities clients. *Vocational Evaluation and Work Adjustment Bulletin*, 1978, *9*, 15–19.

SENGSTOCK, W. L., & STEIN, J. U. Recreation for the mentally retarded: A summary of major activities. *Exceptional Children*, 1967, 491-497.

SMEETS, P. M. Teaching retarded adults monetary skills using an experimental calculator. *Behavioral Engineering*, 1978, *5*, 51–59.

SPRADLIN, J. E., COTTER, J. W., STEVENS, C., & FRIEDMAN, M. Performance of mentally retarded children in pre-arithmetic tasks. *American Journal of Mental Deficiency*, 1974, *78*, 397-403.

STOKES, T. F., BAER, D. M., & JACKSON, R. L. Programming the generalization of a greeting response in four retarded children. *Journal of Applied Behavior Analysis*, 1974, *7*, 599–610.

TRACE, M. W., CUVO, A. J., & CRISWELL, J. L. Teaching coin equivalence to the mentally retarded. *Journal of Applied Behavior Analysis*, 1977, *10*, 85–92.

TWARDOSZ, S., & BAER, D. M. Training two severely retarded adolescents to ask questions. *Journal of Applied Behavior Analysis*, 1973, *6*, 655–661.

TURNER, S. M., HERSEN, M., & BELLACK, A. S. Use of social skills training to teach prosocial behaviors in an organically impaired and retarded patient. *Journal of Behavior Therapy and Experimental Psychiatry*, 1978, *9*, 253-258.

WEHMAN, P. C., & RETTIE, C. Increasing actions on play materials by severely retarded women through social reinforcement. *Therapeutic Recreation Journal*, 1975, *9*, 173–178.

WHITMAN, T. L., MERCURIO, J. R., & CAPONIGRI, V. Development of social responses in two severely retarded children. *Journal of Applied Behavior Analysis*, 1970, *3*, 133–138.

WITT, P. A. A historical sketch of recreation for the mentally retarded. *Mental Retardation*, 1971, *9* (1), 50–53.

WOLFENSBERGER, W. *The principle of normalization in human services*. Washington, D. C.: National Institute on Mental Retardation, 1972.

WUNDERLICK, R. A. Programmed Instruction: Teaching coinage to retarded children. *Mental Retardation*, 1972, *10*, 21–23.

ZAHARIA, R. *Behavior modification and normalization: Process of checks and balances*. Paper presented at Region VII AAMD Conference, October, 1975.

8 Vocational and Social Work Behavior

An Evaluative Review

FRANK R. RUSCH AND RICHARD P. SCHUTZ

INTRODUCTION

A decade ago, a major milestone marking the reform of the human service delivery system for mentally retarded and other developmentally disabled persons was introduced—normalization (Nirje, 1969; Wolfensberger, 1972). The normalization principles has as its most rudimentary tenet the delivery of services in environs and under circumstances (contingencies) that are as culturally normal as possible. Today, interpretation of normalization includes enlarging the scope of programming for mentally retarded individuals to encompass the broad array of services, activities, and events that most nonhandicapped individuals have access to and benefit from.

State and federal statutes enacted during the past decade reflect the impact of the normalization principle. From the Rehabilitation Acts of 1973 (P.L. 93-112) and 1974 (P.L. 93-516), the trends of expanded services and the delivery of services to the more severely handicapped are apparent. Unfortunately, the continuum of services envisioned in ideology and legal mandates remains in its infancy. This state of affairs is particularly evident with services provided at the postsecondary level. Whitehead (1979) indicated that over 200,000 severely handicapped adults are being served by this nation's sheltered workshops, with 30 times that number not receiving appropriate services. Further, work activity centers serving the more severely disabled as "inconsequential producers" have grown by over 600% during the period between 1968 to 1977 (Whitehead, 1979). Unlike the provision of educational services to the school-age population, goals have re-

FRANK R. RUSCH AND RICHARD P. SCHUTZ • Department of Special Education, University of Illinois, Champaign, Illinois 61801.

mained too general, and few specific guidelines have been suggested for use by direct-service personnel serving adults.

Successful integration of persons into a community requires that each individual acquire community-relevant vocational and social survival skills (Schutz, Vogelsberg, & Rusch, 1980). This chapter reviews some extensions of a behavioral approach (Matson & Martin, 1979) to work-related vocational and social skills that has permeated the literature for over two decades. Throughout this chapter, clear references to work conducted in sheltered settings, such as workshops, and more natural, nonsheltered settings, such as restaurants, are made. The focus of this chapter is on all adults labeled mentally retarded. This chapter introduces the concept of survival skills as applied to vocational skills and social skills and includes discussion of such areas as discrimination learning, attention, production, and social interaction. This chapter also examines past efforts aimed at maintaining and generalizing work behavior, and concludes with a statement of the overall consumability of the work behavior research in relation to its internal and external validity.

SURVIVAL SKILLS: A MEASURE OF SOCIAL VALIDITY

Recently, Rusch (1979a) argued that vocational habilitation researchers should direct their efforts toward those behaviors having immediate social value. In contrast, over the past two decades these researchers have largely demonstrated that the mentally retarded adult can acquire production-oriented skills, such as pulling a plunger (Evans & Spradlin, 1966), folding boxes (Loos & Tizard, 1955), dropping marbles (Tramontana, 1972), stuffing envelopes (Brown & Pearce, 1970), and threading labels (Teasdale & Joynt, 1967). Although behavioral techniques have been applied to a wide range of treatment problems, target populations, and settings, the greater part of the work behavior literature has been directed toward training (Bellamy, Inman, & Yeates, 1978) and managing (Brown, Van Deventer, Perlmutter, Jones, & Sontag, 1972) task-production behavior in segregated, sheltered work settings. This approach ignores the behaviors that Rusch and Mithaug (1980) believe to contribute directly to a person's work adjustment: stated simply, if employer-required behavior patterns are not present, Rusch and Mithaug (1980) believe that mentally retarded persons will probably adjust poorly. Accepting this view, one could question the overall value of past, present, and future research efforts directed toward training and managing a single dimension of one's overall work adjustment—for example, the training and management of production-oriented tasks while ignoring potentially critically socially interactive behaviors. Obviously, as the principle of normalization is interpreted to include habilitative efforts in nonsheltered work settings, future research will need to be directed toward a wider range of work-related behaviors, such as conversing during breaks and working continuously during four separate two-hour periods daily.

Applied behavioral research focusing on problems related to integrating mentally retarded persons into the mainstream of society has been directed toward select problems of social value. Increasingly, a broad range of community-relevant, work-related behavior is being addressed by work behavior researchers (see reviews by Rusch & Schutz, 1979; Rusch, Schutz, & Heal, in press). Indeed, the selection of community-relevant problems for investigation is not new to the field of behavior analysis (Baer, Wolf, & Risley, 1968). Today, the technology of behavior analysis has developed to include new methods for evaluating problems of social import (Kazdin, 1977; Wolf, 1978) in such diverse areas as teaching mentally retarded persons to play board games (Wehman, Renzaglia, Berry, Schutz, & Karan, 1978), purchase color-coordinated clothing (Nutter & Reid, 1978), cross partially controlled intersections (Vogelsberg & Rusch, 1979), and ride a bus to and from work (Sowers, Rusch, & Hudson, 1979) and around the community (Marholin, O'Toole, Touchette, Berger, & Doyle, 1979). Applied to work behavior, this measure of social acceptability or social validation has entailed corroboration, by potential consumers, of the relevance of training goals (Rusch, Weithers, Menchetti, & Schutz, 1980), procedures (Schutz, Rusch, & Lamson, 1979), and results (Schutz, Jostes, Rusch, & Lamson, 1980).

The concept of *survival*, as articulated by Rusch (1979a), refers to behavior that is judged by potential consumers, e.g., employers, as acceptable and necessary for entrance into any given setting. In the context of employment, the survival skills concept entails corroboration by employers, supervisors, and co-workers of the goals, procedures, and results which will help others gain acceptance into their community, that is, into a specific work setting. The identification of these skills has been the subject of recent research in vocational (Nelson, 1977) and special (Mithaug & Hagmeier, 1978) education. These studies have focused on identifying the skills thought necessary for admittance into the work force. Given the complexity of work settings, this body of research has only partially delineated the list of social and vocational skills that could have survival value if acquired and maintained.

The process of identifying survival skills extends beyond accepting initial verbal reports and survey results which suggest that certain skills are more important than others. Two empirical methods to obtain these work-related measures of social validation have been outlined by Rusch and Mithaug (1980). The first, descriptive validation assessment, entails collecting job requirement data, as suggested by Nelson (1977) and Mithaug and Hagmeier (1978) from knowledgeable persons, such as employers, supervisors, co-workers and employees; the second, comparative validation assessment, requires that direct measures of acceptable behavior be obtained, also from these knowledgeable persons, in addition to the collection of descriptive data.

The primary difference between these measures is that descriptive measures are obtained primarily via verbal reports and surveys, whereas comparative measures are obtained through direct observation of behavior of persons comprising the normative sample. As mentioned above, investigators have recently reported efforts to obtain descriptive measures to guide their research. Mithaug and Hagmeier (1978) and Johnson and Mithaug (1978) sought to identify those skills which supervisors, from five northwestern states and Kansas, perceived as critical for entry into sheltered workshops. Ideally, consensus about the behavior patterns, both vocational and social, that would need to be acquired for entrance into certain settings would be a measure of validity that could be used in the undertaking of behavioral research and, ultimately, secondary-curricula development (Rusch, Rusch, Menchetti, & Schutz, in press). Mithaug and Hanawalt (1978) also utilized a measure of social acceptability to assess prevocational task preferences in severely mentally retarded young adults. Mithaug and Hanawalt (1978) presented six tasks, including: (1) sorting parts of a flour sifter; (2) placing inserts and envelopes into booklets; (3) folding/stapling/labeling written sheets and stuffing them into envelopes; (4) assembling components of a pulley; (5) assembling components of a flour sifter; and (6) attaching resistors to a circuit board. Each task required discrete behavioral responses, such as sorting, collating, stuffing, and assembling. These tasks were presented two at a time in all possible pairs—collate and stuff, collate and sort, and so on. These results led Mithaug and Hanawalt (1978) to suggest that nonverbal severely handicapped persons do have task preferences and that these preferences should be assessed to allow these persons a choice in selecting which task they would like to perform—an example of descriptive social validation.

A study incorporating comparative assessments has been reported by Rusch, Weithers, Menchetti, and Schutz (1980). They eliminated topic repetitions of one mentally retarded person employed as a kitchen laborer in a nonsheltered setting (a large mid-western dormitory kitchen). Supervisors and co-workers indicated that topic repetitions during lunch and break periods were excessive. Following a baseline measure of the frequency of topics discussed and repeated by both the employee and his co-workers, co-workers were instructed in the use of providing feedback. Results indicated that co-workers were effective in reducing topic repetition only when they were provided feedback by trained follow-up personnel. Data collected on the number of co-worker and employee topic repetitions (the comparative validation assessment) indicated that, following treatment, the mentally retarded employee repeated topics in a quantity equal to the number of topics repeated by co-workers. Of greater importance, however, was the finding that subsequent ratings by co-workers suggested that they believed that the employee did not reduce his repeats—a finding contrary to the direct, comparative-validation measure. Rusch *et al.* (1980) suggested that the measure used by co-workers may have comprised a broader definition than that used by the trained follow-up personnel, and/or that co-workers may have let repetitions during periods other than lunch and break influence their ratings.

Unquestionably, completing one's job is essential to successful work adjustment. However, there are other behaviors that will influence whether one maintains his or her job. Although much of the work behavior reported in the research literature has dealt with training new tasks and changing the rate at which these tasks are performed, a solid body of recent behavioral research has focused on other work-relevant behavior. This section has introduced the survival skills concept and examples of recent research efforts that have suggested methods to obtain a degree of social acceptability when addressing these skills. The concept of survival is an important one when considering mentally retarded persons and current efforts to integrate these individuals into the community. Logically, communities differ with respect to what is considered normal and acceptable. As intimated by Thurman and Fiorelli (1979), "normalcy is a local issue." Therefore, researchers must validate the behaviors that, when acquired, will increase the likelihood of survival in that community. Obtaining measures of social acceptability focuses applied research toward these standards for behavior (survival skills). Advancing the importance of social validation has led recent work behavior research to include descriptive and comparative validation assessments of goals, procedures, and results. The next section, vocational survival skills, further develops the survival skills concept.

VOCATIONAL SURVIVAL SKILLS

For the purposes of this chapter, *vocational survival skills* are defined as employee behaviors directed toward work tasks, such as mopping a floor, moving from one task to another, attending to a task. The term "survival" suggests that the presence of these skills increases the likelihood of entrance into the work force. In this section, four interrelated research areas are presented. The first area is a review of a body of literature focused on training mentally retarded persons to discriminate prominant characteristics of the task in order to promote skill acquisition. This line of inquiry has typically been referred to as discrimination learning. The purpose of reviewing this body of research is that discrimination-learning research, conducted primarily in analog settings throughout the 1960s, has influenced directly the questions posed by researchers throughout the 1970s. Following this review of discrimination-learning research is an overview of studies focused on attentional variables and the relationship between completion of one's job and the amount of time spent attending to task. The third area reviewed is production. Production, in the context of work behavior research, has referred largely to completing a task. Included in the production research is an overview of the traditional line of investigation in sheltered settings and recent research in nonsheltered settings. Finally, this section concludes with a brief overview of research on related vocational survival skills.

Discrimination Learning

Discrimination learning, in general, has stimulated a great deal of research; as early as 1904, Kuhlman indicated that mentally retarded children had difficulty in matching dominoes according to the number of spots. Almost 50 years later, a group of studies on discrimination learning with mentally retarded children was begun by House and Zeaman and their associates. Their work sought to demonstrate the importance of one's attention being directed to relevant dimensions of the stimuli to be discriminated. Further, this line of inquiry suggested that procedures which influence the probability of attending to the relevant dimensions will enhance problem-solving efficiency. Most notable from their earlier work was a study showing that mentally retarded persons with mental ages of 2–4 learned substantially more slowly than 2- to 4-year-old normal children (House & Zeaman, 1958a). This study involved the discrimination of stimulus forms differing in both shape and color (e.g., red triangle vs. black cross). Candy was placed in a dispenser directly below either of the two stimulus forms in random order. The task involved the selection of the stimuli with associated candy during 25 massed trials daily until the criterion of 20 correct out of 25 was attained. Results showed that the 10 subjects elicited approximately 25 times more errors than the matched nonhuman subjects (119 for the mentally retarded subjects as compared with 4 for the monkeys).

These results were questioned because it was not clear that the candy was a reinforcer. Therefore, a second study was conducted (Zeaman, House, & Orlando, 1958) with the same subjects. They were presented a simple "junk" stimulus that differed multidimensionally. "Junk stimuli" refer to objects which differ along many relevant dimensions (e.g., a toy versus a hair brush) compared to objects that differ on a single dimension (e.g., red and green circles). Seven of the eight subjects in this study learned the discrimination between the "junk" stimuli but again failed to make the color/form discrimination. These results suggested that the subjects were motivated enough to learn and that "catching on to the game" could not reasonably be used as an explanation of the original results.

House, Zeaman, Orlando, and Fisher (1957) later included a larger sample of mentally retarded children with essentially the same problem. The findings of this particular study and another conducted soon thereafter (House & Zeaman, 1958b) suggested that IQ was correlated significantly with errors, positing a low IQ deficit in discrimination learning. In this second study, however, a group of mentally retarded children with estimated mental ages of 5 to 6 years learned as rapidly as the matched normal group. This led Zeaman and House to suggest that a low IQ discrimination-learning deficit appeared most pronounced at an IQ level of 50 and below.

Although the data presented by Zeaman and colleagues suggested a relation between IQ and discriminatory learning, other research has been either contradictory or different in relation to IQ level. Most notable are additional studies that have shown little or no difference between mentally retarded and normal subjects matched for mental age (Plenderleith & Postman 1956; Stevenson, 1960; Sevenson & Ziegler, 1957). Research by Girardeau (1959) and O'Connor and Hermelin (1959) indicated a different IQ cutoff from that posed by Zeaman and House. Girardeau, for example, suggested that discrimination learning differed significantly at the IQ level of 40 for 10 "mongoloids" matched for mental age with a normal population.

Zeaman and House (1963) ultimately demonstrated the importance of the subjects' attention being directed toward the relevant stimuli to be discriminated. These results were achieved by determining that there was a characteristic difference in the acquisition phase of learning for mentally retarded children when compared with normal children; but once the mentally retarded population began making the discrimination, the learning curve was very similar to that of a normal population. Inspecting the flat portion of the acquisition phase led Zeaman and House to hypothesize that the process influencing its length was attentional in nature (Zeaman, 1965). They suggested that the mentally retarded child must attend to the relevant dimension (e.g., size) and then determine which stimulus (e.g., large) along that dimension is or was correct. In essence, until the child attends to the relevant dimension he or she will be unable to make the necessary discrimination(s). Finally, it was shown that procedures that influence the probability of the child's attending to the relevant dimension would increase problem-solving proficiency (Heal, Bransky, & Mankinen, 1966).

Since the development of Zeaman and House's attention theory, eight separate areas of research on attention and acquisition have emerged: redundancy (Gold, 1972; Zeaman, 1968), irrelevant cues (Zeaman, 1965); fading (Moore & Goldiamond, 1964; Terrace, 1966), clustering (Bousfield, 1953), overlearning (Belmont, 1966), easy-to-hard sequencing (House & Zeaman, 1960; Zeaman & House, 1963), set failing (Zeaman, 1965), and adding and reducing large cue differences (Irvin & Bellamy, 1977). Because most of these studies occurred in analog settings, only those by Gold (1972; 1974), Gold and Barclay (1973a; 1973b), Irvin (1976), Irvin and Bellamy (1977), and Close, Irvin, Prehm, and Taylor (1978) will be reviewed to exemplify the recent development of discrimination research.

Among those investigators focusing upon attentional variables, Gold (1969) reported the first study using the attention theory of Zeaman and House in an applied setting with mentally retarded subjects. Sixty-four subjects with an average IQ of 47 from four sheltered workshops learned to assemble 15-piece and 24-piece bicycle brakes. Half the subjects learned to assemble a 15-piece bicycle brake attending to form only, while the other half learned to assemble a 15-piece bicycle brake attending to form and color. Color constituted a cue redundancy. Redundancy referred to the use of color as a relevant dimension across all parts (form) of the 15-piece bicycle brake. Later, all subjects were taught with color as the relevant dimension across the 24-piece brake assembly. Results indicated that the group provided with cue redundancy (color coding) on the 15-piece bicycle brake learned the task in an average of 17 trials, as opposed to 33 trials for the group working with the form dimension only. On the 24-piece bicycle brake all subjects learned to make the bicycle brake in an average of 22 trials.

Additional research by Gold and Barclay (1973a,b) demonstrated that mentally retarded adolescents and adults can be taught to make visual discriminations necessary to assemble 15- and 24-piece bicycle brakes. Gold and Barclay (1973a) studied the effects of verbal labels on acquisition and retention of an assembly task. Sixteen moderately and severely mentally retarded subjects were randomly selected from a work activity program. The procedures tried in this investigation were similar to those of Gold (1972). One group received specific verbal cues, such as "The square goes up," and a second group was told simply, "Try another way." It was found that specific verbal cues were more effective than general ones. Further, both groups required less time to learn a similar task, that is, a 24-piece bicycle brake versus a 15-piece bicycle brake. In a second study, Gold and Barclay (1973b) taught 16 adolescents and adults (mean IQ = 58) to sort bolts differing in size. This easy-to-hard discrimination involved sorting four separate bolt lengths. These were 1½ in., 1 in., ⅞ in., and ¾ in. Subjects were assigned to a "hard" or "easy" group. Subject were then provided one-to-one instruction and allowed 750 trials to reach criterion (sorting one pile of 50 bolts without any errors). The "easy" group learned the task when required to sort 1½-in. and ¾-in. bolts, followed by 1-in. and ¾-in, and 1-in. and ⅞-in bolts. The "hard" group did not learn the task of sorting 1-in. and ⅞-in. bolts until they, too, were taught on the 1½-in. and ¾-in. bolts.

In a more recent study, Gold (1974) attempted to train 36 mildly and moderately mentally retarded adolescents and adults selected from a sheltered workshop to assemble a 12-unit coaster brake. The purpose of this study was to investigate the effects of three fading procedures after the task had been learned. The fading procedures consisted of training to criterion on color coded brakes, then switching to non-color-coded brakes and back to training on color-coded brakes until criterion had been reached for three consecutive days. Then the trainer withdrew the color-coded brakes until subjects failed to assemble the non-color-coded brakes for three consecutive trials, at which time subjects were returned to color-coded brakes. Finally, training on color-coded brakes first, and then, when criterion was reached, switching to non-color-coded brakes, was tried. If an error occurred in this final fading attempt, the subject making the error was forced to make a correction involving no color code. No significant difference among the three approaches to fading was found.

Additional research by Irvin (1976) and Irvin and Bellamy (1977) sought to clarify those dimensions that facilitated discrimination of difficult assembly tasks. Irvin (1976) studied the easy-to-hard training procedure applied to 24 moderately and severely mentally retarded adults residing in a state hospital. The task involved learning the discriminations required to assemble lock nuts and bicycle axle posts. In a pilot investigation it was established that these subjects would not learn the task via differential reinforcement alone. Subsequently, all subjects were exposed to four phases of training requiring successively more difficult discriminations. The four phases involved discriminations to be made between a lock nut with a flat face and lock nuts raised 45 cm (phase 1), 30 cm (phase 2), 20 cm (phase 3), and 10 cm (phase 4). Subjects were permitted 700 trials across each of the four training phases. Of the original 24 subjects, 17 learned the discrimination within the 700 trial allotments. Irvin concluded that stimulus control should be established as soon as possible to eliminate trial-and-error learning in the initial stages of acquisition.

In a subsequent investigation, Irvin and Bellamy (1977) assessed the effects of three strategies to promote discrimination learning. They consisted of (1) adding and reducing large cue differences on the relevant shape dimension, (2) adding and fading redundant color dimensions, and (3) combining the two strategies, that is, simultaneous presentation of fading the high salience, redundant color dimension and the large cue differences on the relevant stimulus dimension. Fifty-one severely mentally retarded adults with no visual or physical handicaps were selected from a state institution and randomly assigned to one of three training groups. The criterion task was assembly of a bicycle axle nut and post. Results of this investigation suggested that the combined method produced the most efficient learning. This technique was the most efficient for learning and was found to be sufficiently powerful to train visual discrimination.

Finally, Close *et al.* (1978) assessed the effects of a training strategy applied *after* a discrimination error had been made. This effort is different from those reported above, as each of the studies noted to this point has been directed to antecedent events as necessary conditions to promote or set the occasion for learning. Close *et al.* (1978) employed 70 severely mentally retarded adults randomly selected from two private residential facilities. These adults were then randomly assigned to one of six experimental conditions. Similar to Gold (1972) they utilized general ("try another way") and specific ("flat side in") verbal cues. Subjects were provided either a cue and a gesture, a physical prompt, or repeated practice. The use of repeated practice resulted in significantly less acquisition time, as compared to gestures or prompts. Also, no differences were found between the general and the specific verbal cue.

In this section, several articles addressing discrimination learning have been reviewed. The early work of Gold and Barclay (Gold, 1972; Gold & Barclay, 1973a,b) demonstrated that mildly and moderately mentally retarded adolescents and adults could learn assembly tasks representative of behavior upon which remuneration is based in sheltered workshops. However, each of these studies suffers major methodological weaknesses. For example, in Gold's work the training procedures were contrived and appear limited in general application. Also, the failure to control for practice, history, and sequence effects, and the failure to incorporate checks on whether data reported were reliable, limit interpretation and replication. The general interest in applying a theory from the basic learning research of Zeaman and House, in Gold's work and in subsequent efforts by Irvin (1976) and Irvin and Bellamy (1977), may have prolonged the investigation of stimulus manipulations and types of dimensional shifts; perhaps at the cost of not investigating more basic training procedures that could have suggested methods to employ to arrange environments so that people with lower IQs can become competent members of a community (Brooks & Baumeister, 1977).

The practicality of designing stimulus feature changes to accentuate relevant stimulus characteristics, and fading the added stimulus features as soon as the subject (worker) responds reliably and correctly, appears questionable. A similar problem is evident with the generality of the results in each of the stimulus-manipulation articles reviewed. None of the techniques presented by discrimination-learning researchers worked for all subjects. Perhaps a more promising area of research is the work of Close *et al.* (1978). Their training procedures incorporated verbal cues, gestures, prompts, and, in some cases, repeated practice requiring little in the way of material adaptation. The repeated-practice component was found to be most effective. Referring back to the original discrimination-learning work of Zeaman and House and the eventual development of the "attention theory," one could speculate that the provision of more trials per session on the difficult discrimination may reduce the length of the acquisition period.

Attention

Few studies have reported improvement in performance as a result of direct reinforcement of attending. Conceptually, problems of acquisition have been addressed through manipulation of antecedent events, whereas problems of rate of response have been addressed by manipulating consequent events. The distinction is important, because most vocational habilitation literature is distinguished by efforts directed toward training (acquisition) or producing (rate of responding) tasks. Several studies have suggested a relationship between attention and production. For example, Cohen and Close (1975) reported that adults who spent less time attending to the task also produced more slowly. The results suggested the hypothesis that measures of actual time spent attending related to individual differences in performance.

A recent investigation reported by Jackson (1979) extended Cohen and Close's work. Jackson found that the rate at which one mentally retarded adult cut chain links was increased substantially by differentially reinforcing attending to task behavior. The differential-reinforcement procedure included a component for visual feedback via a light. The light served as a stimulus occasioning the opportunity for reinforcement (the reinforcer consisted of money). Results of this investigation suggested that directly reinforcing attending behaviors results in performance gains.

Rusch (1979b) also reported a relationship between attending to task and production. Six mentally retarded adult males were randomly assigned to two experimental groups and treated in multiple-baseline fashion. Group one received reinforcement for speed of task completion, and group two received reinforcement for time spent attending to task. Subjects who spent more time completing tasks (worked slower) also spent an appreciable percentage of their time attending to the task. The task included 15 separate responses necessary to clean and wipe tables in a restaurant setting. Results of this investigation unequivocally supported the point that when subjects did not attend to task, without exception they did not complete the work. Directly reinforcing speed of task completion resulted in speedier task completion and increased time spent attending to task.

The results reported by Cohen and Close (1975), Jackson (1979) and Rusch (1979b) point to a relationship between attention and production. Further, Rusch (1979b) suggested that contingencies applied to attending or producing result in considerable improvements in collateral measures. Determining which measure, when treated, would be the more economical to address, however, was only conservatively approached in the Rusch study. Rusch (1979b) confirmed that to produce one needs to attend, and inversely implied that attending does not necessarily lead to production, suggesting that both measures are crucial.

Several studies have reported efforts to increase time spent on task. For the most part, these investigations have sought to increase on-task behavior while measuring a second, incompatible behavior. Mithaug (1978a) employed such a strategy with a 20-year-old severely mentally retarded young man. Following inappropriate laughing, time-out was given, whereas time spent on task (attending) was reinforced with chips and juice, resulting in a decrease in the rate of laughing and an increase of time on task, respectively.

Production

The most popular line of inquiry represented in the vocational habilitation literature, to date, is production training conducted primarily in sheltered vocational settings. These production studies have largely addressed the acquisition of specific job skills *and* the improvement of skills performed. The majority of the research specifically addressing acquisition training has been aimed at demonstrating that mentally retarded individuals can acquire a variety of potentially remunerative vocational skills, involving long skill sequences once considered far too complex for them to learn. For example, mentally retarded persons have been trained to perform skill sequences such as the assembly of cable harnesses (Hunter & Bellamy, 1976) and saw chains (O'Neill & Bellamy, 1978). Much of this research has employed task analysis in which the skill to be trained is broken down into discrete components (Crosson, 1969; Gold, 1972; Mithaug, 1979). Efforts are then directed toward sequencing individual responses in a fashion that is appropriate for completing each of these separate steps. Procedures employed to facilitate response sequencing have included verbal instructions paired with modeling (Bellamy, Peterson, & Close, 1975; Clarke & Heremelin, 1955), priming responses and physical guidance (Williams, 1967), positive practice (Wehman, Schutz, Renzaglia, & Karan, 1977), cue redundancy (Gold, 1974; Renzaglia, Wehman, Schutz, & Karan, 1978), and easy-to-hard task sequencing (Gold & Barclay, 1973b; Irvin, 1976).

Vocational habilitation research concerned with the improvement of task performance, or with increased production rates, has included utilizing a more efficient approach to better perform a task or better design a work station (Martin & Flexer, 1975) and strengthening reinforcing contingencies to increase production rates (Crosson, 1969; Huddle, 1967; Zimmerman, Stucky, Garlick, & Miller, 1969). Performance-oriented studies have also examined the improvement found with task analysis (Gold, 1972) and the effectiveness of a variety of positive consequences, such as money (Schroeder, 1972a), music (Cotter, 1971), and choice of work assignment (Zimmerman, Overpeck, Eisenberg, & Garlick, 1969). Other studies have investigated verbal prompts to work faster (Bellamy, Peterson, & Close, 1975; Loos & Tizard, 1955), peer modeling (Brown & Pearce, 1970; Kliebhahn, 1967), and the manipulation of schedules of reinforcement (Schroeder, 1972a). Recent research has also demonstrated that mentally retarded persons can be instructed to decrease interfering behaviors which distract coworkers (Mithaug, 1978a; Schutz, Wehman, Renzaglia, & Karan, 1978). Collectively, this area of work behavior research suggests that even severely mentally retarded persons can acquire vocational skills associated with success in sheltered settings. These studies also indicate that the mentally retarded adult need not be made to perform simple tasks which are not particularly useful to society, such as collating paper. This research further suggests that intelligence levels, learning characteristics, and many standardized vocational evaluation tests are not valid predictors of work potential (Bellamy, Horner, & Inman, 1979; Brolin, 1976).

A recent trend in the vocational habilitation literature is the investigation of procedures which may facilitate the entry of mentally retarded adults into nonsheltered, competitive employment. Similar to studies conducted in sheltered settings, this research has addressed task production issues. Specifically, this area of inquiry has focused on the acquisition and performance of tasks associated with various service occupations, such as janitor (Cuvo, Leaf, & Borakove, 1978), kitchen laborer (Sowers, Thompson, & Connis, 1979), and elevator operator (Wehman, Hill, & Koehler, 1979). For example, continuous effort on designated tasks throughout the entire work day (Rusch, Connis, & Sowers, 1979) and speed of task completion have been trained in nonsheltered settings (Rusch, 1979b).

Different from sheltered-oriented vocational research, competitive-employment-training studies appear to reflect a more comprehensive view of an individual's functioning in relation to environmental demands. Although research efforts have attended to production issues, programmatic efforts have attempted to expand beyond treating single dimensions of behavior to include a broader set of applied issues. For example, several researchers have incorporated maintenance and generalization procedures within the total training package (i.e., Cuvo *et al.*, 1978; Rusch *et al.*, 1979; Schutz *et al.*, 1979). As stated previously, researchers have also incorporated consumers, that is, potential employers, in the habilitative effort to measure the social acceptability of training goals (Rusch, Weithers, Menchetti, & Schutz, 1980), procedures (Schutz *et al.*, 1979) and results (Schutz, Jostes, Rusch, & Lamson, 1980). Finally, training efforts have attempted to address behaviors in addition to task completion, such as topic repetition (Rusch, Weithers, Menchetti, &

Schutz, 1980), time management (Connis, 1979; Sowers, Rusch, Connis, & Cummings, 1980), and appropriate responding to requests by supervisors (Rusch & Menchetti, in press). (Each of these topics will be developed in ensuing sections on social survival skills and maintenance and generalization).

Other Related Work Behaviors

Historically, researchers have focused on the specific factors that influence the employability of mentally retarded persons, vocational evaluation and prediction, and the modification of rates of existing behaviors, that is, increasing productivity (Rusch, Schutz, & Heal, in press). Interestingly, we enter the 1980s with little consensus among researchers concerning correlates of success in work settings, with evaluation and prediction results that generally lack practical significance, and with gross differences between accumulated research results and actual practice in work settings serving mentally retarded persons. Fortunately, studies do show that mentally retarded adults can make successful adjustments in the community and acquire employment. For example, recent articles have suggested that mentally retarded adults can acquire gleaning jobs (Jacobs, 1976, 1978) and jobs as porters (Tomasulo, 1976). Stewart (1977) has also suggested viable training areas for mentally retarded people, including clerical, service stations, and upholstery-related occupations based on a survey of community employers. For the most part, however, a thorough review of the work-related research will point out that investigators have conducted most of their work along a very limited range of vocational skills, in an even narrower range of settings.

One additional area of research that has been reported is the reduction of social behavior incompatible with completion of designated vocational skills. Two recent reports, by Mithaug and Hanawalt (1978) and Mithaug (1978a), exemplify this line of inquiry. Mithaug and Hanawalt (1978) used negative reinforcement to control the aggressive behavior of a severely mentally retarded adolescent in a prevocational secondary classroom. Finger pressure on the inside of the upper biceps area was employed to increase collating work responses. The finger pressure was terminated contingent on the subject's touching the cover of a booklet to begin the collating task. Compared to tapping on the subject's hand to prompt initiating the task and repeating a verbal cue while ignoring aggressive responses, the negative reinforcement procedure not only increased collating rate but also resulted in decreasing and eliminating self-biting and hitting the experimenter. This procedure also promoted increased collating rate and decreased self-biting and hiting when applied by a teacher aide at a different time in the day.

Mithaug (1978a) reported a series of case studies in the management of inappropriate behaviors. These case studies focused on the simultaneous pursuit of skill training and behavior management. The four case studies presented such problem behaviors as excessive out-of-seat and running behaviors, incessant and irrelevant verbal behavior, screaming and shrieking, excessive hysterical laughing, refusal to work, biting, pinching, tantruming, and general noncompliance. The procedures used to reduce these behaviors included shaping, differential reinforcement, ignoring, time-out, and negative reinforcement. The results obtained supported the conclusion drawn by Mithaug (1979a) that a single universal management tactic was not effective for all behaviors across all subjects. Mithaug did argue that "a degree of success in controlling and ultimately eliminating disruptive behaviors was a function of the clients' increased correct responding to instructional task" (p. 143). This concurrent strategy suggests that direct service staff avoid the negative atmosphere created by eliminating inappropriate responding before actual skill training is undertaken.

SOCIAL SURVIVAL SKILLS

Social survival skills refers to behavior of workers that influences the behavior of co-workers. Therefore, social survival skills differ from vocational survival skills in that they refer to interactions between people. One area of investigation reviewed in this section is that of research concerned with improving social interactions between and among co-workers. Although considerable discussion has focused on the overwhelming value of appropriate social behavior, there is a remarkable dearth of available research addressing this class of behavior. The few reports available are directed toward social interactions and critical language functions. Necessarily, this section provides some areas of research that, from the authors' perspective, could have considerable impact on service delivery and, therefore, would appear to be critical areas for future research.

Social Interactions

The ability to exchange information, question positions presented by others, initiate interactions, and continue discussions with co-workers are but a few of the many skills American workers possess. The inability to inter act socially with co-workers on the job will restrict the successful work adjustment of many mentally retarded persons. The use of behavioral techniques such as training co-workers to repeat topics less often (Rusch, Weithers, Menchetti, & Schutz, 1980), administer reinforcement to increase the frequency of interaction (Kazdin & Polster, 1973), and procedures to increase compliant responding (Rusch & Menchetti, in press) are recent innovations.

Kazdin and Polster (1973) increased the social interactions of two mentally retarded adult males in a sheltered workshop setting. Verbal reports were made by the two subjects to the supervisor after each break. Subsequently, the supervisor verified these verbal reports with other clients whose names were mentioned by the two target subjects as persons they interacted with. Tokens were given to the two target subjects for each verified report. A one-token fine was imposed for false reporting, (i.e., telling the supervisor he talked with another person when he did not). Token reinforcement resulted in considerable interaction in comparison with conditions where tokens were not administered. The overall value of this study rests largely on the behaviors targeted, that is, social interactions and efforts to assess response maintenance. This second aspect of the Kazdin and Polster (1973) investigation, maintenance, is detailed in the maintenance and transfer of training section of this chapter.

Rusch and Menchetti (in press) trained a single employee to respond to requests to comply made by supervisors, fellow kitchen laborers, and cooks. In this investigation, the subject was told that he would be "fired for a day" (sent home) if he failed to comply with supervisors and fellow kitchen laborers. During baseline measures the subject grimaced, exchanged abrupt language, or failed to comply altogether. Following warnings and brief practice session on how to respond, the subject complied and interacted appropriately with the requester. After two weeks of compliance and positive social interactions, the subject was fired for one day for negative interactions (yelling several times while complying with the request). Interestingly, after he returned to work positive interactions with supervisors, fellow kitchen laborers, and a third, untreated group of co-workers (cooks), continued.

Finally, Dwinell and Connis (1979) sought to increase the appropriate social interactions of one mentally retarded adult when contingencies were applied to decreasing inappropriate social interactions. The introduction of praise, instructions, and reprimands resulted in the reduction and near elimination of select inappropriate verbal behavior directed toward an experimenter, with concurrent increases in acceptable responses. Conclusions drawn suggested that moderately mentally retarded adults can make complex discriminations regarding their verbal behavior and, therefore, can be effectively trained to interact appropriately in a normal environment—a conclusion supported by the research of Rusch, Weithers, Menchetti, and Schutz (1980), Polster (1973), and Rusch and Menchetti (in press).

Following Directions

For many mentally retarded persons, one of the most critical language functions is following directions. Unfortunately, few studies have addressed this aspect of work-related social behavior. Peripherally, Mithaug (1978b) addressed training generalized instruction-following responses to preposition-noun combinations by training one severely mentally retarded male to respond to instructional requests that included the prepositions "in," "on," "under," and "beside." Prior to combining these prepositions into multiple-work phrases, each preposition and a set of nouns were trained separately to develop appropriate discriminations. Following the training of discriminations between the four prepositions, four direct-object nouns and four prepositional object nouns, the subject was trained to respond to two-word combinations consisting of a direct object and a prepositional object. This initial training produced correct responses to untrained combinations of direct objects, prepositions, and prespositional objects. A second experiment evaluated instruction-following responses when irrelevant cues were added to three-word requests (i.e., "Put the ______ ______ the ______"). Also, pausing between the third and fourth words (i.e., "Put the ______ (pause) ______ the ______") was evaluated. Adding irrelevant cues resulted in a decrease in the subject's accuracy, but pausing resulted in increased accuracy. Mithaug (1978b) suggested that these results indicate "that generalization to new instructional forms may depend upon training in the appropriate responses to relevant and irrelevant verbal cues as well as to different styles of delivering the request" (p. 230).

One aspect of the Mithaug (1978b) investigation led Karlan and Rusch (in press) to investigate the correspondence between acknowledging a request and compliance. Mithaug (1979) indicated that pausing resulted in increased accurate instruction following responses. These increases were interpreted by Karlan and Rusch to be related to the experimenter's requiring a measure of acknowledgment. It is possible that the method of delivering the instructional cue, that is, the pause, and associated methods of measuring both the independent and the dependent variable resulted in increased attention to the instructional cue when pausing was used (Mithaug, 1978b). Perhaps, in Mithaug's study, the subject failed to interpret the intent of the instructional cue presented without a pause because the combination of words was presented before the subject had an opportunity to recognize that an instruction was forthcoming. In the instances of pausing, the initial three words may have served to gain the attention of the subject. Increasing the probability of attending to the experimenter increased the likelihood of correct responding. Karlan and Rusch (in press) required kitchen laborers competitively employed at a large midwestern university to acknowledge requests to perform tasks. The results of this study suggested that increased acknowledgment led to increased compliance.

Two recent studies have investigated instruction following behavior when verbal preinstructions were supplemented with correlated pictorial materials. Connis (1979) trained four mentally retarded adults to change tasks independently throughout a work day. Self-recording the completion of a task by marking below a picture displaying the task was tried in combination with daily preinstruction on the use of the recording forms and photographs. These instructional sessions included modeling appropriate use, inclusion of a rationale for correct use, and acknowledgment from each of the four subjects that they understood the procedure. It was found that the pictorial cues, self-recording procedures, and preinstruction were effective in increasing the criterion behavior.

Sowers, Rusch, Connis, and Cummings (1980) instructed three mentally retarded persons in the correct management of time during lunches and breaks. The combined procedures of preinstruction, a time card, and feedback, were effective in decreasing the number of inappopriate breaks. The time card was 5 × 7 in., with four clock faces drawn on it. Two clock faces were designed to depict the configuration of the clock when it was time to go to lunch or break, and the other two clock faces depicted the configuration for returning from lunch or break.

Future Areas of Social Survival Skills Research

Three areas of research related to social skills that could affect co-worker behavior are grooming and general oral hygiene, leisure, and conversational behaviors. The mentally retarded adult is oftentimes distinguished by his or her grooming, clothing, and general hygienic care. Few readers will dispute that people are distinguishable from others by the style, fit, and appropriate weather match of the clothes they wear. Further, general hygienic care, including bathing, dental care, hair care, using community rest-room facilities, and cosmetology, is a factor to be concerned with on the job as well as in the community. However, the available research literature has only begun to consider these skill areas. For example, Cuvo, Jacobi, and Sipko (1981) trained five moderately mentally retarded adults in appropriate laundry skills. Other studies have explored methods of training the selection of color-coordinated clothing (Nutter & Reid, 1978), the mending of clothing (Cronin & Cuvo, 1979), and the brushing of teeth (Horner & Keilitz, 1975). These investigations collectively suggest that mentally retarded persons, provided the training, can acquire the skills necessary to groom, clothe, and care for themselves. Additional studies addressing the importance of these and related areas to occupational survival appear warranted.

Today there are significant numbers of workers enjoying their leisure time before, during, and after work. Playing racquetball, walking, and running, as well as playing cards, are activities that occupy leisure time. Although the work research literature fails to report efforts directed toward training the mentally retarded adult in leisure time activities in work settings, a growing body of research suggests conclusively that mentally retarded adults can acquire a variety of leisure-relevant behaviors (Wehman, 1976, 1979). Further research should take into account the leisure activities of co-workers on the job and document the approach, methods, and success of training mentally retarded adults to engage in similar activities.

Similar to social interaction, conversation requires that appropriate initiating skills, such as, "Hi, how are you," and answering skills, such as, "Fine, thank you," be acquired. Unlike social interactions, conversation relies on continuing exchanges of information. Typically, nonhandicapped co-workers have the ability to engage each other in social conversations. Many mentally retarded individuals, however, lack even basic conversational skills. Training these skills appears an obvious area of future research. Including co-workers in the actual training, as tried by Rusch, Weithers, Menchetti, and Schutz (1980) in reducing topical repetitiveness, and training appropriate nonverbal and related gestural responses, would be valuable adjuncts to the work-related research literature.

This section has suggested a few areas of inquiry that could bear directly upon the ability of mentally retarded adults to survive in work settings. To date, such a body of literature does not exist; nor is there a limit to what social skills the consumers of research results should include in their habilitative efforts.

Response Maintenance and Transfer of Training

Two major concerns in the evaluation of behavior-change programs are the degree to which behaviors are maintained once a training program is terminated, and the degree to which newly acquired behavior transfers to extra training settings. These concerns are referred to as response maintenance and transfer of training, respectively. Despite the obvious importance of these concerns, they have only recently received attention in behavioral research. For some time it was thought that the "natural environment" would support adaptive behavior change. Consequently, the advice provided practioners was to select a behavior that was likely to be maintained by natural consequences in the environment (e.g., Ayllon & Azrin, 1968).

The behavioral literature does provide examples in which vocational behavior did not completely revert to preprogram levels after withdrawal of an intervention (Zimmerman, Stuckey, Garlick, & Miller, 1969), and examples in which other behavior transferred across situations (Bailey, Timbers, Phillips, & Wolf, 1971; Walker, Mattson, & Buckley, 1971). Despite these examples, maintenance and transfer of training typically do not occur without programming the environment (Kazdin & Polster, 1973; Marholin, Siegel, & Phillips, 1976; Stokes & Baer, 1978; Wahler, 1969; Walker & Buckley, 1972). A reversal of treatment contingencies to baseline conditions has been demonstrated, repeatedly, across a wide range of settings and persons (Kazdin & Bootzin, 1972; Kazdin & Craighead, 1973; O'Leary & Drabman, 1971) to influence loss of stimulus control. Research evidence also suggests that such human learning tends to be situationally specific (Redd & Birnbrauer, 1969). Typically, behavior changes are restricted to the specific setting or time of training (cf. Schutz *et al.*, 1978) and to the presence of those who conducted the program (cf. Lovaas & Simmons, 1969). Transfer of training usually will not occur unless programming is available across settings (Wahler, 1969; Walker & Buckley, 1972). Consequently, if response maintenance and transfer of training are habilitation goals, they must be included in the treatment process (Baer, Wolf, & Risley, 1968).

As indicated throughout this chapter, research studies appearing in the vocational habilitation literature have primarily focused on demonstrating that mentally retarded adults are capable of acquiring specific task-related skills and improving their production. Consequently, an emphasis has been placed on the development and subsequent evaluation of the efficacy of skill acquisition and production-oriented training techniques. However, several procedures that appear to be functionally related to the durability and transfer of behavioral changes have been cited in the work behavior research literature. The evidence for many of these procedures is not sufficiently clear, however, to suggest unequivocal guidelines for direct service. Although it would appear that some procedures are more suited to response maintenance than to transfer of training, in most instances the goals and procedures incorporated are difficult to interpret.

A necessary step toward maintenance and transfer of training entails measuring behavior over extended periods of time and across situations. Bellamy, Inman, and Yeates (1978) conducted one of the few vocational training studies which did address the measurement of work performance over a protracted period. In this study, the effectiveness of a timer contingency, which differentially reinforced higher cable harness production of three severely mentally retarded workers, was assessed over a period of 3 to 7 months.

Cuvo *et al.* (1978) provided an example of vocational skills maintenance and generalization; they taught six moderately mentally retarded adolescents to clean a restroom, using a task analysis containing 181 response components, and demonstrated that acquired skills transferred to a nontreatment setting and performance maintained in the new environment without additional programming. Few habilitation research studies, as noted above, provide similar evidence of generalization to settings different from training.

A number of work behavior research studies have addressed procedures associated with maintenance. One area which has received attention is the relationship between job performance variability and various schedules of reinforcement. Evans and Spradlin (1966) evaluated the difference between a fixed-ratio (piece-rate) and fixed-interval (salary) schedule of reinforcement on the plunger-pulling rates of mildly mentally retarded adults. The results of this investigation indicated that higher production rates were achieved under the fixed-ratio schedule, although the actual difference accounted for only about 10% of total productivity. Similarly, Schroeder (1972a) reported three studies concerning the effects of ratio and interval schedules on the work performance of mildly and moderately mentally retarded adults. The subject's repetitive electronics assembly work was mechanically recorded by measures of tool usage (Schroeder, 1972b). Performance rates under fixed-interval schedules decreased as the frequency of reinforcement was systematically decreased, and performance rates under fixed-ratio schedules increased as the frequency of reinforcement decreased. However, Schroeder (1972a) also obtained results which suggested that the type of contingency may interact with behavioral characteristics required by the tasks. Consequently, these qualified results suggest that the use of ratio rather than interval schedules might be more effective in maintaining behavior when the required response effort is low.

The applicability of these schedule effects to sheltered workshops or competitive employment settings appears limited, because the reinforcers (wages) earned in applied settings are typically delivered on a fixed-interval schedule, that is, biweekly or monthly paychecks. Consequently, manipulation of consequent schedules would appear to be more functionally related to the improvement of work performance rates, with the schedule of reinforcement in the latter phase of training approximating that of the targeted placement. The schedule effects reported above may be limited further by the reliance in this research on short repetitive tasks. Whether similar results would be obtained with longer task sequences has not been addressed.

Several authors have addressed the issue of fading extrinsic reinforcement and instructional cues, and bringing vocational behavior under the control of the schedule of reinforcement that exists in a targeted, posttraining setting (Crosson, 1969; Rusch *et al.*, 1979). For example, Rusch *et al.* (1979) trained an individual to work continuously throughout a six-hour work day, in a restaurant-training setting. The results of this investigation suggested that a combination of praise and feedback (token points) for continuous work, and response cost (loss of points) for discontinuing work, resulted in maximum work performance, as compared to praise or praise and feedback without response cost. Data collected following the gradual withdrawal of the training components (praise, tokens, and response cost) indicated that behavioral gains were maintained. Further, the results indicated that work performance was maintained following the extension of the daily token-point exchange ratio to weekly exchanges and, finally, a weekly paycheck.

Connis, Rusch, Sowers, and Cummings (1977) provided a similar example of maintenance programming which consisted of withdrawing individual components of a larger treatment package. The treatment package, consisting of praise, reprimands, and instruction, was introduced to reduce the inappropriate behavior of three mentally retarded adults in a restaurant-training setting. Following a reduction in such inappropriate behaviors as drooling and noncompliance, the individual components of the intervention package were sequentially withdrawn. Lowered levels of inappropriate behavior were maintained throughout each procedural withdrawal, suggesting that these adults failed to discern which stimuli were present.

Another procedural strategy which has been investigated is the effect of training initially under those contingencies present in targeted posttraining settings. For example, Schutz *et al.* (1979) determined the effectiveness of two employed procedures applied to the verbally abusive behavior of three moderately mentally retarded adults participating in a food-service vocational training program. A warning and a one-day suspension were identified as the procedures a potential employer used when employees were verbally abusive or generally socially inappropriate. Therefore, following the use of warnings alone, Schutz *et al.* (1979) applied a one-day suspension in concert with warnings. The use of the one-day suspension had an immediate impact on the inappropriate behavior of each of the three potential employees. This study suggested the importance and feasibility for individuals enrolled in vocational-training programs to respond, while in training, to the contingencies most likely found in the ultimate placement setting.

The procedures discussed thus far pertain to external control on the part of a significant change agent, such as a trainer or workshop supervisor. If relied on exclusively, external-control procedures could present potential disadvantages for the development of independent vocational behavior (Kazdin, 1973). One problem associated with an external-control approach is that it may preclude the development of self-directed behaviors. This deficit has been recognized as a primary obstacle to the community transition process (Wehman, 1975). Second, change agents may become discriminative stimuli for behaviors to occur rather than those stimuli present in the natural environment (Redd & Birnbrauer, 1969). Consequently, the external-control approach must not be viewed as an end in itself but rather as a means to train an individual to control his or her own behavior and to achieve self-selected goals.

Self-control has been defined as "those behaviors an individual deliberately undertakes to achieve self-selected outcomes" (Kazdin, 1975, p. 192). Self-control training procedures reported in the work-behavior research literature include self-observation, self-reinforcement, and stimulus control. Self-observation has been utilized with the mentally retarded in vocational settings through the use of behavioral graphs (Jens & Shores, 1969; Loos & Tizard, 1955) and daily feedback of work performance from a videotape (DeRoo & Haralson, 1971). Employing these procedures, an individual is trained in work performance awareness through displaying a visual record of his or her work behavior. Jens and Shores (1969) provided evidence that informational feedback may affect work performance without additional incentives. The number of units produced by moderately mentally retarded workers performing either a hinge-mechanism assembly or a packaging task was charted and displayed for each worker during training. The results indicated that the charting procedure effectively changed work performance. However, a similar feedback investigation conducted by Loos and Tizard (1955) indicated that the effects of this procedure may decrease over time. Consequently, research regarding self-observation procedures currently provide inconclusive information about the long-term effects of self-recording procedures.

Wehman, Schutz, Bates, Renzaglia, and Karan (1978) investigated the effects of self-reinforcement as a self-control training strategy. In a series of three studies, they evaluated two components of self-reinforcement, and self-administered reinforcement, and self-determined reinforcement and compared them to the effects of externally controlled reinforcement on the production rates of three severely mentally retarded adults. Results of these studies suggested that severely handicapped workers may be capable of performing equivalent rates of production under externally controlled or self-controlled reinforcement contingencies and across several different tasks. The primary implication of this work is that self-reinforcement training is feasible and may become an integral part of incentive systems in vocational training settings. In turn, the development of self-control on the part of workers may facilitate the durability of behavioral changes, as well as the preparation of individuals to enter a variety of post-training work settings.

Several studies have investigated the efficacy of stimulus control as a self-control strategy. *Stimulus control* refers to specific behaviors being performed in the presence of specific stimuli that serve as discriminative stimuli increasing the probability that the behavior(s), if performed, will be reinforced. Sowers *et al.* (1980) and Connis (1979) demonstrated such an approach. Sowers *et al.* (1980) showed that preinstruction, instructional feedback, and picture cues were effective in producing independent time management responding in three mentally retarded adults. Each individual, participating in a food service vocational-training program, successfully acquired independent time management behaviors despite being unable to tell time. The results of this investigation demonstrated that the subjects successfully went to and from lunches and breaks, independently, by utilizing the time card. Similarly, Connis (1979) noted the use of potential cue effects in controlling task-sequencing behavior.

The existing body of research on maintenance and transfer of training of work behavior reviewed here can be viewed as a relatively positive finding in lieu of the small number of vocational and social behaviors treated. The available evidence suggests that behaviors are difficult to maintain and transfer and that these goals must be included in the habilitative efforts if desired; that environmentally produced cues have transitory effects, and worker-generated cues should be investigated; and that alternative strategies exist to promote maintenance and transfer, suggesting that future research should be directed toward including self-control procedures to maximize treatment effects. Although basic, these suggestions should provide years of inquiry into a socially relevant area, namely, how to preserve the vocational and social skills required for occupational survival.

CONCLUSION

The available literature on work behavior represents a promising area of research, largely owing to the contemporary importance of community integration (Novak & Heal, 1980). This chapter has reviewed several notable work-related behaviors, vocational and social, that have been the focus of research for over two decades. Although the greater part of this research literature has been directed toward training mentally retarded adults to acquire a task and change the rate at which tasks are performed, many recent efforts have investigated a myriad of other vocational and social skills. Further, a growing number of investigators are challenging traditional efforts to address work behavior in sheltered settings, by addressing socially significant behavior in more naturalistic environments. This appears particularly noteworthy, inasmuch as natural environments already have a large-scale incentive system, namely money, which can be used effectively for the purpose of integrating mentally retarded adults into local communities. Therefore, it would appear that artificially introducing reinforcers not normally part of everyday living detracts from habilitative efforts. Simply, if the adult being trained does eventually respond to normally available contingencies, the reinforcement system, payment of wages, does not have to be withdrawn after change has occurred. Increasing employment options for mentally retarded adults in more natural, nonsheltered settings will undoubtedly introduce behavioral scientists to qualitative problems of transferring stimulus control to this system.

Although the work behavior research presented here suggests that diverse skills can be acquired and managed, it is important to consider additional noteworthy limitations of this research. Obviously, the ability of mentally retarded adults to acquire a variety of difficult and potentially marketable work-related behaviors has been amply demonstrated for over two decades. That this literature cumulatively supports the importance of systematic applications of learning principles and behavioral technology cannot be disputed. However, from an ecological perspective, the work behavior research literature is lacking in a number of crucial areas, most notably in scope. Recently, Brooks and Baumeister (1977) made a plea to researchers to consider ecological validity in investigations centered around mental retardation. The basic position that they suggested was that mental retardation can be meaningfully understood only to the extent that ecological validity is assigned prominence in the field's theories and experiments. Certainly the discussion of the relative merits of an ecological perspective is neither new nor confined to mental-retardation theories and experiments (Willems, 1974). In fact, this perspective appears to be a logical extension of recent ecological perspectives in behavior analysis (Rogers-Warren & Warren, 1977)

In an important extension of Campbell and Stanley's (1963) treatise on experimental design, Bracht and Glass (1968) elaborated considerably on the concept of external validity, including population and ecological validity. Related to population validity, the lack of research related to generalization and maintenance strategies in the work behavior research literature has limited the applicablity of findings to the mentally retarded population as a whole, to applied settings, and to the wider variety of jobs available in the working world. For example, most production studies involved subjects who were either involved in university research programs (i.e., Schroeder, 1972a) or were specifically selected for those programs. It is, therefore, difficult to evaluate whether this selectivity has systematically eliminated applicability across individuals whom community vocational-training programs are expected to serve.

Regarding ecological validity, much of the work behavior research has evaluated the relation between supervision procedures and work performance over relatively brief time periods. Therefore, it is questionable whether performance during the first few weeks after a procedure is implemented is representative of performance over several months or years. Several studies have reported changes in rate over time. In many of these, gradual improvement over time appeared to reflect practice or exposure (Brown *et al.*, 1972; Crosson, 1969; Gold, 1973; Kahn & Burdett, 1967). Evidence is also available suggesting that the effectiveness of various contingency arrangements may decrease over time (Loos & Tizard, 1955).

Related to ecological validity, Bracht and Glass (1968) also discussed problems of multiple-treatment interference, Hawthorne effects, novelty effects, experimenter effects, and the measurement of dependent variables over brief periods. Several studies have demonstrated that the effects of a variety of setting characteristics, including both antecedents and consequences, are different depending on other treatments that may have preceeded them (Gordon, O'Conner, & Tizard, 1955; Rusch *et al.*, 1979; Siegel, Williams, & Forman, 1967). These studies suggest that multiple-treatment interference can reduce the generalizability of findings about setting characteristics. Reactive effects of experimental arrangements may also confound generalizability of findings. In work behavior research, these include the presence of observers, the use of short repetive tasks, and the use of the shortened work days during experiments (e.g., Brown & Pearce, 1970; Gold, 1972, Gold, 1976).

Another major problem with the current work behavior research literature is its almost exclusive focus on vocational-skill acquisition and production. Unquestionably, completing one's job and producing at an acceptable rate are regarded as essential. There are, however, certainly other behaviors which affect maintaining one's job (Rusch, 1979a). For example, Mithaug and Hagmeier (1978), in their survey of sheltered workshop supervisor's entry requirements, found that the ability to communicate basic needs, to move safely about the workshop, and to participate, were listed as the three most agree-upon behaviors ensuring workshop entry, whereas the ability to learn new tasks was tied in rank (seventh) with maintaining proper grooming. These data suggest that work behavior researchers have not necessarily addressed the same problems as those identified by the consumers of their efforts—those persons hiring mentally retarded persons in naturalistic settings.

REFERENCES

AYLLON, T., & AZRIN, N. H. *The token economy: A motivational system for therapy and rehabilitation.* New York: Appleton-Century-Crofts, 1968.

BAER, D. M., WOLF, M. M., & RISLEY, T. R. Some current dimensions of applied behavior analysis. *Journal of Applied Behavior Analysis,* 1968, *1,* 91–97.

BAILEY, J. S., TIMBERS, G. D., PHILLIPS, E. L., & WOLF, M. M. Modification of articulation errors of pre-delinquents by their peers. *Journal of Applied Behavior Analysis,* 1971, *4,* 265–281.

BELLAMY, G. T., INMAN, D. P., & YEATES, J. Workshop supervision: Evaluation of a procedure for production management with the severely retarded. *Mental Retardaton,* 1978, *16,* 317–319.

BELLAMY, G. T., HORNER, R. H., & INMAN, D. P. *Vocational habilitation of severely retarded adults.* Baltimore: University Park Press, 1979.

BELLAMY, T., PETERSON, L., & CLOSE, D. Habilitation of the severely and profoundly retarded: Illustrations of compentence. *Education and Training of the Mentally Retarded,* 1975, *10,* 174–186.

BELMONT, J. Long-term memory in mental retardates. In N. R. Ellis (Ed.), *International review of research in mental retardation* (Vol. 1). New York: Academic Press, 1966.

BOUSFIELD, W. A. The occurrence of clustering in the recall of randomly arranged associates. *Journal of General Psychology*, 1953, *49*, 229–240.

BRACHT, G. H., & GLASS, G. V. The external validity of comparative experiements in educational and the social sciences. *American Education Research Journal*, 1968, *5*, 437–474.

BROLIN, D. E. *Vocational preparation of retarded citizens*. Columbus, Ohio: Charles E. Merrill, 1976.

BROOKS, P. H., & BAUMEISTER, A. A., A plea for consideration of ecological validity in the experimental psychology of mental retardation: A guest editorial. *American Journal of Mental Deficiency*, 1977, *81*, 407–416.

BROWN, L., & PEARCE, E. Increasing the production rate of trainable retarded students in a public school simulated workshop. *Education and Training of the Mentally Retarded*, 1970, *5*,15–22.

BROWN, L., VAN DEVENTER, P., PERLMUTTER, L., JONES, S., & SONTAG, E. Effects of consequences on production rates of trainable retarded and severely emotionally disturbed students in a public school workshop. *Education and Training of the Mentally Retarded*, 1972, *7*, 74–81.

CAMPBELL, D. J., & STANLEY, J. C. Experimental and quasi-experimental designs for research on teaching. In N. L. Gage (Ed.), *Handbook of research on teaching*. Chicago: Rand McNally, 1963.

CLARKE, A., & HEREMELIN, F. Adult imbeciles: Their abilities and trainability. *The Lancet*, 1955, *2*, 337–339.

CLOSE, D. W., IRVIN L. K., PREHM, H. J., & TAYLOR, V. E. Systematic correction procedures in vocational-skill training of severely retarded individuals. *American Journal of Mental Deficiency*, 1978, *83*, 270–275.

COHEN, M. E., & CLOSE, D. W. Retarded adults' discrete work performance in a sheltered workshop as a function of overall productivity and motivation. *American Journal of Mental Deficiency*, 1975, *60*, 733–743.

CONNIS, R. T., The effects of sequential pictorial cues, self-recording, and praise on the job task sequencing of retarded adults. *Journal of Applied Behavior Analysis*, 1979, *12*, 355–361.

CONNIS, R. T., RUSCH, F. R., SOWERS, J., & CUMMINGS, L. T. *Programming maintenance through sequential withdrawal of social contingencies*. Paper presented at the Oregon Conference, University of Oregon, Eugene, February, 1977.

COTTER, V. W. Effects of music on performance of manual tasks with retarded adolescent females. *American Journal of Mental Deficiency*. 1971, *76*, 242–248.

CRONIN, K., & CUVO, A. J. Teaching mending skills to mentally retarded adolescents. *Journal of Applied Behavior Analysis*, 1979, *12*, 401–406.

CROSSON, J. A. A technique for programming sheltered workshop environments for training severely retarded workers. *American Journal of Mental Deficiency*, 1969, *73*, 814–818.

CUVO, A. J., LEAF, R. B., & BORAKOVE, L. S. Teaching janitorial skills to the mentally retarded. Acquisition, generalization, and maintenance. *Journal of Applied Behavior Analysis*, 1978, *11*, 345–355.

CUVO, A. J., JACOBI, E., & SIPKO, R. Teaching laundry skills to mentally retarded students. *Education and Training of the Mentally Retarded*, 1981, *16*, 54–64.

DEROO, W., & HARALSON, H. Increasing workshop production through self-visualization on videotape. *Mental Retardation*, 1971, *9*, 22–25.

DWINELL, M. A., & CONNIS, R. T. Reducing inappropriate verbalizations of a retarded adult. *American Journal of Mental Retardation*, 1979, *84*, 87–92.

EVANS, G., & SPRADLIN, J. Incentives and instructions as controlling variables in productivity. *American Journal of Mental Deficiency*, 1966, *71*, 129–132.

GIRADEAU, F. L. The formation of discrimination learning sets in mongoloid and normal children. *Journal of Comparative Physiological Psychology*, 1959, *52*, 566–570.

GOLD, M. The acquisition of a complex task of retarded adolescents. Final Report, Project No. 8-8060, University of Illinois, Champaign-Urbana Library, 1969.

GOLD, M. Stimulus factors in skill training of the retarded on a complex assembly task: Acquisition, transfer, and retention. *American Journal of Mental Deficiency*, 1972, *76*, 517–526.

GOLD, M. Factors affecting production by the retarded: Base rates. *Mental Retardation*, 1973, *11*, 9–11.

GOLD, M. Redundant cue removal in skill training for the retarded. *Education and Training of the Mentally Retarded*, 1974, *9*, 5–8.

GOLD, M. Task Analysis of a complex assembly task by the retarded blind. *Exceptional Children*, 1976, *43*, 78–84.

GOLD, M., & BARCLAY, C. R. *The effects of verbal labels on the acquisition and retention of a complex assembly task*. Childrens Research Center, University of Illinois, 1973. (a)

GOLD, M., & BARCLAY, C. R. The learning of difficult visual discrimination by the moderately and severely retarded. *Mental Retardation*, 1973, *11*, 9–11. (b)

GORDON S., O'CONNER, N., & TIZARD, J. Some effects of incentive on the performance of imbeciles on a repetitive task. *American Journal of Mental Deficiency*, 1955, *60*, 371–377

HEAL, L. W., BRANSKY, M. L., & MANKINEN, R. L. The role of dimensional preference in reversal and non-reversal shifts of retardates. *Psychonomic Science*, 1966, *6*, 509–510.

HORNER, D. R., & KEILITZ, I. Training mentally retarded adolescents to brush their teeth. *Journal of Applied Behavior Analysis*, 1975, *8*, 301–309.

HOUSE, B. J., & ZEAMAN, D. A. Comparison of discrimination learning in normal and mentally defective children. *Child Development*, 1958, *29*, 411–415. (a)

HOUSE, B. J., & ZEAMAN, D. A. Visual discrimination learning in imbeciles. *American Journal of Mental Deficiency*, 1958, *63*, 447–452. (b)

HOUSE, B. J., & ZEAMAN, D. A. Transfer of a discrimination from object to patterns. *Journal of Experimental Psychology*, 1960, *59*, 298–302.

HOUSE, B. J., ZEAMAN, D. A., ORLANDO, R., & FISHER, W. *Learning and transfer in mental defectives*. Progress Report No. 1. Research Grant M-1099 NIMH, 1957.

HUDDLE, D. Work performance of trainable adults as influenced by competition, cooperation, and monetary reward. *American Journal of Mental Deficiency*, 1967, *72*, 198–211.

HUNTER, J., & BELLAMY, T. Cable harness constructin for severely retarded adults: A demonstration of a training technique. *AAESPH Review*, 1976, *1*, 2–13.

IRVIN, L. K. General utility of easy to hard discrimination training procedures with the severely retarded. *Education and Training of the Mentally Retarded*, 1976, *11*, 247–250.

IRVIN, L. K., & BELLAMY, G. T. Manipulation of stimulus features in vocational skill training of the severely retarded: Relative Efficacy. *American Journal of Mental Deficiency*, 1977, *81*, 486–491

JACKSON, G. M. The use of visual orientation feedback to facilitate attention and task performance. *Mental Retardation*, 1979, *17*, 281–284.

JACOBS, J. W. Retarded persons as gleaners. *Mental Retardation*, 1976, *14*, 42–43.

JACOBS, J. W. Gleaning: Sheltered employment for retarded adults in rural areas. *Mental Retardation*, 1978, *16*, 118–122.

JENS, K., & SHORES, R. Behavioral graphs as reinforcers for work behavior of mentally retarded adolescents. *Education and Training of the Mentally Retarded*, 1969, *4*, 21–26.

JOHNSON, J. L., & MITHAUG, D. E. A replication of sheltered workshop entry requirements. *AAESPH Review*, 1978, *3*, 116–122.

KAHN, R. L., & BURDETT, A. D. Interaction of practice and rewards on motor performance of adolescent mental retardates. *American Journal of Mental Deficiency*, 1967, *72*, 422–427.

KARLAN, G. R., & RUSCH, F. R. Analyzing the relationship between acknowledgement and compliance in a non-sheltered work setting. Education and Training of the Mentally Retarded, in press.

Kazdin, A. E. Toward a client administered token reinforcement program. *Education and Training of the Mentally Retarded*, 1973, *8*, 4–11.

Kazdin, A.E. *Behavior modification in applied settings*. Homewood, Ill.: Dorsey Press, 1975.

Kazdin, A. E. Assessing the clinical or applied importance of behavior change through social validation. *Behavior Modification*, 1977, *1*, 427–451.

Kazdin, A. E., & Bootzin, R. R. The token economy: An evaluation review. *Journal of Applied Behavior Analysis*, 1972, *5*, 343–372.

Kazdin, A. E., & Craighead, W. E. Behavior modification in special education. In L. Mann & D. A. Sabatino (Eds.), *The first review of special education* (Vol. 2). Philadelphia: Buttonwood Farms, 1973.

Kazdin, A. E., & Polster, R. Intermittent token reinforcement and response maintenance in extinction. *Behavior Therapy*, 1973, *4*, 386–391.

Kliebhahn, J. Effects of goal setting and modeling on job performances of retarded adolescents. *American Journal of Mental Deficiency*, 1967, *72*, 220–226.

Kuhlman, F. Experimental studies in mental deficiency. *American Journal of Psychology*, 1904, *15*, 391–446.

Loos, F. M., & Tizard, J. The employment of adult imbeciles in a hospital workshop. *American Journal of Mental Deficiency*, 1955, *59*, 395–403.

Lovaas, O. I., & Simmons, J. Q. Manipulation of self-destruction in three retarded children. *Journal of Applied Behavioral Analysis*, 1969, *2*, 143–157.

Marholin, D., Siegel, L. J., & Phillips, D. Transfer and treatment: A search for empirical procedures. In M. Hersen, R. M. Eisler, & P. M. Miller (Eds), *Progress in behavior modification* (Vol. 3). New York: Academic Press, 1976.

Marholin, D., Touchette, P., Berger, P., & Doyle, D. "I'll have a Big Mac, large fries, large coke, and apple pie,"... or teaching adaptive community skills. *Behavior Therapy*, 1979, *10*, 236–248.

Martin, A.S., & Flexer, R. W. *Three studies on training work skills and work adjustment with the severely retarded*. Lubbock, Texas: Research and Training Center in Mental Retardation, Texas Tech University, 1975.

Matson, J., & Martin, J. A. A social learning approach to vocational training of the severely retarded. *Journal of Mental Deficiency Research*, 1979, *23*, 9–17.

Mithaug, D. E. Case studies in the management of inappropriate behaviors during prevocational training. *AAESPH Review*, 1978, *3*, 132–144. (a)

Mithaug, D. E. Case study in training generalized instruction-following responses to preposition-noun combinations in a severely retarded young adult. *AAESPH Review*, 1978, *3*, 94–115. (b)

Mithaug, D. E. The relation between programmed instruction and task analysis in the prevocational training of severely and profoundly handicapped persons. *AAESPH Review*, 1979, *4*, 162–178.

Mithaug, D. E., & Hagmeier, L. D. The development of procedures to assess provocational competencies of severely handicapped young adults. *AAESPH Review*, 1978, *3*, 94–115.

Mithaug, D. E., & Hanawalt, D. A. The validation of procedures to assess provocational task preferences in retarded adults. *Journal of Applied Behavior Analysis*, 1978, *11*, 153–162.

Moore, R., & Goldiamond, J. Errorless establishment of visual discrimination using fading procedures. *Journal of the Experimental Analysis of Behavior*, 1964, *7*, 269–272.

Nelson, R. E. Perceptions of secondary school personnel concerning the teaching of occupational survival skills. *Illinois School Research and Development*, 1977, *13*, 57–61.

Nirje, B. The normalization principle and its human management implications. In R. Jugel & W. Wolfensberger (Eds.), *Changing patterns of residential services for the mentally retarded*. Washington, D. C..: President's Committee on Mental Retardation, 1969.

NOVAK, A. R., & HEAL, L. W. (EDS.). *Community integration of developmentally disabled individuals*. Baltimore: Paul H. Brookes, 1980.

NUTTER, D., & REID, D. H. Teaching retarded women a clothing selection skill using community norms. *Journal of Applied Behavior Analysis*, 1978, *4*, 475–487.

O'CONNOR, M., & HERMELIN, B. Discrimination and reversal learning in imbeciles. *Journal of Abnormal Social Psychology*, 1959, *59*, 409–412.

O'LEARY, K. D., & DRABMAN, R. Token reinforcement programs in the classromm: A review. *Psychological Bulletin*, 1971, *75*, 379–398.

O'NEILL, C. T., & BELLAMY, G. T. Evaluation of a procedure for teaching sawchain assembly to a severely retarded women. *Mental Retardation*, 1978, *16*, 37–41.

PLENDERLEITH, M., & POSTMAN, L. Discrimination and verbal habits in incidental learning. *American Journal of Psychology*, 1956, *69*, 236–243.

REDD, W. H., & BIRNBRAUER, J. S. Adults as discriminative stimuli for different reinforcement contingencies with retarded children. *Journal of Experimental Child Psychology*, 1969, *7*, 440–447.

RENZAGLIA, A., WEHMAN, P., SCHUTZ, R., & KARAN, O. Use of cue redundancy and positive reinforcement to accelerate production in two profoundly retarded workers. *British Journal of Social and Clinical Psychology*, 1978, *17*, 183–187.

ROGERS-WARREN, A., & WARREN, S. F. (EDS.). *Ecological perspectives in behavior analysis*, Baltimore: University Park Press, 1977.

RUSCH, F. R. Toward the validation of social/vocational survival skills. *Mental Retardation*, 1979, *17*, 143–145. (a)

RUSCH, F. R. A functional analysis of the relationship between attending and producing in a vocational training program. *The Journal of Special Education*, 1979, *13*, 399–411. (b)

RUSCH, F. R., & MENCHETTI, B. M. Increasing compliant work behaviors in a non-sheltered setting: *Mental Retardation*, in press.

RUSCH, F. R., & MITHAUG, D. E. *Vocational training for mentally retarded adults; A behavior analytic approach*. Champaign, Ill.: Research Press, 1980.

RUSCH, F. R., & SCHUTZ, R. P. Non-sheltered competitive employment of the mentally retarded adult: Research to reality? *Journal of Contemporary Business*, 1979, *8*, 85–98.

RUSCH, F. R., CONNIS, R. T., & SOWERS, J. A. The modification and maintenance of time spent attending using social reinforcement, token reinforcement and response cost in an applied restaurant setting, *Journal of Special Education Technology*, 1979, *2*, 18–26.

RUSCH, F. R., WEITHERS, J. A., MENCHETTI, B. M., & SCHUTZ, R. P. Social validation of a program to reduce topic repetition in a non-sheltered setting. *Education and Training of the Mentally Retarded*, 1980, *15*, 208–215.

RUSCH, F. R., SCHUTZ, R. P., & HEAL, L. W. The impact of setting on non-sheltered work behavior: A recommendation. In K. Kernan & R. B. Edgerton (Eds.), *Impact of specific settings on behavior and development*. Baltimore: University Park Press, in press.

RUSCH, F. R., RUSCH, J. C., MENCHETTI, B. M. & SCHUTZ, R. P.Survey-train-place: Developing a school-aged vocational curriculum for the severely handicapped student. In R. Dubose (Ed.), *Recommended practices manual for severely handicapped learners*. Springfield: Illinois State Department of Public Instruction, in press.

SCHROEDER, S. R. Parametric effects of reinforcement frequency, amount of reinforcement, and required response force on sheltered workshop behavior. *Journal of Applied Behavior Analysis*, 1972, *5*, 431–441. (a)

SCHROEDER, S. R. Automated transduction of sheltered workshop behaviors. *Journal of Applied Behavior Analysis*, 1972, *5*, 523–525. (b)

SCHUTZ, R., WEHMAN, P., RENZAGLIA, A., & KARAN, O. Efficacy of contingent social disapproval on inappropriate verbalizations of two severely retarded males. *Behavior Therapy*, 1978, *9*, 657–662.

SCHUTZ, R. P., RUSCH, F. R., & LAMSON, D. C. Evaluation of an employer's procedure to eliminate unacceptable behavior on the job. *Community Services Forum*, 1979, *1*, 4–5.

SCHUTZ, R. P., VOGELSBERG, R. T., & RUSCH, F. R. A behavioral approach to community integration of mentally retarded persons. In A. R. Novak & L. W. Heal (Eds.), *Community integration of developmentally disabled individuals.* Baltimore: Paul H. Brookes, 1980.

Schutz, R. P., Jostes, K. F., Rusch, F. R., & Lamson, D. S. Acquisition, transfer, and social validation of two vocational skills in a competitive employment setting. *Education and Training of the Mentally Retarded*, 1980, *15*, 306–311.

SIEGEL, P., WILLIAMS, J., & FORMAN, C. Instrumental behavior in the retardate in relation to qualitative variation in the incentive. *American Journal of Mental Deficiency*. 1967, *72*, 450–454.

SOWERS, J., RUSCH, F. R., & HUDSON, C. Training a severely retarded young adult to ride the city bus to and from work. *AAESPH Review*, 1979, *4*, 15–22.

SOWERS, J. THOMPSON, L. E. & CONNIS, R. T. The food service vocational training program. In G. T. Bellamy, G. O'Connor, & O. C. Karan (Eds.), *Vocational rehabilitation of severely handicapped persons.* Baltimore: University Park Press, 1979.

SOWERS, J. A., RUSCH, F. R., CONNIS, R. T., & CUMMINGS, L. E. Teaching mentally retarded adults to time-manage in a vocational setting. *Journal of Applied Behavior Analysis*, 1980, *13*, 119–128.

STEVENSON, H. W. Learning of complex problems by normal and retarded subjects. *American Journal of Mental Deficiency*, 1960, *64*, 1021–1026.

STEVENSON, H. W., & ZEIGLER, E. F. Discrimination learning and discrimination reversal in normal and feebleminded individuals. *Journal of Personality*, 1957, *61*, 699–711.

STEWART, D. M. Survey of community employer attitudes. *Mental Retardation*, 1977, *15*, 30–31.

STOKES, T. F., & BAER, D. M. An implicit technology of generalization. *Journal of Applied Behavior Analysis*, 1978, *10*, 349–367.

TEASDALE, R., & JOYNT, D. Some effects of incentives on the behavior of adolescent retardates. *American Journal of Mental Deficiency*, 1967, *71*, 925–930.

TERRACE, H. S. Stimulus control. In W. K. Honig (Ed.), *Operant behavior: Areas of research and application.* New York: Appleton-Century-Crofts, 1966.

THURMAN, S. K., & FIORELLI, J. S. Perspectives on normalization. *The Journal of Special Education*, 1979, *13*, 339–346.

TOMASULO, D. J. An economical approach to the development of a training program for porters. *Mental Retardation*, 1976, *14*, 12–13.

TRAMONTANA, J. Social versus edible rewards as a function of intellectual level and socioeconomic class. *American Journal of Mental Deficiency*, 1972, *77*, 33–38.

VOGELSBERG, R. T., & RUSCH, F. R. Training three severely handicapped young adults to walk, look and cross uncontrolled intersections. *AAESPH Review*, 1979, *4*, 264–273.

WAHLER, R. G. Setting generality: Some specific and general effects of child behavior therapy. *Journal of Applied Behavior Analysis*, 1969, *2*, 239–246.

Walker, H. M., & Buckley, N.K. Programming generalization and maintenance of treatment effects across time and across settings. *Journal of Applied Behavior Analysis*, 1972, *5*, 209–224.

WALKER, H. M., MATTSON, R. H., & BUCKLEY, N. R. The functional analysis of behavior within an experimental class setting. In W.C. Becker (Ed.), *An empirical basis for change in education.* Chicago: Science Research Associates, 1971.

WEHMAN, P. Behavioral self-control with the mentally retarded. *Journal of Applied Rehabilitation Counseling*, 1975, *6*, 27–34.

Wehman, P. *Helping the mentally retarded acquire play skills: A behavioral approach.* Springfield, Ill.: Charles C Thomas, 1976.

WEHMAN, P. (ED.), *Recreation programming for developmentally disabled persons.* Baltimore: University Park Press, 1979.

WEHMAN, P., SCHUTZ, R. RENZAGLIA, A., & KARAN O. The use of positive practice training in work adjustment with two profoundly retarded adolescents. *Vocational Evaluation and Work Adjustment Bulletin*, 1977, *14*, 14–22.

WEHMAN, P., RENZAGLIA, A., BERRY, G., SCHUTZ, R., & KARAN, O. Developing a leisure skill repetoire in severely and profoundly handicapped persons. *AAESPH Review*, 1978, *3*, 162–172.

WEHMAN, P., SCHUTZ, R. BATES, P., RENZAGLIA, A., & KARAN, O. Self-management programs with mentally retarded workers: Implications for developing independent vocational behavior. *British Journal of Social and Clinical Psychology*, 1978, *17*, 57–64.

WEHMAN, P., HILL, J. W., & KOEHLER, F. Placement of developmentally disabled individuals into competitive employment: Three case studies. *Education and Training of the Mentally Retarded*, 1979, *14*, 268–276,

WHITEHEAD, C. Sheltered workshops in the decade ahead: Work and wages, or welfare. In G. T. Bellamy, G. O'Connor, & O. C. Karan (Eds.), *Vocational rehabilitation of severely handicapped persons*. Baltimore: University Park Press, 1979.

WILLEMS, E. P. Behavioral technology and behavioral ecology. *Journal of Applied Behavior Analysis*, 1974, *7*, 151–165.

WILLIAMS, P. Industrial training and remunerative employment of the profoundly retarded. *Journal of Mental Subnormality*, 1967, *13*, 14–23.

WOLF, M. M. Social validity: The case for subjective measurement or how applied behavior analysis is finding its heart. *Journal of Applied Behavior Analysis*, 1978, *11*, 203–214.

WOLFENSBERGER, W. *Normalization: The principle of normalization in human services*. Toronto: National Institute on Mental Retardation, 1972.

ZEAMAN, D. Learning process of the mentally retarded. In S. Osler & R. Cooke (Eds.), *The biosocial basis of mental retardation*. Baltimore: The Johns Hopkins University Press, 1965.

ZEAMAN, D. *The law of redundancy*. Paper presented at the Gatlinburg Conference on Research and Theory in Mental Retardation, Gatlinburg, Tennessee, March 1968.

ZEAMAN, D., & HOUSE, B. J. The role of attention in retardate discrimination learning. In N. R. Ellis (Ed.), *Handbook of mental deficiency*. New York: McGraw-Hill, 1963.

ZEAMAN, D., HOUSE, B. J., & ORLANDO, R. Use of special training conditions in visual discrimination learning with imbeciles. *American Journal of Mental Deficiency*, 1958, *63*, 453–459.

ZIMMERMAN, J., OVERPECK, C., EISENBERG, H., & GARLICK, B. Operant conditioning in a sheltered workshop. *Rehabilitation Literature*, 1969, *30*, 323–334.

ZIMMERMAN, J., STUCKEY, T., GARLICK, B., & MILLER, M. Effects of token reinforcement on productivity in multiply handicapped clients in a sheltered workshop. *Rehabilitation Literature*, 1969, *30*, 34–41.

9 Language Acquisition

James F. McCoy and Joseph A. Buckhalt

Introduction

For years, deficiencies in language acquisition have been recognized as a primary problem associated with mental retardation (Jordon, 1967). Although "normal" children acquire language from naturally occurring interactions with their respective language environments, many retarded children, particularly those functioning in the severe and profound ranges of retardation, fail to acquire even the most rudimentery language skills. During the past 20 years, increasing research attention has been devoted to the discovery of environmental variables that will accomplish for retarded children what the natural environment has failed to provide—a useful language repertoire.

The purpose of this chapter is to review some of the major developments in the area of language acquisition with mentally retarded children. Behavioral procedures, derived primarily from principles of operant conditioning, have had a tremendous impact, but other theoretical perspectives have made a substantial contribution to current language acquisition approaches. In view of the enormous amount of attention devoted to this general area over recent years, our review must necessarily be abbreviated in covering some topics, and detailed in others. We have chosen to present more detailed description and discussion of techniques which demonstrate a greater degree of methodological advancement, while presenting other topics in a more general manner.

First, a general discussion of some historical events in language acquisition and modification of language behavior will be presented. This review will be followed by a description of language acquisition models and training procedures. Some space will be devoted to a discussion of stimulus control, generalization, and generativity, not only because of their importance, but also because of the frequent inconsistent use of these concepts. Next, training procedures and considerations, and detailed descriptions of several important studies organized around receptive and expressive language and the relationship

James F. McCoy • Department of Psychology, Auburn University, Auburn, Alabama 36849.
Joseph A. Buckhalt • Department of Counselor Education, Auburn University, Auburn, Alabama 36849.

between the two modalities, will be presented. Finally, we have chosen two topics from the several potentially important current issues for inclusion: parental factors and nonvocal language systems.

Historical Overview

A considerable body of knowledge is accumulating regarding how best to facilitate the acquisition of various language skills in mentally retarded children. Several fairly discrete training models now exist which differ along many dimensions, such as degree of reliance on orthodox operant technology, incorporation of psycholinguistic structure as content to be taught, perceived importance of different prerequisites, and many others. Before discussing these training models, it might be useful to review some of the foundations which have led to their development.

Although neither Skinner's (1957) *Verbal Behavior* nor Chomsky's subsequent review (1959) contained any empirical data or even many suggestions as to how language might be practically facilitated, the works were important for at least two reasons. First, Skinner was perhaps the first to suggest that, although language is one of man's most complex and sophisticated behaviors, it should nevertheless be amenable to explanation by principles which have been shown to govern other behaviors. This mere suggestion may have been incentive enough for some researchers to attempt to modify language when they might have otherwise been satisfied to study more elementary behaviors. The most important outcome, however, seems to have been the enormous theoretical controversy generated by the two works, which practically begged for empirical studies that might confirm one hypothesis or the other about how language is acquired. In the early 1960s, quite a number of studies were done, primarily as demonstrations that language, like other behaviors, could indeed be modified with operant methods (e.g., Isaacs, Thomas, & Goldiamond, 1965; Sherman, 1963; Wolf, Risley, & Mees, 1964). Several of these first studies were done with psychotic adults or with children who had previously used language but had become mute. Through the application of reinforcement schedules, effects which were termed "reinstatement" of language were obtained. Part of the rationale for selecting language deficient populations for these first studies may have come from the realization of practical needs, but theoretical concerns may have also played a part. One might argue that if language can be initiated, shaped, and controlled via operant methods in the most severely impaired persons, then less severe impairments should pose fewer training problems.

Whereas behaviorists have typically chosen to attempt to remediate language in atypical individuals as a demonstration that language can be taught in a didactic fashion, psycholinguists have chosen to conduct more naturalistic, observational studies of nonhandicapped children. Their studies have been aimed at showing the structure and regularity of how children learn to speak in many different cultural contexts. And, of course, their intent has been to demonstrate that language development can be advanced in children without any intentional efforts on the part of adults to teach it with the application of reinforcement principles. Of course, one might reasonably argue that, in addition to working with different strategies of research, the two groups of researchers have been studying essentially different problems. Whereas the psycholinguists have been concerned with how language naturally occurs in average children, the behaviorists have been more interested in how language can be taught to children who have failed to acquire it in the "normal" course of development. It seems that, even though procedures may be developed to facilitate the acquisition of some language skills by a previously nonverbal mentally retarded child, those procedures may have nothing to do with the way a nonretarded child learns those same skills in his natural environment. Conversely, a comprehensive description of the structure and sequence of normal language development may or may not be particularly useful in teaching language to individuals for whom the normal environmental circumstances have been insufficient.

Even though the behaviorists and psycholinguists appear to be operating in different realms, there is now evidence that language training programs are using the research produced by both groups. These areas of integration, discussed in general terms by Staats (1974) and Lynch and Bricker (1972), will be mentioned with respect to how they are applied in actual training models in later sections.

One of the first comprehensive language programs based on behavior modification principles was contained in Bereiter and Englemann's (1966) work which was concerned with preschool disadvantaged children. By today's standards, the program was more explicit in the content of the curriculum to be taught than in the specific teaching methods used. Also, some degree of language usage (although assumed to be nonstandard) was expected of the children entering the program. Significant improvements in general training-program models did not come about until the early to mid-1970s, and these models depend heavily on a great amount of study done in the interim.

In a number of studies, the smallest definable unit of syntax, the morpheme, was chosen for training. Guess, Sailor, Rutherford and Baer (1968), for example, trained a mentally retarded child in the use of plural morphemes. A subsequent series of studies showed moderate degrees of success in using reinforcement techniques to teach proper use of very limited grammatical rules, such as singular and plural endings and present and past tense of verbs (Baer & Guess, 1971, 1973; Guess, 1969; Sailor, 1971; Schumaker & Sherman, 1970). The theoretical rationale for choosing an area of training with such little apparent immediate relevance may have been twofold. First, the choice of elementary morphemic usage derives from the propensity of operant researchers to subdivide complex tasks into their simplest discrete units for training in an analytic fashion. That logic would demand that the simplest grammatical element would be a starting place. Another reason, however, might have come from the previously mentioned controversy with the linguists. To demonstrate that true syntax could be taught directly through operant methods was to discredit much of what linguists were claiming about the way in which syntax is acquired.

As time progressed, more ambitious goals were accomplished by behavioral researchers. As early as 1970, Wheeler and Sulzer documented the training of complete sentences by a child whose speech had previously been telegraphic. Garcia, Guess, and Byrnes (1973) showed that a severely retarded girl previously not using sentences could be taught to do so through the use of modeling and reinforcement of imitation. Some degree of generalization to untrained sentences of similar form to those trained was also obtained. Stremel (1972) presented results of a training study in which three retarded children were taught subject–verb–object constructions with shaping and reinforcement techniques.

Some of the work done during this period was aimed not so much at building language skills in children who had none as at reducing the frequency of inappropriate language before training appropriate language. One general paradigm, pioneered by Lovaas (1966) with echolalic autistic children, has been to remove positive reinforcement for echolalic responses, punish the responses in some instances, and bring verbalizations under more appropriate environmental stimulus control through prompting and selective reinforcement. Several subsequent successful efforts at eliminating echolalia were reported by Risley and Wolf (1967), Johnston (1968), Tramontana and Shivers (1971), and others. Other inappropriate speech forms, such as diminished volume (Jackson & Wallace, 1974), perseverative speech (Butz & Hasazi, 1973), bizarre, schizophrenic-like speech (Barton,

1970), and elective mutism (Nolan & Pence, 1970), have been successfully remediated through operant procedures.

One purpose in referring to a small portion of the studies done during this period is to illustrate the piecemeal and somewhat haphazard fashion in which behavioral studies of language training with language-deficient individuals progressed for some time. Since behavioral researchers tended to view the complexities of human language as an aggregation of discrete and simple individual skills, success at training the individual component skills was first necessary before comprehensive training could be accomplished. In retrospect, although behavioral researchers may have suffered somewhat from inadequate knowledge of the structure and sequence of language development in designing their first training studies, their work did serve to demonstrate that certain aspects of language could indeed be modified via behavioral technology. Also, to be fair, the field of developmental psycholinguistics was relatively undeveloped when the behavioral studies began, so knowledge about how language develops in children was very limited initially, and has paralleled the growth of knowledge in behavioral training methods.

By the early to mid-1970s, a few researchers had become interested in piecing together information from the many individual training studies into comprehensive models of language training. By this time, not only were many individual demonstrations of the effectiveness of operant methodology available, but enough observational data had been gathered by developmental psycholinguists (e.g., Bloom, 1970; Brown, 1973) to give a clearer idea of how children's language is structured and how it changes. Not surprisingly, training models which were initiated then, and now have continued to evolve, have some different orientations. The model prompted by Guess, Sailor, and Baer (1974, 1978) follows orthodox behavioral theory and method more closely than any others. Other models vary in the degree to which they incorporate psycholinguistic and cognitive-developmental theories. Miller and Yoder (1972, 1974), for example, were among the first to suggest that the structure and sequence of material to be taught to mentally retarded children should be the same as that observed in children of normal intelligence as reported, for example, by Bloom (1970), Brown (1973), and Schlesinger (1971). Bricker and Bricker (1974), in addition to agreeing that psycholinguistic studies might well dictate the content to be taught, stated that cognitive prerequisites such as the sensorimotor skills discussed by Piaget should also be entered into a language-training curriculum for retarded children. A review of the basic components of several of the broad training models now follows.

Current Language Intervention Models

Several comparative reviews of language intervention models have been published recently. The review of Guess, Sailor, and Keogh (1977) is perhaps the most extensive in scope, summarizing research in language prerequisites and direct individual training studies, as well as comprehensive models. The basic components of 12 different training models are outlined by Guess *et al.* (1977). A second recent work which includes a comparative look at several different models is that of McLean and Snyder (1977). In their work, several models are discussed with regard to how they relate to their own theoretical framework, termed a "transactional" model. Mahoney, Crawley, and Pullis (1979) do not attempt to describe the models extensively, but instead classify them according to several dimensions, including characteristics of target group, theoretical orientation, and instruction-and-response modality. All three of these recent reviews also include some discussion of relevant conceptual and practical issues which are as yet unresolved by any of the current models.

Perhaps the most obvious means of classifying current language intervention programs is according to their theoretical orientation. As mentioned in the previous section, although the Guess, Sailor, and Baer (1974, 1978) model follows traditional learning theory for both content and instructional method, many other programs (Bricker, Dennison, & Bricker, 1976; Carrier & Peak, 1975; Miller & Yoder, 1974; Stremel & Waryas, 1974) now advocate the incorporation of knowledge of the structure and sequence of normal-child language development as the content for teaching language-impaired children. At the same time, some of the programs retain operant techniques as the primary instructional method (especially Bricker, Dennison, & Bricker, 1976), while others suggest the use of techniques such as imitation and expansion, which some claim is a major part of the informal "training" that adults give to all children learning language (Miller & Yoder, 1974). Theoretical rationale has become an imprecise criterion for classifying intervention programs, however, because almost none of them are "pure" in the sense of deriving *all* components from either behavioral or linguistic theory. Even the most behaviorally oriented group (Guess, Sailor, & Baer, 1974) has conceded that findings from developmental psycholinguistics are helpful in determining program content, and, conversely, almost all the linguistically oriented persons (e.g., Miller & Yoder, 1974) not only admit that behavioral teaching strategies have been effective in many instances, but also include certain behavioral principles in their suggested methodology.

The various models differ to some degree in the characteristics of the group to whom they are addressed. These target group differences appear to have little theoretical justification, but appear to be the result of rather arbitrary choices. Etiology of target group has simply not been seen as a primary consideration. Cromer's (1974) review appears to have convinced most that the *process* of language acquisition by retarded persons carrying different etiological labels is basically the same. Much less attention, therefore, has been paid to diagnostic categories, or even levels of retardation, than to level of linguistic development at the beginning of training. In fact, many programs are described as suitable not only for mentally retarded persons, but for any person whose language is deficient or delayed. Several of the models claim to offer teaching paradigms for individuals who have no verbal-communication skills at all (Bricker, Dennison, & Bricker, 1976; Carrier & Peak, 1975; Guess, Sailor, & Baer, 1974), whereas others seem to require that the individual taught already be speaking in at least two-word utterances (Miller & Yoder, 1974; Stremel & Waryas, 1974). Two programs (Bereiter & Englemann, 1966; Dunn, Horton, & Smith, 1965) appear to be different from the others in that they are geared more to language *enrichment* exercises for children who already possess a fair amount of basic language skills, but whose language is nonstandard or impoverished because of cultural or social disadvantage.

Another target group difference is that the behavioral programs appear to have been developed with older, more severely retarded, and institutionalized persons, while most of the models now suggest the initiation of training as early as a handicap can be identified. Whereas the Bereiter and Englemann (1966) model assumed language deficits in disadvantaged children as early as preschool age (4–5 years) many current models now advocate beginning language intervention around the age that normal children begin to use expressive language (e.g., Bricker, Dennison, & Bricker, 1976), and there are even suggestions that training directed to nonverbal communication and/or cognitive prerequisites might be advisable shortly after birth.

Some Major Language Programs

A number of different language-training "programs," "models," or "curricula" have evolved. These programs differ along a number of dimensions, including target group addressed, theoretical underpinnings, specific techniques espoused, content to be taught, generalization methods recommended, and many others. As previously mentioned, some comparative reviews are available, the best of which to date was done by Guess, Sailor, and Keogh (1977). Guess *et al.* (1977) selected programs to summarize according to the criteria of (1) program visibility or notoriety, (2) terminal goal (spontaneous use of speech and language for purposes of communication), and (3) "comprehensiveness," which they mean to refer to programs addressing more than one component of language training. We shall sketch briefly the best known of the programs of those included in their comparative review.

Guess, Sailor, and Baer (1974, 1978)

This program is one in which operant techniques are embodied in the theory as well as the specific methods of training. Basing the program around a general learning-theory model, the authors have developed step-by-step training techniques which follow what they term a "functional" or "remedial" rather than a "developmental" model. The authors disavow any need to include any content or methods deriving from developmental psycholinguistic research and theories. The format of the approach is a linear, algorithmic sequence of a great number of discrete training steps. Two of the interesting aspects of the program are the emphasis on teaching functional communication skills (e.g., language which gets immediate social results) to children very early so that the benefits of learning language may be realized, and the emphasis on teaching children strategies which will elicit from adults language-training interactions (e.g., "What's that?").

Non-SLIP (Carrier & Peak, 1975; Hollis & Carrier, 1978)

The non-SLIP program was specifically designed to teach severely and profoundly retarded persons very basic forms of communication. Prerequisite skills for persons entering the training sequence are fine-motor abilities, ability to make shape, color, and pattern discriminations, and ability to perform match-to-sample exercises. Persons are then taught to communicate by manipulating plastic symbols through a system devised by Premack (1972) in his work with chimpanzees.

Miller and Yoder (1972, 1974)

Miller and Yoder were perhaps the first to attempt to incorporate psycholinguistic theory and data into a language-training model for mentally retarded children. Among the concepts they adopted from psycholinguistics is the idea that the "curriculum" or content of those specific language forms to be used in teaching retarded children should come from our observations of language development in children of normal intelligence. Another notion prevalent in their model is that semantics should precede syntax in the curricular sequence. They rely on the characterization of children's utterances in terms of case relations which correspond roughly to functions outlined by Schlesinger (1971) and others. Their training suggestion is that one first observe the child in his home environment to see which functions can be matched accordingly. Miller and Yoder's model has remained at primarily a conceptual level, since specific steps are described for some phases of training while steps for other phases are not yet readily available. No systematic training manual is available for this model.

Bricker and Bricker (Bricker & Bricker, 1974; Bricker, Dennison, & Bricker, 1976)

The Brickers' program is unique in its integration of operant techniques, psycholinguistic theory, and the cognitive-developmental theory of Piaget. In their description of an early-language-training model considered appropriate for any language-delayed child, heavy reliance is made on direct instruction in Piaget's sensorimotor skills. Their idea is that for children to develop language, which is a referent system for relations to the environment, the concepts or relations must be learned first. Explicit in the Brickers' work is their belief that training should begin as early as possible. Operant techniques are recommended as the instructional means, with the end being development of expressive language as described by psycholinguistic research. Although much of the Brickers' research has been conducted in laboratory settings, they have consistently advocated extensive parental involvement, and they recommend expanding the scope of the training environment to every extent possible.

Stremel and Waryas (Stremel, 1972; Stremel & Waryas, 1974)

This model was developed primarily with mentally retarded adults who were institutionalized. It, like the Brickers' model, relies on psycholinguistic data for the goals of training, and operant techniques for training specific language behaviors. There are different stages of the program, depending on entry level skills possessed by the trainee, but the prerequisites at the simplest stage exclude children who are nonverbal, under poor instructional control, and unable to imitate. The program has much in common conceptually with Miller and Yoder's model, but the training techniques are delineated with much greater specificity.

Kent (1974)

Kent has termed her model the Language Acquisition Program. It is a highly structured "clinical" approach to training, and the training manual contains very clear and direct steps. The program has three stages—preverbal, verbal-receptive, and verbal-expressive—which are taught successively with the use of standard operant procedures such as attention training, modeling and imitation, shaping, and reinforcement. The model was developed for use with severely mentally retarded children, and is somewhat rare in its alleged suitability even for those persons who are initially completely nonverbal.

MacDonald (MacDonald, 1976; MacDonald & Blott, 1974)

The Environmental Language Strategy devised by MacDonald was designed for children already using single words. Psycholinguistic data are used to determine content to be taught, and, as in several other programs, Schlesinger's (1971) functional case relations are relied on. In addition to the emphasis on semantics and teaching functions, MacDonald advocates training particular language functions concurrently with different methods. Conversational training and structured play are often used concurrently with imitation training.

TRAINING PROCEDURES

The major language acquisition programs use operant procedures in teaching their respective curricula, content, or target behaviors. Although there are differences between programs in the degree of precision in applying procedures, the structure of the training setting, and the extent of systematic tracking of behaviors, there is a general consensus that, for the present, operant conditioning procedures are the most effective training tactics available. The procedures most typically mentioned are positive reinforcement, differential reinforcement, aversive consequences, correction procedures, prompting, physical guidance, modeling, imitation, fading, shaping, chaining, and discrimination training. These procedures will be briefly described. Detailed description of these procedures may be found in general behavior modification texts (e.g., Craighead, Kazdin, & Mahoney, 1976; O'Leary & Wilson, 1975; Redd, Porterfield, & Andersen, 1979), child behavior texts (e.g., Gelfand & Hartmann, 1975; Sulzer-Azaroff & Mayer, 1977), and publications devoted specifically to operant language training (e.g., Kent, 1974; Lovaas, 1977; Sloane & MacAulay, 1968).

Positive reinforcement consists of immediate presentation of a positive reinforcer contingent on specified behavior, which results in an increase in or maintenance of the behavior. Reinforcers may be scheduled continuously (i.e., for each occurence of behavior), or intermittently, usually on a variable-ratio schedule where a varied number of responses are required for each reinforcer. The predominant reinforcers in language training have been edible, actually portions of meals or treats such as soda pop, ice cream, sugar cereals, chips, fruit, etc., and tokens, which are exchangeable for a variety of tangible items or privileges immediately following training sessions. The most important requirements for edibles are that small portions function effectively and that consumption be rapid (e.g., Risley & Wolf, 1967). The most effective reinforcers may be those specifically related to the target behaviors. Guess *et al.* (1977) suggest, for example, that vocalization of the phonemes "ju" and "ce" could be reinforced with sips of juice rather than M & Ms. An alternative suggested by Striefel, Wetherby, and Karlan (1978) is a reinforcer selection procedure where each reinforcing event consists of presentation of an ice tray with each compartment containing a different reinforcer, and the child then selects each time from multiple reinforcers. Differential reinforcement combines positive reinforcement and extinction procedures, so that responses which meet clearly specified requirements are reinforced, and those which rail to meet requirements are extinguised by withholding reinforcers. Most instances in the literature reporting the use of reinforcement procedures have consisted of differential reinforcement operations, unless some active, presumed aversive consequence is applied to behaviors failing to meet criterion. Aversive consequences for incorrect language responses have typically consisted of social punishment or disapproval and brief time-out where the therapist says "No" and turns away from the child for 10–20 sec. Variations of these consequences for incorrect responses have been termed correction procedures and consist of the therapist saying "No," demonstrating the correct response, and presenting the same problem after a short delay. Whether a time-out or a correction procedure is used, attention should be given to the possibility that contingent delays in task presentation could function as negative reinforcement for some children and increase rather than decrease incorrect responses (see, e.g., Solnick, Rincover, & Peterson, 1977).

Prompting refers to the procedure of using additional assistance prior to the occurrence of a desired response in order to increase the probability that the response will be made. Prompts may be nonverbal or verbal, depending on the characteristics of the target behavior. For example, a prompt for pointing to an object just labeled by a therapist could consist of sliding the object toward the child, or a prompt for labeling an object when asked the question, "What is this?" could be the therapist saying, "Cup, say cup." In both cases, the desired terminal behavior is a child's identification of an object by pointing to a verbally labeled object or by articulating the label of an object when shown an object and asked what it is. Prompts, then, are additional, artificial, antecedent stimuli or aids which initially function to bring about the desired behavior. Fading refers to the gradual removal of prompts so that control of the desired response shifts from prompts to control by appropriate task stimuli.

Physical guidance has been used extensively in training attending behaviors, motor imitations, and instruction following. Physical guidance initially consists of manually guiding the child so that the desired response occurs. For example, for the response of tapping on a table, the therapist would grasp the child's hand, mold it into a fist, and tap the child's knuckles on the table. Gradually the amount of guidance would be faded as the child performed more of the response, until guidance would be unnecessary. Usually physical guidance involves a task analysis of the terminal behavior and breaking it into discrete steps or components with the nature and amount of physical guidance for each component clearly specified. Striefel and Wetherby (1973) present an example of a task analysis for a motor response of raising an arm.

Modeling and imitation have been used most extensively in language training. Modeling refers to the demonstration of some behavior, and imitation refers to engaging in behavior which matches the behavior of the model. In two important studies (Baer & Sherman, 1964; Baer, Peterson, & Sherman, 1967) imitations were shown to be members of a response class where similarity between the model's behavior and the imitative behavior, not just specific imitative behaviors, becomes discriminative for reinforcement. These generalized imitations may be explicitly trained by reinforcing a series of imitative behaviors which match modeled behaviors.

Shaping refers to gradually increasing the topographical (form, intensity, etc.) requirements a behavior must meet for reinforcement. Initially, behaviors which only remotely resemble or approximate the desired behavior may be reinforced, and gradually behaviors which successively come closer and closer to the desired behavior are required for reinforcement. Shaping procedures can be used on any language target behavior. The only requirements are that approximations to the desired behavior occur at some minimal frequency and that steps or approximations toward the desired behavior be identifiable and differentially reinforcable.

Chaining involves combining already existing simple behaviors into more complex behavioral units. For example, a child may vocalize the phonemes "ce" and "ju," but not combine them to make the word juice. Chaining procedures would involve reinforcement for sequencing the "ju" and "ce" phonemes in close temporal proximity.

Discrimination training consists of differential reinforcement in the presence of two or more stimuli. Responses to the presence of one stimulus (S^D or S+) are reinforced, and responses in the presence of another stimulus (S^Δ or S−) are not reinforced. Discrimination-training procedures are used to teach the meaning of language units. For example, the goal may be to train the receptive meaning of an object. The object (e.g., cup) would be an S^D for the response of pointing to it when the therapist says, "Point to cup," and all other objects would be SΔs for the pointing response. Each time the child pointed to cup a reinforcer would be delivered, and each time another object was pointed to the reinforcer would be withheld.

Stimulus Control, Generalization, and Generativity

The terms stimulus control, generalization, and generativity are invariably used in conceptual discussions of language acquisition or descriptions of language intervention procedures and results. Unfortunately, there has not been a consistent use of these terms, particularly among authors of differing theoretical perspectives. A brief discussion of stimulus control, generalization, and generativity should clarify the process and procedures of language intervention programs.

Both stimulus control and generalization have developed from basic research in learning theory and have received considerable emphasis in operant language programs. Stimulus control refers to a functional relationship between a discriminative stimulus (S^D) and a behavior. One type of evidence for a functional relationship involves the observation of a high probability of a response when an S^D is present, and a low probability of response when the S^D is absent. Thus, stimulus control is descriptive of the phenomenon traditionally labeled stimulus discrimination, which is often the result of discrimination training (Terrace, 1966). In language development, stimulus control is directly related to semantics, or the acquisition of meaning, and discrimination learning underlies this process. For example, Lovaas (1977) views the development of appropriate stimulus control over verbal behavior as consisting of two basic discriminations. With expressive language the S^D is nonverbal and the response is verbal, as in labeling objects, and describing actions or relationships. With receptive language the S^D is verbal and the response is nonverbal, as in following instructions or understanding others. Of course, as Lovaas notes, complex combinations of these two types of discrimination usually exist in most language situations.

Generalization refers both to behavioral phenomena and to procedures which produce those phenomena. As phenomena, generalization may be categorized in three types: (1) concurrent occurrence of trained behaviors under nontraining conditions, that is, different settings, experimenters, and other variables which may be specified and controlled, (2) the persistence of trained behaviors after training procedures are removed, and (3) the concurrent emergence of untrained behaviors that are usually related to those directly trained. These phenomena have been identified as generalization across settings, or stimulus generalization; generalization across time, or maintenance effects; and generalization across responses, or side effects of treatment, or behavioral covariation. Of course, these types of generalization may occur either singularly or in combination.

The term "generativity" originated in psycholinguistics rather than in learning theory, and refers to the expression and understanding of an unlimited number of utterances, many of which are novel, that follow the unifying rules or regularities of appropriate grammar. Thus, specific instances of generative language would consist of extensions of a grammatical rule from trained to untrained exemplars, that is, novel utterances. Learning theory, particularly operant, approaches to language acquisition have been criticized by psycholinguists on numerous grounds (Chomsky, 1959). A main focus of these criticisms has centered around generative language. For both theoretical and practical reasons, operant researchers have concentrated on developing procedures to analyze and produce generative language. On a theoretical level, generative language is viewed by psycholinguists as emanating from deep structures of transformational grammar which are hypothesized to arise from a human genetic propensity for language. Thus, psycholinguists argue that generative language entails much more than can be owing to direct experience, and remain skeptical of the role of imitation and differential reinforcement in language development. An empirical demonstration of training generative speech in nonverbal children (even if it is limited to surface grammar), would bolster an operant theory of language. On the practical side, establishing generative speech with replicable procedures would have two distinct advantages: the utilization of the technology with other nonverbal children, and the providing of children with a language-expanding skill that enables them to organize their current and future repertoire.

From an operant perspective, generative language has been defined as expression and understanding of novel and grammatically correct utterances or sentences. The concept of response class provides a parsimonious conceptual framework for understanding the emergence of new language behaviors. Baer and his colleagues (Baer, Guess, & Sherman, 1972; Guess & Baer, 1973; Guess, Sailor, & Baer, 1978) have noted that the psycholinguistic concept of generative language and the operant concept of response class are conceptually similar, since both encompass the emergence of novel forms of behavior. A response class is comprised of a large, even unlimited, number of individual responses or members that are related in the sense that all members of the class are affected similarly by the same environmental operation. Thus, reinforcement of one member indirectly strengthens other members of a response class, and reinforcement of some members is sufficient to maintain all members of the response class. An early illustration of the concept of response class in language acquisition was reported by Salzinger, Feldman, Cowan, and Salzinger (1965). A child was reinforced for articulating the phrase "Give me candy," which increased the frequency of that phrase but also of other members of the response class consisting of "Give me ______," with a multitude of new words substituted for "candy."

An early example of the experimental analysis of generative language which was conducted by Guess *et al.* (1968) may be used to illustrate further the concepts of stimulus control, generalization, and generativity as a response-class phenomenon in language development. This study warrants detailed discussion. A severely retarded 10-year-old girl served as the subject. Previously, the same authors had eliminated disruptive behavior and established an expressive vocabulary consisting of singular labels of common objects. The purpose of their present experiment was to examine the role of imitation and differential reinforcement in the development of expressive use of the plural morpheme and to determine whether direct training was necessary for establishing each instance of correct plural usage. The same common objects were used for a given session, and different objects were used across sessions. Daily sessions consisted of three phases. In each phase a correct response was reinforced with food, and incorrect responses resulted in the experimenter's saying, "No," modeling a correct response, and presenting the next trial after a brief delay. In the first phase, one object was placed on a table in front of the subject, and she was asked, "What do you see?" Following three consecutive correct singular labels, the second phase was begun, which consisted of presenting two of the same objects used in the first phase. Again, the criterion of three consecutive correct plural responses had to be met before progressing to the next phase. In the third phase, the single objects and pairs of the objects were presented in a random fashion, and the session was terminated after six consecutive correct responses consisting of three singular and three plural usages.

The first noteworthy result was a demonstration with an ABA reversal design that singular and plural usage were controlled by the training procedures. Initially, use of the singular form for one object and the plural form for pairs of objects was reinforced, then use of the singular form for pairs of objects and plurals for singular objects was reinforced, which was followed by a reinstatement of the initial contingencies. Responding was clearly controlled by the contingencies as appropriate use of singular/plural forms was initially produced, followed by gradual acquisition of a high level of accuracy for reversed singular/plural forms, followed by a rapid discovery of appropriate singular/plural forms when the original contingency was reinstated.

The most noteworthy aspect of the experiment was evidence for the generative or generalized use of the plural morpheme, which was provided by two measures, the correct use of pluralization on the first presentation of pairs of objects (Trial 1 in Phase 2), and the percent correct responses in all three phases. Both measures reflected a high degree of generative use of the plural morpheme. That is, once a singular label was learned, there was a consistent usage of correct pluralization, although that specific example of the plural form had not previously been reinforced. In fact, after only three plural labels were directly trained, correct pluralization occurred to pairs of objects. There are two additional findings which further point to the fact that the training procedures produced acquisition of a surface grammatical rule which the subject could use on new exemplars. The first of these concerned responses to four objects originally learned under the reversed contingency of reinforcement for pluralization to single objects. The question was, would the subject make the previously learned responses, or operate under the correct rule which was then in effect? In all four instances, appropriate singular and plural usage occurred. The second manipulation involved presentation of trios, rather than the typical pairs of objects. Again, appropriate pluralization occurred, indicating that the subject's appropriate use of the plural morpheme was not limited to labeling the configurations used previously in training pairs of objects.

Now the results of this study will be described from the conceptual perspective of stimulus control, generalization, and generativity. In terms of stimulus control, a single object was or became and S^D for verbalization of the label for the object in singular form. Two objects became an S^D for affixing the plural morpheme, usually consisting of /s/ and /z/ sounds, to the singular label. Interestingly, the subject responded with appropriate pluralization to trios of objects, which suggests that pairs of objects did not exert complete discriminative control over appropriate use of the plural form. There are two possibilities for this effect. First, it is possible that the controlling S^D for plurals consisted of a stimulus class defined by the property of "more than one," and any member of the stimulus class set the occasion for plural responses. Second, it is possible that the only functional S^D was the presence of single objects, which set the occasion for singular responses, and that when this S^D was absent, material presented, and the question "What do you see" asked, then plural responses were given.

The term "generative" was used by Guess *et al.* (1968) to describe generalization of the plural morpheme to untrained examples. Since this precedence, the use of the term by operantly oriented researchers usually has been in reference to generalization within a response class. From this perspective, an aspect of language (e.g., a grammatical rule) is specified and conceptualized as a response class, and direct training is conducted on a series of exemplars, eventuating in correct responding to novel, untrained members within the response class. This type of generalization or generalized responding has been consistently obtained with retarded children, and should not be confused with the problems of measuring and programming generalization, which has been a focal issue in recent reviews (e.g., Cooke, Cooke, & Apolloni, 1976; Garcia & DeHaven, 1974; Harris, 1975). These authors have been most concerned with generalization to nontraining settings, that is, the natural environment.

RECEPTIVE LANGUAGE

"Receptive language," for the purposes of this chapter, refers to motoric responses under the discriminative control of combinations of verbal/nonverbal stimuli, such as, given an array of objects, pointing to a particular object when requested to identify it, and opening a door when given the instruction to do so. In both instances, a complex discrimination is involved which consists of at least three components. The verbal stimuli must be decoded, the nonverbal stimuli located, and the motoric behavior given which corresponds to the combination of verbal/nonverbal stimuli. In the case of object identification, the number of nonverbal and verbal stimuli are restricted, and the motoric response is uniform. In the case of instruction following, the nonverbal stimuli are embedded in the environment, and the motoric response is varied.

Rationale

The rationale for an intervention program which concentrates on the establishment and expansion of receptive language is twofold. First, much of daily living involves following directions or requests of others (Striefel *et al.*, 1978), and the ability to respond to verbal stimuli appropriately could enhance development of other adaptive behaviors, facilitate positive interactions with significant others, and minimize the need to rely on nonverbal directives, such as physical guidance. Second, language acquisition programs which initially focus on the establishment of expressive or productive language require an entry skill of generalized vocal imitation or must first train such a skill. Many severely handicapped children are deficient in vocal imitation responses, and the current technological sophistication of vocal imitation training indicates a substantial failure rate and extremely slow progress for children with no vocal-imitation skills. For example, Guess *et al.* (1978) indicate that of entry variables, verbal imitation is the most predictive of success. They cite a 40% failure rate of children without vocal-imitation skills in a total sample of 400 subjects trained with their program. In addition, they state that most of the successful subjects (60%) took almost two years to be trained to the desired entry level of generalized vocal imitation. Needless to say, there are distinct advantages, reviewed elsewhere in this chapter, to focusing on establishing productive language first. However, this goal remains an important question to consider for the professional embarking on a language intervention project with children who do not vocally imitate. More immediate and frequent success, as well as increases in adaptive behavior, may ensue with an emphasis on establishing generalized instruction following.

Prerequisite Skills

Prerequisite skills for receptive-language training include attention to the trainer and task, the absence of severe interfering and incompatible behaviors, and acceptance of physical guidance. For training in instruction following, the ability to engage in generalized motor imitation is a desirable prerequisite.

Attention training is included in most language acquisition programs, either formally or informally. For structured one-to-one or group training, the child must learn to stay seated in a chair and visually fixate on the therapist and/or training materials. One of the first systematic attention-training programs was reported by Lovaas, Berberich, Perloff, and Schaeffer (1966). Their target behavior was to have the child fixate on the trainer's mouth. Initially brief and gradually longer periods of visual fixating were required for food reinforcement. Training continued until the child was looking at the trainer's mouth for 50% of the session. The Lovaas *et al.* program progressed next to the establishment of prerequisites for expressive language and vocal imitation. However, the procedure could easily be adapted for other target behaviors, such as visually fixating on an array of objects, pictures, etc. Harris's (1975) review details variations of this procedure which include individual versus group training, absence or presence of a verbal command to "Look at ________," and edible versus conditioned reinforcement.

Interfering behaviors that are incompatible with structured training, such as temper tantrums, self-injurious/self-stimulatory behavior, grabbing or mouthing materials, aggression, etc., decrease the probability of successful training. Procedures for handling such problems effectively are reviewed by O'Brien, by Repp, and by Schroeder and his co-authors in their respective chapters. It should be emphasized that interfering behaviors are minimized by a careful structuring of the training environment in terms of competing stimuli and activities, selection and effective usage of positive reinforcers, consideration of the task, duration and frequency of the session, and so forth.

Physical guidance is a means by which to communicate correct and desired responses to nonverbal children. To be maximally effective, physical guidance should be administered without resistance on the part of the child and should involve minimal pressure from the theraoist. Children who resist physical contact should be given exposure to graduated physical guidance and positively reinforced for their cooperation. Establishment of responses such as pointing or handing objects to the therapist, as well as motor imitation, is greatly facilitated by the use of physical guidance.

Nouns

In a series of studies, the Brickers (Bricker, 1972; Bricker & Bricker, 1970, 1971; Bricker, Vincent-Smith, & Bricker, 1973) have investigated development of a single-word receptive vocabulary consisting of learning the labels of objects. The basic arrangement is a two-choice, simultaneous-discrimination paradigm. A set of common objects are selected, and these are presented to the subject in pairs, with the experimenter saying the word that names one of the two objects. The subject's response in the Bricker's research has consisted of picking up the object, since they have employed a Wisconsin General Test Apparatus (WGTA) for testing and training. Over trials the position of correct choices and pairing of objects can be systematically manipulated or randomized. Bricker and Bricker (1974) have noted the advantage of using two-choice discrimination problems. They note that response rates may be analyzed in terms of the binomial expansion, which allows identification of the point in training where better-than-chance correct responding consistently occurs as well as detecting position preferences and other inappropriate response strategies.

In one of their early studies (Bricker & Bricker, 1970), 50 severely retarded, institutionalized children served as subjects. Twenty-five small replicas of common objects—five each from the categories of food, people, vehicles, clothing, and utensils—were presented during a pretest. Each of the 25 objects was presented 10 times, five times as the named stimulus and five times as the distracting stimulus, in a WGTA for a total of 125 trials. On each trial, an experimenter said, "Take the ________," raised a door on the apparatus to expose the two objects, and repeated, "Take the ________" twice. If the subject responded by taking the named object within 15 sec, a token or edible reinforcer under the named object was collected, but taking both objects or the unnamed (distracting stimulus) object, as well as no response, were scored as errors, and the reinforcer was withheld. Ten of the 50 subjects were eliminated because of 80% or greater correct responding during the pretest. The remaining 40 subjects were randomly assigned to two training and two control groups, which were further subdivided into "learner" groups (those who improved during the pretest) and "nonlearner" groups (those who did not improve during the pretest). One of the training conditions—random training—consisted of random presentation of the five objects in each of the five categories, until criterion of 92% correct, or until five sessions were conducted for those items. The second training condition consisted of sequential presentation of one object until five consecutive correct responses occurred; then a second object was trained, etc. The two control conditions involved a no-contact group given only pre- and posttesting, and an attentional control group where subjects spent 25 sessions interacting with an experimenter, playing with the objects, being told their names, and receiving noncontingent reinforcers. In addition to receiving a posttest identical to the pretest, all 40 subjects received a generalization test on 10 similar and 10 dissimilar objects from training objects. Although the design of this study is rather complex, the major results are simple and clear. One half of the subjects improved significantly during the pretest, and training (regardless of which of the two types) was necessary to maintain this improvement. Thus, for these subjects, simple differential-reinforcement procedures were sufficient to establish rapidly and maintain a single-word receptive vocabulary. However, these procedures were not sufficient even with extended (i.e., 25 sessions) training in improving the receptive vocabulary of the other subjects. Given that this study has generality, a therapist interested in establishing a receptive vocabulary of noun labels should first assess (train) with a two-choice discrimination paradigm and reinforce correct responses. Many of the children will master receptive use of nouns in short order, and these noun labels can be used to establish instruction following for noun–verb combinations. On the other hand, more involved procedures than differential reinforcement would be indicated for those children who do not rapidly master receptive labels for objects.

A more intensive procedure was developed by Bricker (1972) and involved the establishment of motor movements for each of the objects. Subjects were 26 severely retarded, institutionalized children, with 13 in a training group ($\bar{X}$ CA = 12.7 years and $\bar{X}$ Vineland SQ = 32.09) and 13 in a no-training control group ($\bar{X}$ CA = 11.62 and $\bar{X}$ Vineland SQ = 30.23). Each subject received a pretest on 30 items, each of which was presented three times for a total of 90 trials, and an identical posttest on the same 30 items. Training consisted of dividing the 30 objects into six blocks of five objects each and progressing through the following three phases. First, subjects were trained in motor imitations specific to each object, such as a pouring motion for a pitcher, chopping motion for an ax, etc. Using standard imitation procedures, the experimenter said, "Do this," and modeled the motor movement with physical prompts and fading where necessary. Movements for each of the five objects were established sequentially. Second, subjects were trained to engage in the motor movements when the label for the object was substituted, such as "Do ax," again using imitation-training procedures as needed until motor movements were under the control of the auditory cues. Third, subjects were presented with the actual object along with the verbal prompt, "Do ______," and modeling of the movement specific to the object. Probe tests were administered after each of the three phases within training blocks, and after training was complete on all six blocks of five objects posttests were administered. Significantly greater overall posttest performance occurred for the training group as well as for the probe tests following final training on each of the six blocks of five objects. Although training such as this may appear involved, time investments ranged from 1½ to 8 hours across subjects.

However, two subjects had to be eliminated for failure to meet criterion on training for the first block of objects. Obviously, more procedures need to be developed for establishing receptive labels. Kent, Klein, Falk, and Guenther (1972) and Kent (1974) have outlined a detailed program which integrates training in receptive and expressive language acquisition. The initial stage involves basic receptive language, consisting of training the child to point to body parts, objects, and parts of the room.

Instruction Following

The next area of receptive-language acquisition to receive systematic research attention has been instruction-following behavior. Most of the work has concentrated on establishing motor responses to verb–noun combinations, although some progress has occurred in training responses to verb–adjective–noun combinations. These studies have evolved toward the goal of developing procedures to establish generalized instruction-following behavior, defined as appropriate responses to untrained combinations of verb–noun instructions within a training setting.

One of the first studies on instruction-following was conducted by Whitman, Zakaros, and Chardos (1971) with two mentally retarded children, one a 4½-year-old male and the other a 7-year-old female with a Vineland SQ of 37. Both were diagnosed as severely retarded. All sessions were conducted in a small training room equipped with two chairs, a table, and items used in some of the instructions, which were placed on the table. Twenty-two instructions were used with the first subject, and 20 different instructions were used with the second subject. Half the instructions for each subject were directly trained, and half served as generalization instructions and were never trained. Training instructions consisted of items such as "stand up," "point to your nose," "give me the pencil," "pick up the jacket," "go to the door," and examples of generalization instructions were "come here," "point to your ear, mouth, arm," "pick up the toy." The experimental design consisted of an ABAB withdrawal design for both subjects, with five sessions of baseline, 20 or 35 sessions of training, 5 or 15 sessions of reinstatement of baseline (withdrawal of training), and 15 or 10 sessions of reinstatement of training. During baseline, each instruction was presented twice, always in the same order, with training instructions first and then generalization instructions. Correct responses had to occur within 15 sec, and instructions were presented once without any additional prompts or consequences. In each training session an instruction was given which had previously been performed correctly, and each correct response was reinforced with edibles and praise. Following four or five correct responses, a second instruction was trained. If the subject did not respond, physical guidance was used by the experimenter to the extent necessary to prompt the correct response. Gradually the guidance was lessened, and each guided or unguided response was reinforced. The only specific criterion used in training was to return to a previously learned instruction if three consecutive incorrect responses occurred. Each of the 10 or 11 training instructions was presented sequentially over training sessions. At the termination of each training session, measurement of instruction-following for all 20 or 22 instructions was conducted in the same fashion as for baseline sessions. Results for both subjects showed increases in instruction-following during the initial training condition relative to initial baseline, a decrease during return to baseline, and an increase with the final reinstatement of training, thus demonstrating the role of the physical guidance and reinforcement procedures. The interesting aspect of the results was that correct responses to novel instructions increased along with response to trained instructions, and this increase corresponded to differences existing between training items and generalization items during the initial baseline. For example, for one subject an average of 3 of 22 and 2 of 22 training and generalization instructions, respectively, were followed in the initial baseline, and an average of 12 of 22 and 9 of 22 correct responses for trained and generalization instructions, respectively, occurred for the last block of five training sessions. More recent research (Striefel & Wetherby, 1973) suggests that this generalization effect to untrained instructions was owing to motivational factors. That is, the subjects were capable of following the instructions prior to training, and reinforcement produced a generalized effect of greater compliance.

Striefel and Wetherby (1973) studied instruction-following behavior in an 11-year-old profoundly retarded male. Similar instructions to those used by Whitman *et al.* (1971) were employed with 25 directly trained instructions and 10 nontrained generalization instructions. Each generalization item consisted of recombinations of nouns and verbs used on training items. For example, training instructions of "lift block" and "push car" were converted to "lift car" for a generalization item. The experimental design was a multiple baseline-across-behaviors (instructions) design, with probe data collected before and during training sessions. Training procedures consisted of physical guidance and reinforcement procedures similar to those used by Whitman *et al.* An added feature of Striefel and Wetherby's study was the detailed presentation of training procedures and the training and probe assessment sequence. All but two of the trained instructions were correctly followed on the last assessment. However, none of the untrained generalization instructions (a verb from one training item and a noun from another training item) was followed correctly. Since this lack of generalized instruction-following is common, more recent work by Striefel and his colleagues has been directed toward finding an efficient strategy for producing generalized instruction-following to novel combinations of trained verbs and nouns. These studies will be reviewed following the description of an alternative training procedure to physical guidance for initially establishing instructional control.

Instruction-following behavior may be conceptualized as appropriate motoric responses under the discriminative stimulus control of auditory or verbal stimuli. If a child has developed sufficient skills in imitating motoric responses, then these motoric responses are considered to be under the discriminative-stimulus control of movements engaged in by the model (i.e., visual stimuli). Striefel, Bryan, and Aikens (1974) used a transfer of stimulus control or fading procedure to shift discriminative control over motoric responses from imitative stimuli to verbal instructions. Three severely language-deficient persons served as subjects. Their ages were 11, 15, and 12, with reported IQs on the Peabody Picture Vocabulary Test of 20, 13, and 18. Subjects had been previously trained to imitate a variety of motor responses. A multiple-baseline across behaviors design was used to evaluate a transfer of stimulus control procedure originally described by Touchette (1971). The transfer procedure consisted of gradually increasing a time delay between giving the instruction and modeling the appropriate response. Specifically, the subjects were given imitation-training trials on one behavior, consisting of the experimenter's saying, "Do this," and modeling the response; each correct imitation was reinforced with praise and edibles, and incorrect responses resulted in social punishment (Experimenter saying, "No") and complete physical guidance of the movement. Following three consecutive correct imitations, the experimenter said the verbal instruction (instead of "Do this") and simultaneously modeled the correct response. Each correct response resulted in increasing delays of 0.5 sec between giving the verbal instruction and modeling the response, with incorrect responses resulting in decreases in the delay and the consequence for incorrect imitations (i.e., "No" and complete physical guidance). If correct response occurred during the delay interval, modeling was not presented.

The delay procedure proved to be an effective technique for training specific instruction-following behaviors in all three subjects. As in the previous study, generalization to recombinations of verbs and nouns was again totally absent in all subjects. The most noteworthy aspect of the study was the demonstration that the delay procedure is an alternative to physical guidance and fading of physical guidance. The results suggest that the delay procedure is more efficient than fading of physical guidance, since fewer trials were necessary for subjects to respond to instructions. For all three subjects, the median delay interval reached before responses occurred to instructions was .5 sec, or the first delay interval. Additional advantages of the delay procedure noted by Wetherby and Striefel (1978) are its ease of implementation and the lack of a need to develop a task analysis for the motoric components of each instruction.

Three more recent publications have focused on producing generalized instruction-following (Striefel, Wetherby, & Karlan, 1976, 1978; Wetherby & Striefel, 1978). The studies reported in these publications have been organized around the framework of a miniature linguistic system which was originally developed by Esper (1925). A miniature linguistic system is a two-dimensional-matrix approach involving two stimulus dimensions where each

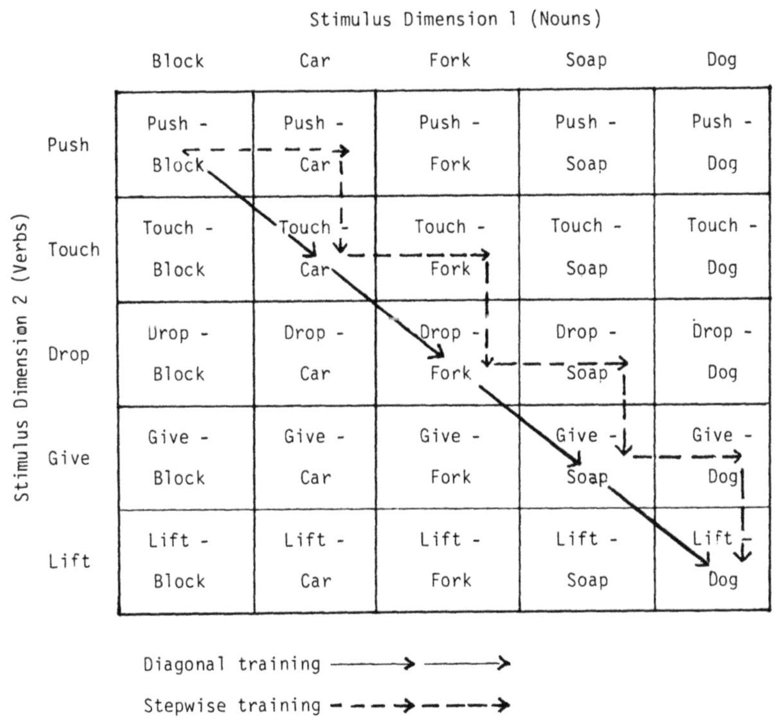

Figure 1: Matrix for diagonal and stepwise training.

stimulus from each dimension controls separate responses. However, each stimulus from one dimension can combine with those from the other dimension, generating a unique response for each cell in the matrix. For example, a 5 × 5 matrix where verbs comprise one stimulus dimension and nouns the other would involve five separate responses to verbs (actions) and five separate responses to nouns (labels). Each possible combination of nouns and verbs would yield 25 unique responses. Such a 5 × 5 matrix could be as seen in Figure 1.

If the goal of language training is to produce appropriate instruction-following responses to all combinations of verbs and nouns without direct training on each combination, several training strategies are available. The first strategy reported was to train one verb sequentially with each noun, then the next verb with each noun, and so forth (Striefel *et al.*, 1976). Two 12-year-old institutionalized severely mentally retarded males served as subjects. Expressive repertoires consisted of a few one-word echolalic responses in the case of one subject, and a few phonemes for the other. Both had been trained in making motor imitations and following several instructions. Twelve nouns (common objects, e.g., car, ball, comb) and 12 verbs (e.g., push, blow on, point to) were used, resulting in a possible 144 different noun–verb combinations. Each session consisted of reinforced probes before and after training, and each instruction was given with four objects placed on a table. It was found that with each successive verb, fewer nouns had to be trained before correct responding occurred to untrained nouns combined with that particular verb. For example, by the eighth verb for one subject, only one noun had to be directly trained before correct responding occurred to the other 11 novel nouns combined with that verb. Correct responding after the first noun was trained occurred with the 10th verb for the other subject. The amount of all the 144 verb–noun combinations which did not need direct training (generalization) was 78% for one subject and 65% for the other.

Striefel, Wetherby, and Karlan (1978) and Wetherby and Striefel (1978) have presented multiple experiments which have focused on identifying the most efficient sequence of training verb–noun combinations to produce a generative repertoire of responding to untrained combinations. Among variables investigated were prior training on verbs and nouns separately, combining new verbs with nouns already trained within a matrix and vice versa, and diagonal and stepwise progression through the matrix. Diagonal training in the example matrix would be to train push-block, touch-car, drop-fork, give-soap, and lift-dog. Stepwise training would be to train push-block, push-car, touch-car, touch-fork, drop-fork, and so forth. In general, the tentative conclusion from these experiments is that stepwise training is the most efficient and effective in producing generalized instruction-following. The advantage of stepwise training noted by Wetherby and Striefel (1978) is the required mastery of a discrimination between two stimuli within a dimension for each new instruction. The effect of this arrangement is to produce control by both components of the instruction.

EXPRESSIVE LANGUAGE

Rationale

The most persuasive argument for first attempting to train expressive language is that expressive language allows the child to control the environment to a much greater extent than receptive language. Guess, Sailor, and Baer (1978) point out that initially training expressive labels for children to communicate their needs is the most direct way to emphasize to children that they can use language to their advantage. As they note, expressive language allows children to control others rather than be controlled. Thus, the child's use of expressive language should be inherently more reinforcing. Although data from psycholinguistic researchers indicate that receptive language precedes expressive language in normal child development, successful results have been obtained in programs which initially target expressive skills (e.g., Guess, Sailor & Baer, 1976a; Lovaas, 1977). In addition, one of the critical training components in programs emphasizing expressive speech—generalized vocal imitation—requires receptive discriminative abilities, and mastery of all expressive units are soon followed by receptive training.

Prerequisite Skills

In order for a child to profit from expressive language training in a structured tutorial setting, it is necessary that the child (1) attend to the therapist and/or instructional materials, and (2) engage in a minimum of incompatible or disruptive or interfering behaviors. Additionally, some form of vocalizations should be in the child's repertoire. Ideally, the child should engage in generalized vocal imitation (Baer, Peterson, & Sherman, 1967). However, if the child vocalizes even a limited number of phonemes, or is echolalic, then training in expressive language could prove fruitful, and an attempt is warranted.

Attention training consists of establishing or increasing the child's remaining seated in a chair and visually fixating on a therapist. Lovaas *et al.* (1966) established eye contact in the following manner. The child was seated directly in front of the therapists, and the therapists used their legs to assist the child in remaining seated. Food reinforcers were used by therapists to increase the rate at which the child visually fixated on the therapist's mouth. This training continued until the child was visually fixating for 50% of the session. Risley and Wolf (1967) prompted eye contact by having the therapists hold food reinforcers in front of their faces. As soon as the children shifted visual fixation from the reinforcer to the therapists' faces, they were reinforced. Gradually the reinforcer was held lower and lower, and the children made eye contact rather than fixating on the food. This same prompting procedure was used by Risley and Wolf to establish attention to pictures and objects.

Interfering behaviors such as tantrums, self-stimulation, grabbing materials, etc. should be eliminated or reduced by positively reinforcing the incompatible behaviors of remaining seated and attending to the therapists or materials. Additional response suppression procedures may be necessary and are reviewed by Repp and Brulle in Chapter 6 of this volume.

The most desirable prerequisite skill for expressive-language training is generalized vocal imitation, that is, the ability to imitate sounds the first time they are modeled. For those children who are not adept vocal imitators, several programs and procedures have been devised. One of the most frequently cited set of procedures is that developed by Lovaas and colleagues (Lovaas, 1977; Lovaas *et al.*, 1966; Lovaas & Newsom, 1976). Four phases are involved. During the first phase, a variety of attempts is made to elicit vocalizations, such as keeping the child content, tickling or fondling the child, and prompting vigorous physical activity. Essentially, any positive activity which could enhance squeals or other vocal sounds is used. During this phase, all vocalizations and visual fixations toward the therapist are reinforced, usually with food. Following acceleration of vocalizations to the rate of about 10 per min in the absence of deliberate prompts and increasing eye contact to about half the session, the second phase is begun. The therapist modeled a verbalization every 10 sec and differentially reinforced any vocalization by the child occurring within 5 sec. This training continued until the child's vocal responses within 5 sec of the therapist's verbalizations were three times greater than during initial sessions of this phase. Phase 3 marked the beginning of requiring approximations to the sound modeled by the therapist. One sound was used, which met the following criteria: (1) a sound emitted frequently by the child during phase 1, (2) a sound which exaggerated visual components of lip placement, and (3) a sound which could be physically prompted by manually molding the child's lips. The sound was modeled every 10 sec, and closer approximations by the child in imitating the sound were gradually required for reinforcement. Following 10 consecutive correct imitations on the first sound, phase 4 was initiated. In phase 4, discrimination training for imitation of sounds began. A second sound was chosen, which met the additional criterion of being very different from the sound of phase 3. The two sounds were randomly presented, and the same prompting and reinforcement procedures were used. Ten consecutive correct imitations were required before adding a third sound, and this process continued, with each new sound or word requiring a finer and finer discrimination.

Other investigators (Baer *et al.*, 1967; Sloane, Johnston, & Harris, 1968) have first trained gross motor imitations, followed by fine motor imitations, and then motor imitations involving mouth and tongue movements before adding vocal components to the mouth and tongue imitations. The training of vocal imitations has been the primary method to establish a repertoire of phonemes. Other procedures to establish initial imitation of phonemes have been provided by McKenna-Hartung and Hartung (1973), who suggest that vocal components be added to a chain of motor movements, and Sherman (1965), who suggests initial approximations such as blowing out a match, then blowing out with the match absent, then imitating a hissing sound while blowing, etc. Once good control over imitation of phonemes is established, training focuses on semantics, the development of meaning of words, objects, or events (nouns), actions (verbs), attributes of objects (adjectives), and temporal and spatial relationships (prepositions and adverbs). The process involves establishing word labels as referents for the real objects, actions, etc., and is typically accomplished by shifting discriminative control from a model's verbalization (imitative stimulus) of the word to the actual object, action, attribute, etc.

Several authors have described imitation, differential reinforcement, and fading procedures for semantical development in expressive language (Cook & Addams, 1966; Guess *et al.*, 1976a,b; Hewett, 1965; Lovaas, 1977; Marshall & Hegrenes, 1970; Risley & Wolf, 1967; Sloane *et al.*, 1968). For example, Lovaas's (1977) procedure involved initially holding up a food object with the therapist verbally modeling the label (prompt) when the child visually fixated on the object. Imitations were reinforced with bites of the food object, and the therapist's verbal prompt was faded until the child was labeling the object when presented without the prompt. Several other objects were trained to criterion and interspersed with already trained objects. In Risley and Wolf's (1967) procedure, the therapist held up an object and said, "What is this?" As soon as the child looked at the object, the therapist immediately modeled the verbal label and reinforced an imitation. Gradually the time between object presentation and modeling a verbal response was lengthened. Then the verbal response was modeled partially and more and more softly until the child responded on the basis of the object and question alone. The same procedure was repeated with new objects, and presentations of already learned objects were interspersed.

Morphological Grammar

Morphology in psycholinquistics refers to the forms and grammatical inflections of words as they are modified for tense, number, case, person, etc. (Carroll, 1961). Morphological grammar is a set of rules which specify slight phonemic variations in words by addition of suffixes to change meanings. Several studies have shown convincingly that training with imitation and differential-reinforcement procedures on a few exemplars of using a morphological rule results in the use of that rule with untrained exemplars. Guess *et al.* (1968) and Sailor (1971), working with institutionalized severely retarded children (ages 10, 8, and 15) showed that imitation and differential reinforcement of plural morphemes for pairs of objects produced pluralization for pairs of objects not directly trained. Baer and Guess (1973) extended this work to noun suffixes. Four severely retarded children (ages 16, 16, 13, and 11), who had modest expressive vocabularies but were screened and found to have no expressive use of noun suffixes, were the subjects. Pictures depicting a person engaging in activities were used as training stimuli according to the following format. The experimenter showed a picture to the child while labeling, for example, "This man farms. He is a ________?" Initially the response "farmer" was modeled, and imitation was differentially reinforced. The children rapidly began applying the /er/ and /ist/ suffix to new verbs and used the suffix currently undergoing training, whether appropriate, for example, thinker, or inappropriate, for example, thinkist.

Schumaker and Sherman (1970) used similar procedures to train expressive usage of present-tense and three classes of past-tense verb inflections, those requiring a /d/, /t/, and /ed/ form. Three severely retarded adolescents participated as subjects, and the three past-tense-verb classes were trained in a multiple-baseline fashion with probes on trained and untrained verbs. Again, results showed that subjects learned a morphological grammar which generalized to untrained verbs within classes.

The theoretical implications of these studies as well as details of training and appropriate experimental controls may be found in Guess and Baer (1973). These studies were critical because they demonstrated that training procedures rule-governed language behavior which extended beyond the specific exemplars used in training.

Syntax

The work on morphology has been concerned with one-word units as the focus of training and analysis. A few researchers have expanded the unit of analysis to syntactical forms. However, much of the recent work on these more complex language behaviors are encompassed as components in more extensive language programs. Two-word combinations were investigated by Jeffree, Wheldall, and Mittler (1973), who worked with two young retarded children (4 years old) with a diagnosis of Down's Syndrome. Single-word labels of objects were first trained for both subjects. Then one subject was trained to combine these nouns with one verb, "gone," by initially socially reinforcing imitations of combinations and later spontaneous combinations. Results indicated an increase in two-word combinations for this subject but not the control subject, and the combining of untrained nouns with the verb.

Wheeler and Sulzer (1970) investigated imitation and reinforcement procedures in establishing use of articles (e.g., "the") and auxiliary verbs (e.g., "is") to form complete sentences. An 8-year-old retarded boy who had a sufficient vocabulary to express complete sentences but did not do so served as the subject. He was shown pictures and asked, "What do you see?" During baseline and reversal phases, the subject omitted articles and auxiliary verbs. Training consisted of modeling and reinforcing responses of complete sentence forms, and results showed increased use of articles and auxiliary verbs, which also occurred to nontrained probe pictures. In this study, the use of reinforcement procedures to produce chaining of already existing response units into grammatically appropriate complete sentences was demonstrated.

A similar study was conducted by Clark and Sherman (1975), whose unit of analysis was also complete sentences but whose training focused on appropriate use of past, present participle, and future verb tenses when subjects were asked questions about events. Three severely retarded, institutionalized children (ages 15, 16, 17) served as subjects. The three verb forms were trained sequentially in a multiple-baseline fashion, and responses to nontrained generalization probes were assessed following each of the three training phases. Examples of the three verb forms are as follows. For future tense, the experimenter would say, "He is a farmer. What will he do tomorrow?" and then model and reinforce the response of "Tomorrow he will farm"; for past tense, "What did he do yesterday?" with a correct response of "Yesterday he farmed"; and for present participle, "What is his job?" with a correct response of "His job is farming." Results showed the training procedures produced correct complete sentence form with generalization to nontrained items within each verb-tense class.

Collectively, these and other similar studies (e.g., Bennett & Ling, 1972; Stevens-Long & Rasmussen, 1974) illustrate that retarded children with existing repertoires of semantically appropriate vocabularies can be trained with modeling, prompting, imitation, and reinforcement procedures in expressive usage of syntactical units.

RECEPTIVE AND EXPRESSIVE LANGUAGE

Studies reviewed in the previous two sections were concerned with either receptive- or expressive-language acquisition, and not both. With naturally occurring language development of normal or retarded children and in comprehensive language-training programs for retarded children, there is an interplay between acquisition of receptive (comprehension or understanding) and expressive (production) forms. All language-acquisition programs in practice train both, but the question arises, which modality should be given emphasis and in what sequence? Surveying the total field of language acquisition provides substantial support for the positions that receptive training should precede expressive training, and vice versa, and that it makes no difference (Guess *et al.*, 1977). With the plethora of theoretical arguments and data, the best suggestion is that training in both modalities should be conducted concurrently or in close sequential proximity, but with emphasis given to expressive training. However, this recommendation has two qualifications; one is that the child should have a rudimentary expressive repertoire, and the other is that the target behaviors are fairly simple. Three illustrative studies which have examined generalization across receptive and expressive modalities with mentally retarded subjects and which supports this emphasis will now be reviewed.

Guess (1969) investigated receptive/expressive acquisition of the plural morpheme in two severely retarded subjects (ages 13 and 14) diagnosed as cases of Down's Syndrome. Training involved placing one object and a pair of the same objects from an item pool of 30 objects on a table. Each session consisted of three phases. During the first phase, the experimenter verbally labeled the object in the singular form, and the subject was required to point to the single object, for which he received token reinforcers. During the second phase, the plural form was verbalized and the subject was required to point to the pair. During the third phase, singular and plural forms were randomly presented. Following criterion responding, six consecutive correct uses of singular and plural forms, probe trials for expressive singular and plural usage were administered for the just trained and to be trained objects. The subject was shown either one object or a pair of objects, and asked, "What do you see?" Reinforcers were never delivered during probes. After receptive training, expressive training was conducted on the same 30 objects, following the same three-phase format, but no probes were administered. Finally, subjects received reversed receptive training, according to the three-phase format, followed by expressive probes. That is, when presented with a singular label, subjects were required to point to pairs for reinforcement, and vice versa.

Results for both subjects showed acquisition of correct plural and singular receptive usage during reinforcement for normal usage, with no generalization in expressive probes (both subjects labeled single objects and pairs with singular labels). Second, both subjects showed rapid acquisition of the plural morpheme in expressive training. Third, both subjects showed rapid development of reversed usage of receptive plural and singulars but continued to respond with normal singular and plural forms on the expressive probes. Thus, there was carry-over from the previous expressive training, and the currently reinforced pluralization rule in effect for receptive form was not utilized on the expressive probes.

Guess and Baer (1973) extended this study to ascertain whether training in receptive form facilitated acquisition in the expressive modality, and vice versa, rather than producing generalization across modalities. Two classes of plural morphemes were used, /s/ and /es/ sounds, and they were trained concurrently in expressive and receptive forms. Four severely retarded subjects (ages 11, 21, 20, and 13) were screened and found to label all objects used, and to articulate the /s/ and /es/ phonemes; but they did not use correct pluralization expressively or receptively. Sessions followed the same three-phase format and probe procedure just described. Expressive /s/ plurals and receptive /es/ plurals were trained for two subjects, and the reverse combinations were trained for the other two subjects. If receptive training was for objects with /es/ sounds, then expressive probes were conducted for the same objects with /es/ sounds, and in the same session expressive training was given for objects with /s/ sounds and receptive probes for the same objects. The absence or weak and variable generalization during nonreinforced probes for three or the four subjects was found. This pattern was the case for both training in expressive (e.g., /s/ sounds) and probes in receptive (same object and /s/ sound) modalities and vice versa, training in receptive (e.g., /es/ sounds), and probes in expressive (same object and /es/ sound) modalities. For one subject, generalization from receptive training to expressive probes and from expressive training to receptive probes gradually developed across sessions. Interestingly, for this subject there was more rapid generalization from expressive training to receptive probes than from receptive training to expressive probes. Also, the three subjects not showing generalization during non-reinforced probes were exposed to the identical training conditions and given reinforced probes instead. Reinforced probes produced generalizations in all subjects. However, overall generalization from productive training to receptive probes was achieved more easily than generalization from receptive training to productive probes.

These same results were obtained in a more recent study with noun labels. Keller and Bucher (1979) trained six mentally retarded children to label pictures either receptively or expressively, and assessed generalization to the untrained modalities with nonreinforced probes. Four sets of five pictures each were used. First, subjects were trained to label expressively each of the five pictures with receptive probes after learning each picture. Then the second set of five pictures was trained receptively with expressive probes after each picture, and these two phases were then replicated with two more sets of five pictures. Results were that five out of six subjects demonstrated highly accurate performance on receptive probes after expressive training. accurate performance on receptive probes after expressive training. However, performance on expressive probes was poor after receptive training, with frequent articulation and mislabeling errors. These results also suggest that training expressive forms produces greater generalization to, or greater ease in acquisition of, receptive counterparts.

SELECTED CURRENT ISSUES

There are several issues which are currently receiving considerable research and theoretical attention in the area of language acquisition of the mentally retarded. These include generalization, emphasis on early intervention, cost-benefit or cost-efficacy analysis, parental factors, sequence of normal developmental language content, and nonvocal language systems. Problems in generalization of training effects to the natural environment were highlighted in three separate reviews some five years ago (Cooke, Cooke, & Apolloni, 1976; Garcia & De Haven, 1974; Harris, 1975). Some, but not enough, progress has been made in developing generalization procedures (Stokes & Baer, 1977). Parental factors may be important in improving generalization strategies, as well as promoting early intervention tactics (this topic will be covered). Another area which undoubtedly will become more important as the technology for establishing vocal language improves but continues to fail for some children is the design of nonvocal language systems. This area will be briefly discussed by outlining some of the antecedent factors and major nonvocal systems under development.

Nonvocal Language Systems

The current interest in the design and implementation of nonvocal language intervention systems for mentally retarded persons is a result of the convergence of several different areas of thought and research. It is quite possible that the earliest formal attempts to teach nonvocal communication skills to mentally retarded individuals were made by teachers of the deaf and the hearing impaired. Especially in the early history of our institutions and programs for the deaf, when diagnostic procedures were even less precise than they are today, it is probable that mentally retarded persons either deaf or presumed deaf were taught sign language. It is even possible that, as diagnostic procedures became more sophisticated and the differentiation of deafness from mental retardation became more prevalent, some mentally retarded persons were actually *prevented* from learning to communicate more effectively by their placement in mental institutions rather than in training schools for the deaf.

Although the foregoing link may seem remote to some, what is obvious is the tremendous intellectual and practical debt owed by those currently applying sign-language systems with mentally retarded populations to those who have developed teaching techniques primarily with nonretarded deaf and hearing-impaired persons for many years. Not only is the concept of teaching a nonverbal communication system a borrowed one, but it is also true that many of the specific techniques and entire systems are extrapolated and applied to mentally retarded persons. Of course, it should likewise be acknowledged that some of the earlier work in this area was devoted to those persons who are *both* mentally retarded and deaf (e.g., Berger, 1972; Hall & Talkington, 1970; Hoffmeister & Farmer, 1972).

An area of contribution perhaps equally important to that made by professionals working with deaf persons is the work begun by several groups of investigators in the late 1960s and early 1970s teaching language to chimpanzees. Drawing from previous work by Kellogg (1968) and others, the Gardners (Gardner & Gardner, 1969), the Premacks (Premack & Premack, 1972), Fouts (1972), and Rumbaugh (Rumbaugh, Gill, & Von Glaserfeld, 1973) all began similar work with chimpanzees within a relatively short time. The differences in approach by these groups of investigators are as fascinating as the similarities. Whereas the Gardners and Fouts focused on teaching traditional sign language systems, Premack developed a system based on plastic symbols, and the Rumbaugh group pioneered in computer-assisted instruction. By now the results and implications of this aggregate research have reached an exceedingly large professional and lay audience. No doubt the widespread attention paid to this work is owing to many factors, including the implications about interspecies similarities and differences, implications for theories of language development, and the seemingly natural interest shown by the public (this being both a product and a result of attention by the communications media); and, most important for present purposes, the implications for language intervention with mentally retarded persons which were apparent from the outset.

A third area of thought which perhaps integrates all the foundations for the current work in nonvocal systems of training is the idea that nonverbal modes are fundamental to all of human communication. The primacy of nonverbal communication can be supported in a number of ways. First, ethologists generally believe that human speech originally evolved from nonspeech communication. Even within the relatively recent period of man's recorded history, nonverbal signs and symbols hold great historical significance. Siger (1968) provides a brief but illuminating historical review of the use of nonverbal signs in communication. Aside from the evolutionary and phylogenetic implications, there are also ontogenetic implications for the role of nonverbal factors. Many persons interested in the development of language from infancy now believe that verbal language is "mapped" onto a nonverbal communication and conceptual system which infants acquire first (e.g., MacNamara, 1972). Finally, even in adult communication, many nonverbal mechanisms, such as facial expressions and gestures, are universally employed.

Since the late 1960s and early 1970s, a sizable number of articles has been published describing nonverbal communication skills taught to mentally retarded adults and children. Although a comprehensive review of these studies is not within the scope of this chapter, three studies indicative of the diversity of research in this area will be reviewed.

Duncan and Silverman (1977) used American-Indian Sign Language (AMERIND) in a total communication program for moderately retarded children. After obtaining some encouraging results, including some degree of spontaneous generalization, the authors suggest that for mentally retarded persons AMERIND is preferable to American Sign Language, because of its greater concreteness and intelligibility to untrained persons. In another representative study, Reid and Hurlbut (1977) taught severely physically disabled and mentally retarded adults to use a head pointer in order to identify word–picture combinations in response to a verbal label. In the third experiment reported, the subjects were taught to communicate their preferred choice of leisure activity to persons who previously were unable to understand their attempts at communication. Deich and Hodges (1977) reported a series of studies in which profoundly retarded young children were taught communication skills using Premack's system. Not only were children able to learn to use the plastic symbols to communicate, but some children also began to vocalize spontaneously during the studies.

Although the proliferation of articles detailing diverse methods for training nonverbal communication has been extremely useful, only recently has anyone provided a theoretical and practical organizational framework for determining which methods are likely to be successful with which populations of language-deficient individuals. In Hollis and Carrier's (1978) recent chapter, such a theoretical framework is offered, and the numerous nonverbal communication modes are classified. The authors then offer cogent arguments for why certain modes are suited to particular populations. Among the modes discussed are manual, such as American Sign Language, fingerspelling, and Signing Exact English, and graphic, such as Braille, Bliss (Bliss, 1965), Rebus (Woodcock, 1965), and Non-SLIP (Carrier & Peak, 1975). In addition to providing organization with regard to *mode* of teaching, Hollis and Carrier (1978) also present a comprehensive communication-training model with consideration given to structure of language taught and specific teaching method.

Of all the systems discussed by Hollis and Carrier (1978) the Non-SLIP program developed by Carrier and Peak (1975) is the only comprehensive nonspeech communication system yet devised specifically for severely and profoundly retarded individuals. A very basic functional communication program is taught, beginning with a lengthy period of training prerequisites (matching to sample with the plastic symbols), progressing to rote sequencing of symbols into "symbol class" slots corresponding to parts of speech, and finally reaching a stage in which symbols are matched to pictures of things and events. Carrier and Peak's system, as described by themselves (Carrier, 1974; Carrier & Peak, 1975; Hollis & Carrier, 1978) and summarized by others (Guess *et al.*, 1977), is a functional-analysis model which approaches language structure and sequencing from a "logical" and functional position, rather than using developmental data from studies of normal language acquisition. As Guess *et al.* (1977) point out, the model's advantages include effectiveness and speed in giving severely handicapped persons communicative ability, but its major limitation is that generalization is a problem because so few persons know and use the plastic symbol language.

Parental Factors in Language Acquisition

Attempts to involve parents directly in the training of language skills in their mentally retarded children have been rare, especially relative to other child problems where parents have frequently served a primary role in treatment. Typically, researchers have trained language skills in the laboratory and clinic, checking then for generalization of that training to the home environment. Garcia and De Haven's (1974) review, for example, catalogues the mixed results which have been obtained with such a research paradigm. Rather than summarize all the studies which have included generalization to the home, perhaps one example may be used in illustration. Garcia, Bullet, and Rust (1977) conducted a study specifically aimed at fostering generalization of training across settings, from classroom to home. After training mentally retarded children through the use of imitation and reinforcement procedures to label pictures with complex sentences in a classroom, the use of these sentences at home was measured. It was discovered that the children did not begin to use the trained sentences at home until some of the sentences were actually trained in the home setting.

Some of the shortcomings of behavioral language intervention programs as they have been described may be due to overreliance on highly skilled intervention "experts" as primary trainers, and attempts to teach language out of its natural physical and social context. It is our contention that greater success may be achieved, including more effective generalization of training, if greater emphasis is given toward parent-mediated training programs. In this section, we will attempt to outline some of the forms this redirection might take.

The Social Context of Language Acquisition

With such a firm historical foundation of concern for the functional aspects of behavior, it is surprising that many behavioral-intervention models appear to have lost sight of the natural functions of language. Language behaviors are acts which are fundamentally social in purpose. Stated differently, our production and reception of language primarily serve social functions. Although it is undeniably true that language also serves some individual, private functions, as in the case of self-guided behavior, most of its functions occur in interactions among two or more persons in reciprocal communication. One advocate of relocating language-training programs within their natural social context has been Mahoney, who has described an "ecological" model of training (Mahoney, 1975; Mahoney, Crawley, & Pullis, 1979; Mahoney & Seely, 1976).

An assumption of the ecological model is that language training can best be accomplished within the context of the child's daily activities and interactions within its caregiver, usually the mother. For example, if a goal of language training is to get the child to express the utterance "go out" when he wishes to do so, the best time to teach it is when he actually wishes to go outside, the best place to teach it is the context of his familiar surroundings, and the best person to teach it is probably his most frequent caregiver. It would be difficult to envision a clinical teaching situation more desirable than that just described. Many training programs have been overly "trainer oriented," with the trainer initiating all teaching exercises and disregarding what the child may actually be intending or interested in at any particular moment. One effect of such training is the high degree of stimulus control over language exerted by the trainer and the structured training environment.

As stated, an assumption of the ecological model is that the child's caregiver is the best person to implement a language-training program. Since it seems apparent that it is hardly feasible to develop all parents whose children are in need of language training into sophisticated operant therapists, simpler ways of training parents must be found. What follows is a discussion of some areas which must be explored before we can do a more effective job of parent training.

Parent–Child Communication

The way in which parents and their young children communicate both verbally and nonverbally must be understood more fully. If one assumes with MacNamara (1972) that language communication is preceded by, and dependent on, much social dialogue between parent and infant which is nonverbal, understanding all aspects of this process seems critical. A great deal of evidence already exists in support of the notion that very early parent–child communication occurs. Kagan's (1967) research with infants and facial schemata suggests that infants have the ability to discriminate human faces during the first few months of life. Research also suggests that infants can differentially process speech sounds at a very early age (Morse, 1974). Although these two areas document the infant's receptive-communication potential, more evidence suggests that infants' capacity for productive communication is also present at a very early age. Among the behaviors capable of acquiring early communicative function are crying, smiling and other facial gestures, babbling, eye contact, and numerous motor behaviors. Shaffer's (1971) early investigations into infants' so-called "signaling" ability, including smiling, have been of particular benefit, as have Bell's (1968, 1974) summaries of the numerous ways in which the active participation of the infant can affect the infant–caregiver interaction.

On the parent side of the interaction, evidence exists that, long before reciprocal language becomes important in parent–infant communications, parents are able to discriminate some of their infants' signals. As an example, some investigators have contended that parents could in some circumstances differentiate varying emotional states of their infants by listening to the infant's cry independent of contextual cues (Wolff, 1969). Other evidence exists that parents modify their speech in characteristic ways when addressing preverbal infants (e.g., Phillips, 1970), and it does not take a linguist to determine that "baby talk" is fundamentally different from speech addressed to other adults.

Although it seems obvious that looking at early parent–child communication is a good idea, many questions regarding the application to intervention programs remain unanswered. For example, can the interaction dialogue be described in qualitative terms? Can it be determined what the discriminative features of "good" and "poor" communicative dialogues are? Are infants differentially effective in their ability to receive messages (discriminate different speech sounds, for instance) and to send messages (communicate different intents by crying or smiling)? If deficiencies in the quality of early interactions between parent and infant can be detected, then two of the biggest questions seem to be, can these interactions be improved, and would the improvement have any bearing on facilitating later language development?

Besides modifying their speech to infants, there are other ways in which parents may modify their responses to children learning language. Persons interested in the modification of language in children have long been concerned with whether parents actively reinforce children's utterances. The issue of whether or not parents reinforce increasing grammaticality in children's language became an early question which linguists investigated as a critical test of behavioral versus linguistic theories of language development. It should be apparent by now, however, that the notions of reinforcement entertained by linguists in their early studies (e.g., Brown & Bellugi, 1964) were fairly unsophisticated. The early claims of linguists were that, because parents were not found to reward children in the general sense of socially praising or tangibly rewarding grammatical utterances, parental reinforcement was not a relevant factor in language development. If positive reinforcers are used in their more accurate sense as any consequence following a child's behavior which tends to increase the probability of that behavior's recurrence, it is easy to imagine how parental reinforcement of child language operates. What reinforces a child's utterance is often any action or word on the part of the parent indicating understanding of the child's communicative intent. Children's messages which are uninterpretable are not likely to produce the desired effect, whereas those that are clear are likely to receive positive feedback, not necessarily in the form of social praise ("good girl") or tangible reward ("I'll give you some juice for that"), but more often in some communication that the message has been received and understood. This communication back to the child could take many forms, including expansion of the utterance, modeling, performing some requested act, a nonverbal acknowledgment, and, yes, even giving social praise or a tangible reward.

Parental Speech to Mentally Retarded Children

Much research with nonretarded children indicates that adults adjust the complexity of their language when speaking to children (Broen, 1972; Phillips, 1970, 1973; Snow, 1972). In general, the speech addressed by adults to children has been found to be slower, more repetitive, more grammatical, of lower linguistic complexity, and characterized by fewer hesitations and broken sentences when compared with speech addressed to other adults. Although parents do not typically think of themselves as consciously teaching language to children, their language undoubtedly serves as a model for children who are learning to understand and speak. The adjustments made by adults, therefore, are likely to be critical in the provision of a model appropriate to the child's ability at the time.

Recently, a group of studies has been conducted to investigate specifically the characteristics of adult speech addressed to mentally retarded children. Since mentally retarded children are almost always delayed in language development, observation of the language models provided for them may be helpful for designing environments more facilitative for language development. One of the earlier studies was conducted by Marshall, Hegrenes, and

Goldstein (1973), who found that mothers of 3- to 5-year-old mentally retarded children used more "mands" than did mothers of nonretarded children when speaking to them. Manding consists of demanding, commanding, requesting, and asking, and is based on Skinner's (1957) classification of verbal operants. Several other studies have since been completed, and additional findings indicate that parents of mentally retarded children apparently regulate the complexity of their language according to the *perceived* competence of the child (Buckhalt, Rutherford, & Goldberg, 1978; Buium, Rynders, & Turnure, 1974; Rondal, 1977). These studies have shown that when groups of mentally retarded children are compared with groups of nonretarded children of comparable age, significant differences in parental language appear, but when groups are more comparable in mental ability, those differences are diminished. Among the questions left unanswered are how the parent assesses the child's competence to understand language, and how the parental language is then matched to the child's ability. Of course, a primary question underlying much of the research is how can an optimal match be achieved which allows for maximum understanding by the child but at the same time exposes him to new language forms and thus encourages development. In all probability, communication problems exist between some parents and their mentally retarded children which prevent optimal development of language.

The work of Fraiberg (1974, 1977) with blind infants and their mothers may provide a model useful for the design of facilitative language interventions for mentally retarded infants. Fraiberg first observed that the communication system between mother and child was not optimal, because of the blind infants' deficiencies in the normal ways in which infants signal various messages. For example, she found that the absence of eye contact and the delayed smiling responses of blind infants tended to cause mothers to misinterpret their emotional states and feel rebuffed by the infants. One result was the provision of fewer verbal interactions, and this state of affairs may have contributed to later delays in language development. When mothers were trained to be more aware of the blind infants' motoric patterns, which often were responsive to maternal stimulation when smiling and eye contact were absent, mothers reported more positive feelings and importantly changed their styles of interacting with the infants. If the ecological model is correct in assuming that a healthy communication system is critical to language development, perhaps parents of mentally retarded infants could be sensitized to their child's communication signals, which may be less pronounced, slower in development, or more idiosyncratic than those of a similar-aged non retarded infant.

Suggestions for Parent-Oriented Language Intervention

In conclusion, the following suggestions are offered as possible directions that language-intervention programs might take to improve their overall effectiveness.

1. Make the locus of language intervention the home and other places where the child spends much time, instead of the clinic or the laboratory. Make the parents the primary language interventionists, with speech therapists and other professionals serving as consultants.

2. Make better use of the linguistic knowledge the parent already possesses as a native speaker of the language. Also, to the extent possible, make the content and methods of intervention as close as possible to the "natural" methods and content of language acquisition, so that parents feel more comfortable and less like technicians applying esoteric principles.

3. Diagnose and remediate difficulties in communication between parents and child, attending first to interactions taking place before the child begins to speak, including verbal and nonverbal interactions. Teach parents to be sensitive to the child's attempts at communication, which may differ from those of a nonretarded child. Teach effective forms of responsiveness and reciprocal communication.

4. Concentrate on giving parents simple, rather than complex, instructional guidelines and rely on their knowledge of the child and of the language to shape the specific course of intervention. An example would be to give parents simple and general notions of how their language complexity should be adjusted to the child's competence and how reinforcement should take many specific forms when applied to the child's utterances.

An excellent intervention study has been reported recently which clearly exemplifies the final suggestion (Cheseldine & McConkey, 1979). In that study, parents of young mentally retarded children were given simple language-training objectives based on their child's level of language development. Some parents were remarkably successful in designing their own training strategies based on the guidelines given to them. Although some similarities existed among parents who were most successful in achieving the objectives, a more interesting aspect was the variety of strategies used, suggesting some accommodation to the individual children, possibly based on knowledge of the children which parents would be in the best position to have.

Another study which seems to add support to this general idea was conducted by Heifetz (1977), who compared the effectiveness of an extensive classroom training program for parents of mentally retarded children with a condition in which parents were merely given the instruction manuals. To the surprise of the author, the manuals-alone format was as effective as other training formats in producing skill acquisition by the children.

The ideas expressed in this section have much congruence with the work of MacDonald (MacDonald, 1976; MacDonald & Blott, 1974; MacDonald, Blott, Gordon, Spiegel, & Hartmann, 1974), who has explicitly called for parents to be considered primary figures in language intervention efforts. For example, in his description of the Environmental Language Intervention Model, MacDonald (1976) suggests that language therapists alter their role to one of the "prescriptive consultant" to parents and teachers.

Finally, the chapter published recently by Schumaker and Sherman (1978), though providing no new empirical support for the positions taken here, is supportive in the sense that a similar training philosophy is espoused. In addition to containing an excellent presentation of the rationale for making parents central figures in language-training programs, a great number of suggestions are offered for specific ways in which parents can promote the language development of their language-delayed children.

ACKNOWLEDGMENT

The authors are gratefully appreciative of the clerical and editorial assistance of Patricia Watson in the preparation of this chapter.

REFERENCES

BAER, D. M., & GUESS, D. Receptive training of adjectival inflections in mental retardates. *Journal of Applied Behavior Analysis*, 1971, *4*, 129–139.

BAER, D. M., & GUESS, D. Teaching productive noun suffixes to severely retarded children. *American Journal of Mental Deficiency*, 1973, *77*, 498–505.

BAER, D. M., & SHERMAN, J. A. Reinforcement control of generalized imitation in young children. *Journal of Experimental Child Psychology*, 1964, *1*, 37–49.

BAER, D. M., PETERSON, R. F., & SHERMAN, J. A. The development of imitation by reinforcing similarity to a model. *Journal of the Experimental Analysis of Behavior*, 1967, *10*, 405–416.

BAER, D. M., GUESS, D., & SHERMAN, J. A. Adventures in simplistic grammar. In R. L. Schiefelbuch (Ed.), *Language of the mentally retarded*. Baltimore: University Park Press, 1972.

BARTON, E. S. Inappropriate speech in a severely retarded child: A case study in language conditioning and generalization. *Journal of Applied Behavior Analysis*, 1970, *3*, 209–217.

BELL, R. Q. A reinterpretation of the direction of effects in studies of socialization. *Psychological Review*, 1968, *75*, 81–95.

BELL, R. Q. Contributions of human infants to caregiving and social interaction. In M. Lewis & L. A. Rosenblum (Eds.), *The effect of the infant on its caregiver*. New York: Wiley, 1974.

Bennett, C. W., & Ling, D. Teaching a complex verbal response to a hearing impaired girl. *Journal of Applied Behavior Analysis,* 1972, *5,* 321–327.
Bereiter, C., & Engelmann, S. *Teaching disadvantaged children in the preschool.* Englewood Cliffs, N. J.: Prentice-Hall, 1966.
Berger, S. L. A clinical program for developing multimodal responses with atypical deaf children. In J. E. McLean, D. E. Yoder, & R. L. Schiefelbusch (Eds.), *Language intervention with the retarded: Developing strategies.* Baltimore: University Park Press, 1972..
Bliss, C. K. *Semantography—Blissymbolics.* Sydney, Australia: Semantography Publications, 1965.
Bloom, L. *Language development: Form and function in emerging grammars.* Cambridge, Mass.: MIT Press, 1970.
Bricker, D. D. Imitative sign training as a facilitator of word-object association with low-functioning children. *American Journal of Mental Deficiency,* 1972, *76,* 509–516.
Bricker, D., Vincent-Smith, L., & Bricker, W. A. Receptive vocabulary: Performances and selection strategies of delayed and nondelayed toddlers. *American Journal of Mental Deficiency,* 1973, *77,* 579–584.
Bricker, D., Dennison, L., & Bricker, W. A. A language intervention program for developmentally young children. *MCCD Monograph Series,* 1976, No. 1.
Bricker, W. A., & Bricker, D. Development of receptive vocabulary in severely retarded children. *American Journal of Mental Deficiency,* 1970, *74,* 599–607.
Bricker, W. A., & Bricker, D. Receptive vocabulary as a factor in the discriminative performance of low functioning children. *American Journal of Mental Deficiency,* 1971, *5,* 599–605.
Bricker, W. A., & Bricker, D. D. An early language training strategy. In R. L. Schiefelbusch & L. L. Lloyd (Eds.), *Language perspectives: Acquisition, retardation, and intervention.* Baltimore: University Park Press, 1974.
Broen, P. The verbal environment of the language learning child. *American Speech and Hearing Association Monographs,* 1972, No. 17.
Brown, R. *A first language: The early stages.* Cambridge, Mass.: Harvard University Press, 1973.
Brown, R., & Bellugi, U. Three processes in the child's acquisition of syntax. *Harvard Educational Review,* 1964, *34,* 133–151.
Buckhalt, J., Rutherford, R., & Goldberg, K. Verbal and nonverbal interactions of mothers with their Down's Syndrome and nonretarded infants. *American Journal of Mental Deficiency,* 1978, *82,* 337–343.
Buium, N., Rynders, J., & Turnure, J. Early maternal linguistic environment of normal and Down's Syndrome language-learning children. *American Journal of Mental Deficiency,* 1974, *79,* 52–58.
Butz, R. A., & Hasazi, J. E. The effects of reinforcement on perseverative speech in a mildly retarded boy. *Journal of Behavior Therapy and Experimental Psychiatry,* 1973, *4,* 167–170.
Carrier, J. K. Application of functional analysis and a nonspeech response mode to teaching language. *American Speech and Hearing Association Monographs,* 1974, No. 18.
Carrier, J. K., & Peak, T. *Nonspeech language initiation program.* Lawrence, Kans.: H & H Enterprises, 1975.
Carroll, J. B. Language development in children. In S. Saporta (Ed.), *Psycholinguistics.* New York: Holt, Rinehart & Winston, 1961.
Cheseldine, S., & McConkey, R. Parental speech to young Down's Syndrome children: An intervention study. *American Journal of Mental Deficiency,* 1979, *83,* 612–620.
Chomsky, N. Review of B. F. Skinner. *Verbal behavior. Language,* 1959, *35,* 26–58.
Clark, H. B., & Sherman, J. A. Teaching generative uses of sentence answers. *Journal of Applied Behavior Analysis,* 1975, *8,* 321–330

COOK, C., & ADAMS, H. E. Modification of verbal behavior in speech deficient children. *Behavior Research and Therapy*, 1966, *4*, 265–271.

COOKE, S., COOKE, T. P., & APOLLONI, T. Generalization of language training with the mentally retarded. *Journal of Speech Education*, 1976, *10*, 299–304.

CRAIGHEAD, W. E., KAZDIN, A. E., & MAHONEY, M. J. *Behavior modification: Principles, issues, and applications*. Boston: Houghton Mifflin, 1976.

CROMER, R. F. Receptive language in the mentally retarded: Processes and diagnostic distinctions. In R. L. Schiefelbusch & L. L. Lloyd (Eds.), *Language perspectives: Acquisition, retardation, and intervention*. Baltimore: University Park Press, 1974.

DEICH, R. F., & HODGES, P. M. *Language without speech*. New York: Brunner/Mazel, 1977.

DUNCAN, J. L., & SILVERMAN, F. H. Impact of learning American Indian Sign Language on mentally retarded children: A preliminary report. *Perceptual and Motor Skills*, 1977, *44*, 1138.

DUNN, L. M., HORTON, K. B., & SMITH, J. O. *Manual for the Peabody Language Development Kit*. Minneapolis: American Guidance Services, 1965.

ESPER, E. A. A technique for the experimental investigation of associative interference in artificial linguistic material. *Language Monographs*, 1925, No. 1.

FOUTS, R. S. Use of guidance in teaching sign language to a chimpanzee. *Journal of Comparative and Physiological Psychology*, 1972, *80*, 515–522.

FRAIBERG, S. Blind infants and their mothers: An examination of the sign system. In M. Lewis & L. A. Rosenblum (Eds.), *The effect of the infant on its caregiver*. New York: Wiley, 1974.

FRAIBERG, S. *Insights from the blind: Comparative studies of blind and sighted infants*. New York: New American Library, 1977.

GARCIA, E. E., & DEHAVEN, E. Use of operant techniques in the establishment and generalization of language: A review and analysis. *American Journal of Mental Deficiency*, 1974, *79*, 169–178.

GARCIA, E. E., GUESS, D., & BYRNES, J. Development of syntax through imitation of a model. *Journal of Applied Behavior Analysis*, 1973, *6*, 299–310.

GARCIA, E. E., BULLET, J., & RUST, F. P. An experimental analysis of language training generalization across classroom and home. *Behavior Modification*, 1977, *1*, 531–550.

GARDNER, R. A., & GARDNER, B. T. Teaching sign language to a chimpanzee. *Science*, 1969, *165*, 664–672.

GELFAND, D. M., & HARTMANN, D. P. *Child behavior analysis and therapy*. New York: Pergamon, 1975.

GUESS, D. A functional analysis of receptive language and productive speech: Acquisition of the plural morpheme. *Journal of Applied Behavior Analysis*, 1969, *2*, 55–64.

GUESS, D., & BAER, D. M. Some experimental analyses of linguistic development in institutionalized retarded children. In B. B. Lahey (Ed.), *The modification of language behavior*. Springfield, Ill.: Charles C Thomas, 1973.

GUESS, D., SAILOR, W., RUTHERFORD, G., & BAER, D. An experimental analysis of linguistic development: The productive use of the plural morpheme. *Journal of Applied Behavior Analysis*, 1968, *1*, 225–235.

GUESS, D., SAILOR, W., & BAER, D. M. To teach language to retarded children. In R. L. Schiefelbusch & L. L. Lloyd (Eds.), *Language perspectives: Acquisition, retardation, and intervention*. Baltimore: University Park Press, 1974.

GUESS, D., SAILOR, W., & BAER, D. M. Functional speech and language training for the severely handicapped. Part I: Persons and things. Lawrence, Kans.: H & H Enterprises, 1976. (a)

GUESS, D., SAILOR, W., & BAER, D. M. Functional speech and language training for the severely handicapped. Part II: Action with persons and things. Lawrence, Kans.: H & H Enterprises, 1976. (b)

Guess, D., Sailor, W., & Keogh, W. *Language intervention programs and procedures for handicapped children: A review of the literature.* Final Project Report, U.S. Office of Education, Division of Mental Health and Mental Retardation of the Social and Rehabilitation Services Department of the State of Kansas, 1977.

Guess, D., Sailor, W., & Baer, D. M. Children with limited language. In R. L. Schiefelbusch (Ed.), *Language intervention strategies.* Baltimore: University Park Press, 1978.

Hall, S. M., & Talkington, L. W. Evaluation of a manual approach to programming for deaf retarded. *American Journal of Mental Deficiency,* 1970, *75,* 376–378.

Harris, S. L. Teaching language to nonverbal children with emphasis on problems of generalization. *Psychological Bulletin,* 1975, *82,* 565–580.

Heifetz, L. J. Behavioral training for parents of retarded children: Alternative formats based on instruction manuals. *American Journal of Mental Deficiency,* 1977, *82,* 194–203.

Hewett, F. M. Teaching speech to an autistic child through operant conditioning. *American Journal of Orthopsychiatry,* 1965, *35,* 927–936.

Hoffmeister, R. J., & Farmer, A. The development of manual sign in mentally retarded deaf individuals. *Journal of Rehabilitation of the Deaf,* 1972, *6,* 19–26.

Hollis, J. H., & Carrier, J. K., Jr. Intervention strategies for non-speech children. In R. L. Schiefelbusch (Ed.), *Language intervention strategies.* Baltimore: University Park Press, 1978.

Isaacs, W., Thomas, J., & Goldiamond, I. Application of operant conditioning to reinstate verbal behavior in mute psychotics. *Journal of Abnormal Psychology,* 1965, *70,* 155–164.

Jackson, D. A., & Wallace, R. F. The modification and generalization of voice loudness in a fifteen-year-old retarded girl. *Journal of Applied Behavior Analysis,* 1974, *7,* 461–471.

Jeffree, D., Wheldall, K., & Mittler, P. Facilitating two-word utterances in two Down's Syndrome boys. *American Journal of Mental Deficiency,* 1973, *78,* 117–122.

Johnston, M. K. Echolalia and automatism in speech: A case report. In H. N. Sloane, Jr., & B. D. MacAulay (Eds.), *Operant procedures in remedial speech and language training.* Boston: Houghton Mifflin, 1968.

Jordon, T. E. Language and mental retardation: A review of the literature. In R. L. Schiefelbusch, R. H. Copeland, & J. C. Smith (Eds.), *Language and mental retardation: Empirical and conceptual considerations.* New York: Holt, Rinehart & Winston, 1967.

Kagan, J. The growth of the "face" schema: Theoretical significance and methodological issues. In J. Hellmuth (Ed.), *Exceptional infant* (Vol. 1). New York: Brunner/Mazel, 1967.

Keller, M. F., & Bucher, B. D. Transfer between receptive and productive language in developmentally disabled children. *Journal of Applied Behavior Analysis,* 1979, *12,* 311.

Kellogg, W. N. Communication and language in the home-raised chimpanzee. *Science,* 1968, *162,* 423–427.

Kent, L. R. *Language acquisition program for the retarded or multiply impaired.* Champaign, Ill.: Research Press, 1974.

Kent, L. R., Klein, D., Falk, A., & Guenther, H. A language acquisition program for the retarded. In J. E. McLean, D. E. Yoder, & R. L. Schiefelbusch (Eds.), *Language intervention with the retarded: Developing strategies.* Baltimore: University Park Press, 1972.

Lovaas, O. I. A program for the establishment of speech in psychotic children. In J. K. Wing (Ed.), *Childhood autism.* Oxford: Pergamon, 1966.

Lovaas, O. I. *The autistic child.* New York: Irvington, 1977.

Lovaas, O. I., & Newsom, C. D. Behavior modification with psychotic children. In H. Leitenberg (Ed.), *Handbook of behavior modification and behavior therapy.* Englewood Cliffs, N. J.: Prentice-Hall, 1976.

Lovaas, O. I., Berberich, J. P., Perloff, B. F., & Schaeffer, B. Acquisition of imitative speech in schizophrenic children. *Science,* 1966, *151,* 705–707

LYNCH, J., & BRICKER, W. A. Linguistic theory and operant procedures: Toward an integrated approach to language training for the mentally retarded. *Mental Retardation*, 1972, *10*, 12–17.

MACDONALD, J. D. Environmental language intervention. In F. B. Withrow & C. J. Nygren (Eds.), *Language, materials, and curriculum management for the handicapped learner*. Columbus, Ohio: Charles E. Merrill, 1976.

MACDONALD, J. D., & BLOTT, J. P. Environmental language intervention: A rationale for a diagnostic and training strategy through rules, context, and generalization. *Journal of Speech and Hearing Disorders*, 1974, *39*, 244–256.

MACDONALD, J. D., BLOTT, J. P., GORDON, K., SPIEGEL, B., & HARTMANN, M. An experimental parent-assisted treatment program for preschool language delayed children. *Journal of Speech and Hearing Disorders*, 1974, *39*, 395–415.

MACNAMARA, J. Cognitive basis of language learning in infants. *Psychological Review*, 1972, *77*, 282–293.

MAHONEY, G. An ethological approach to delayed language acquisition. *American Journal of Mental Deficiency*, 1975, *80*, 139–148.

MAHONEY, G., & SEELY, P. The role of the social agent in language acquisition: Implications for language intervention. In N. R. Ellis (Ed.), *International review of research in mental retardation* (Vol. 8). New York: Academic Press, 1976.

MAHONEY, G. J., CRAWLEY, S., & PULLIS, M. Language intervention: Models and issues. In B. K. Keogh (Ed.), *Advances in special education* (Vol. 1). Greenwich, Conn.: JAI Press, 1979.

MARSHALL, N. R., & HEGRENES, J. R. Programmed communication therapy for autistically mentally retarded children. *Journal of Speech and Hearing Disorders*, 1970, *35*, 70–83.

MARSHALL, N., HEGRENES, J., & GOLDSTEIN, S. Verbal interactions: Mothers with their retarded children versus mothers and their nonretarded children. *American Journal of Mental Deficiency*, 1973, *77*, 415–419.

MCKENNA-HARTUNG, S., & HARTUNG, J. R. Establishing verbal imitation skills and functional speech in autistic children. In B. B. Lahey (Ed.), *The modification of language behavior*. Springfield, Ill.: Charles C Thomas, 1973.

MCLEAN, J. E., & SNYDER, L. K. *A transactional approach to early language training: Derivation of a model system*. Final Project Report. Nashville, Tenn.: George Peabody College for Teachers, 1977.

MILLER, J. F., & YODER, D. E. A syntax teaching program. In J. E. McLean, D. E. Yoder, & R. L. Schiefelbusch (Eds.), *Language intervention with the retarded: Developing strategies*. Baltimore: University Park Pres, 1972.

MILLER, J. F., & YODER, D. E. An ontogenetic language teaching strategy for retarded children. In R. L. Schiefelbush & L. L. Lloyd (Eds.), *Language perspectives: Acquisition, retardation, and intervention*. Baltimore: University Park Press, 1974.

MORSE, P. A. Infant speech perception: A preliminary model and review of the literature. In R. L. Schiefelbusch & L. L. Lloyd (Eds.), *Language perspectives: Acquisition, retardation, and intervention*. Baltimore: University Park Press, 1974.

NOLAN, J. D., & PENCE, C. Operant conditioning principles in the treatment of a selectively mute child. *Journal of Consulting and Clinical Psychology*, 1970, *35*, 265–268.

O'LEARY, K. D., & WILSON, G. T. *Behavior therapy: Application and outcome*. Englewood Cliffs, N. J.: Prentice-Hall, 1975.

PHILLIPS, J. Syntax and vocabulary of mother's speech to young children: Age and sex comparisons. *Child Development*, 1973, *44*, 182–185.

PHILLIPS, J. R. *Formal characteristics of speech which mothers address to their children*. (Doctoral dissertation, The Johns Hopkins University, 1970). Ann Arbor, Mich.: University Microfilms, 1970.

PREMACK, A. J., & PREMACK, D. Teaching language to an ape. *Scientific American*, 1972, *227*, 92–99.

Redd, W. H., Porterfield, A. L., & Andersen, B. L. *Behavior modification: Behavioral approaches to human problems.* New York: Random House, 1979.
Reid, D. H., & Hurlbut, B. Teaching nonvocal communication skills to multihandicapped adults. *Journal of Applied Behavior Analysis,* 1977, *10,* 591–603.
Risley, T. R., & Wolf, M. M. Establishing functional speech in echolalic children. *Behavior Research and Therapy,* 1967, *5,* 73–88.
Rondal, J. A. Maternal speech in normal and Down's Syndrome children. In P. Mittler (Ed.), *Research to practice in mental retardation.* Baltimore: University Park Press, 1977.
Rumbaugh, D. M., Gill, T. V., & Von Glaserfeld, E. C. Reading and sentence completion by a chimpanzee. *Science,* 1973, *182,* 731–733.
Sailor, W. Reinforcement and generalization of productive plural allomorphs in two retarded children. *Journal of Applied Behavior Analysis,* 1971, *4,* 305–310.
Salzinger, K., Feldman, R., Cowan, J., & Salzinger, S. Operant conditioning of verbal behavior of two young speech-deficient boys. In L. Krasner (L. P. Ullman (Eds.), *Research in behavior modification.* New York: Holt, Rinehart, & Winston, 1965.
Schlesinger, I. M. Production of utterances and language acquisition. In D. I. Slobin (Ed.), *The ontogenesis of grammar.* New York: Academic Press, 1971.
Schumaker, J., & Sherman, J. A. Training generative verb usage by imitation and reinforcement procedures. *Journal of Applied Behavior Analysis,* 1970, *3,* 273–287.
Schumaker, J. B., & Sherman, J. A. Parent as intervention agent: From birth onward. In R. L. Schiefelbusch (Ed.), *Language intervention strategies.* Baltimore: University Park Press, 1978.
Shaffer, H. R. *The growth of sociability.* Baltimore: Penguin, 1971.
Sherman, J. A. Reinstatement of verbal behavior in a psychotic by reinforcement methods. *Journal of Speech and Hearing Disorders,* 1963, *28,* 398–400.
Sherman, J. A. Use of reinforcement and imitation to reinstate verbal behavior in mute psychotics. *Journal of Abnormal and Social Psychology,* 1965, *70,* 155–164
Siger, L. C. Gestures, the language of signs, and human communications. *American Annals of the Deaf,* 1968, *113,* 11–28.
Skinner, B. F. *Verbal behavior.* New York: Appleton-Century-Crofts, 1957.
Sloane, H. N., & MacAulay, B. D. (Eds). *Operant procedures in remedial speech and language training.* Boston: Houghton Mifflin, 1968.
Sloane, H. N., Johnston, M. K., & Harris, F. R. Remedial procedures for teaching verbal behavior to speech deficient or defective young children. In H. N. Sloane & B. D. MacAulay (Eds.), *Operant procedures in remedial speech and language training.* Boston: Houghton Mifflin, 1968.
Snow, C. Mothers' speech to children learning language. *Child Development,* 1972, *43,* 549–565.
Solnick, J. V., Rincover, A., & Peterson, C. R. Some determinants of the reinforcing and punishing effects of timeout. *Journal of Applied Behavior Analysis,* 1977, *10,* 415–424.
Staats, A. W. Behaviorism and cognitive theory in the study of language: A neopsycholinguistics. In R. L. Schiefelbush & L. L. Lloyd (Eds.), *Language perspectives: Acquisition, retardation, and intervention.* Baltimore: University Park Press, 1974.
Stevens-Long, J., & Rasmussen, M. The acquisition of simple and compound sentence structure in an autistic child. *Journal of Applied Behavior Analysis,* 1974, *7,* 473–479.
Stokes, T. S., & Baer, D. M. An implicit technology of generalization. *Journal of Applied Behavior Analysis,* 1977, *10,* 349–367.
Stremel, K. Language training: A problem for retarded children. *Mental Retardation,* 1972, *10,* 47–79.
Stremel, K., & Waryas, C. A behavioral-psycholinguistic approach to language training. In L. McReynolds (Ed.), Developing systematic procedures for training children's language. *American Speech and Hearing Monographs,* 1974, No. 18.

American Speech and Hearing Monographs, 1974, No. 18.

STRIEFEL, S. & WETHERBY, B. Instruction-following behavior of a retarded child and its controlling stimuli. *Journal of Applied Behavior Analysis*, 1973, *6*, 663–670.

STRIEFEL, S., BRYAN, K. S., & AIKENS, D. A. Transfer of stimulus control from motor to verbal stimuli. *Journal of Applied Behavior Analysis*, 1974, *7*, 123–135.

STRIEFEL, S., WETHERBY, B., & KARLAN, G. R. Establishing generalized verb-noun instruction-following skills in retarded children. *Journal of Experimental Child Psychology*, 1976, *22*, 247–260.

STRIEFEL, S., WETHERBY, B., & KARLAN, G. Developing generalized instruction-following behavior ion severely retarded people. In C. E. Meyers (Ed.), *Quality of life in severely and profoundly mentally retarded people: Research foundations for improvement*. Washington, D. C.: American Association on Mental Deficiency, 1978.

SULZER-AZAROFF, B., & MAYER, G. R. *Applying behavior-analysis procedures with children and youth*. New York: Holt, Rinehart, & Winston, 1977.

TERRACE, H. S. Stimulus control. In W. K. Honig (Ed.), *Operant behavior: Areas of research and application*. New York, Appleton-Century-Crofts, 1966.

TOUCHETTE, P. E. Transfer of stimulus control: Measuring the moment of transfer. *Journal of the Experimental Analysis of Behavior*, 1971, *15*, 347–354.

TRAMONTANA, J., & SHIVERS, O. Behavior modification with an echolalic child: A case note. *Psychological Reports*, 1971, *29*, 1034.

WETHERBY, B., & STRIEFEL, S. Application of miniature linguistic system or matrix-training procedures. In R. L. Schiefelbusch (Ed.), *Language intervention strategies*. Baltimore: University Park Press, 1978.

WHEELER, A. J. & SULZER, B. Operant training and generalization of a verbal response form in a speech-deficient child. *Journal of Applied Behavior Analysis*, 1970, *3*, 139–147.

WHITMAN, T. L., ZAKAROS, M., & CHARDOS, S. Effects of reinforcement and guidance procedures on instruction-following behanior of severely retarded children. *Journal of Applied Behavior Analysis*, 1971, *4*, 283–290.

WOLF, M. M., RISLEY, T. R., & MEES, H. Application of operant conditioning procedures to the behavior problems of an autistic child. *Behavior Research and Therapy*, 1964, *2*, 305–312.

WOLFF, P. H. The natural history of crying and other vocalizations in early infancy. In B. M. Foss (Ed.), *Determinants of infant behavior* (Vol. 4). London: Methuen, 1969.

WOODCOCK, R. W. *The Rebus reading series*. Nashville, Tenn.: Institute on Mental Retardation and Intellectual Development, George Peabody College for Teachers, 1965.

10 Academic Training

Paul Weisberg, Richard A. Packer,
and Roberta S. Weisberg

Introduction

The contents of instructional programs must be specified in sufficient detail so that they can be followed and delivered in a consistent and coherent manner by all teachers. Just as an instructional designer would like to account for academic improvement partly as a result of the program's clear specification, the designer must also be ready to accept blame for academic failure partly or wholly because of ambiguity in specificity. The emphasis on procedural detail is most important for the mentally retarded or the low-performing individual. These individuals are highly dependent on what occurs in the classroom for their initial and continuing source of academic information in traditional content areas. A program that permits and encourages wide latitude in teacher presentation in effect prevents consistent coverage of material and does the low performer and the technology of instruction a great injustice. Without being able to reconstruct fairly precisely what was taught to the low performer, and how it was taught, one is unable to account for and begin to modify the instructional variables causing any academic setbacks. Further, to ask the teacher to return to earlier and presumably easier formats for correcting present learning difficulties is impossible with programs lacking instructional detail. Although these factors seem obvious, it is surprising how many behavior analysts called into the classroom to reconcile academic difficulties fail to search curriculum material and teacher manuals for completeness in instructional specificity.

An instructional regime can be meticulously descriptive, and yet fail to develop the academic concepts and operations it states as its long-term objectives. Despite clear and elaborate specification of certain details, a rhyming format may not enable the learner to classify words in a particular rhyming group, largely because a number of examples of words belonging to this

Paul Weisberg and Richard A. Packer • Department of Psychology, University of Alabama, Tuscaloosa, Alabama 35401. Roberta S. Weinberg • Tuscaloosa City Schools, Tuscaloosa, Alabama 35405.

group were never modeled by the teacher. A program designed to develop oral reading by teaching the letter names of the alphabet or the discrimination between consonants and vowels will not succeed if these skills are not critical to the actual decoding of words, no matter how easy the training program is to follow. Thus, aside from the aspect of program specificity, the programming logic must be scrutinized. Although there is much debate among educational programmers about what are the relevant component skills for teaching traditional academic operations, such as concept application, decoding of words, addition, spelling, handwriting, etc., and what are the most efficient instructional strategies for the low performer, the programming principles and teaching techniques of some programmers, notably Engelmann and his colleagues (Engelmann, 1969, Engelmann & Carnine, 1980), are admittedly appealing and will form the basis for many of the conceptualizations in this chapter.

Engelmann has been the major contributor to a commercial program known as DISTAR (Direct Instruction Systems for Teaching and Remediation). There are separate programs for language, reading, and arithmetic, each divided into three levels usually corresponding for use in the first three years of school. All these programs are distinquished by their logical and empirical analysis of the prerequisite skills for building complex behavior, preferably through strategy or rule-governed behavior, as well as for a complete specification of instuctional details.

The DISTAR programs are used extensively in special-education classrooms and for low performers in the regular classroom, although the programs are valid for average and advanced performers. The program has been part of a large-scale educational-intervention project, known as Follow Through, the purpose of which was to determine whether the academic performance of high-risk disadvantaged children typically falling in the 20th percentile or lower on achievement tests could be appreciably raised. DISTAR was compared with eight major programs running the gamut of educational practice—Piagetian, Child Development, Behavior Analysis, Language Experience, Parent Education Model, Responsive Education, Bilingual Education and the Open Classroom. Over 9,000 intervention children and 6,000 comparison controls from across the United States were taught in the primary grades (K-3) and evaluated for academic and other performance at the end of third grade. The data were independently evaluated by ABT Associates (1976, 1977). DISTAR was clearly the most effective model in comparison with control groups, national norms, and the eight other intervention models. On the Metropolitan Achievement Test (MAT), DISTAR raised achievement in total reading to the 41st percentile, in total math to the 48th, in spelling to the 51st, and in language to the 59th. Except for MAT spelling by the Behavior Analysis model, none of the other programs came close to normative levels, and many never improved achievement beyond the 20th percentile. DISTAR was also ranked at the top in self-esteem scores, as evaluated by the Coopersmith Self Esteem, Intellectual Achievement Responsibility Scale.

Maggs (Bracey, Maggs, & Morath, 1975a,b; Maggs & Morath, 1975, 1976) has extended the use of DISTAR and related programs to a range of problem learners in Australia. Among the results found were: (1) institutionalized moderately and severely retarded children (IQ between 20 and 30) trained by DISTAR language program were able to gain 22½ mental-age (MA) months on the Stanford-Binet IQ test in the 24 months of the program, which means that the children were progressing at almost a normal rate (controls gained 7½ MA months in 2 years); (2) moderately retarded children (IQ 35 to 50) using the arithmetic program made significant gains in basic computational skills, and another group of nonreading children (IQ 30 to 40) using the Reading program were able to develop effective reading skills; (3) a large group of moderately and severely mentally retarded children given all three DISTAR programs made significant gains in problem-solving skills and on IQ test scores, with the gains made related to the amount of time the schools allowed for instruction (½ hour to 2½ hours daily); and (4) the rate of learning by children in the upper levels of moderate mental retardation, who had been in a special school using various DISTAR programs for an average of 10 years, changed as a function of time in the program. Learning in the beginning stages of DISTAR usage was at the rate of two language-age months gained for each five calendar months, but, after several years of school instruction with DISTAR, it advanced to 34 months for 32 months of instruction.

The significance of reinforcement variables toward the advancement of academic achievement needs briefly to be addressed. There is no doubt that providing sources of appropriate information about the correctness or incorrectness of new performances will contribute greatly toward their future improvement, and providing intermittent reinforcement for already practiced performances is also necessary for maintenance. However, it is also true that reinforcement contingencies, in and of themselves, will not undo the harm created by poorly designed and implemented curriculum materials and instructional programs. Although these facts seem obvious, behavior analysts working in academic settings have attempted to institute reinforcement contingencies without first taking a hard look at the composition, teaching, and sequencing of instructional materials, which will be one of the primary objectives of this chapter.

Reinforcement variables will have a major impact on the "won't-do" learner, one who has the necessary conceptual and response repertoires for attending to and completing academic tasks but, for some reason, fails to do so. The bulk of successfully engineered reinforcement studies in the classroom by behavior analysts are in this realm. However, for the individual currently without these repertoires—the "cant-do" learner—no amount of reinforcement will rectify the problem if its basis stems from inadequate learning owing to instructional variables. For example, assume that two students, given worksheets containing reading-comprehension questions, both demonstrate the same high degree of off-task behaviors. The can't-do learner, never taught efficient strategies for decoding regular words or perhaps because the worksheet features a number of unfamiliar conceptual analogies, gives up working the items after a few false starts, and "acts up." The won't do learner, on the other hand, who is able to handle the material, acts inappropriately possibly because past worksheets have been infrequently graded, and then several weeks have passed before they were returned. A reinforcement system would certainly benefit the won't do learner but not the can't do individual.

Illustrations like these are real and commonplace in educational settings. They should serve to remind the classroom-behavior analyst that the first order of business, before resorting to elaborate reinforcement systems, is the analysis of educational design and programming practices. That programming logic and principles can substantially influence academic performance over and above well-founded and existing reinforcement systems comes from the Follow Through data. Both the DISTAR and Behavior Analysis models made heavy use of reinforcement systems—in fact, the teachers of both models were trained together in the design and use of contingencies of reinforcement (Becker & Carmine, 1980), yet there were major outcome differences in the academic scores of the two models, which must be attributed largely to the use of different curricula material and the mode of presentation.

This chapter will begin with instructional-design features for teaching basic concepts, then will discuss the selection of activities for the expansion, sequencing, and integration of these concepts. Following this will be a rather extensive analysis of the component variables and teaching procedures used in commercial reading programs.

TEACHING CONCEPTS: SOME CONSIDERATIONS

Positive and Negative Concept Instances

The bulk of the research literature surveyed on instructional methods for mentally retarded individuals has dealt with procedures for teaching basic discriminations not easily taught through verbal rules or elaborate definitions. This is understandable, considering that it would be next to impossible for an instructionally naive individual to learn about purple from the dictionary meaning in terms of wavelength location on the spectrum or about slantedness from a verbal description of the various non-90° or -180° angles a flat object can assume.

The preoccupation with teaching basic concepts is well founded. Since basic discriminations are vital building blocks for more complex cognitive concepts, academic programs must do a creditable job in teaching the basics if the learner is to advance steadily to the complex. What is more, instructional formats must teach basic concepts in the most expeditious and efficient manner, particularly to those individuals who are distinguished as lagging behind their age peers in their understanding of these very concepts. Indeed, much curricula material for the mentally retarded does nothing but emphasize the prerequisites for future learning. (Guess, Sailor, & Baer, 1976).

Advanced learners, such as the readers of this chapter, often cannot appreciate the difficulties the instructionally naive have in understanding the meaning of basic concepts. When the learner doesn't understand, concept failure is commonly attributed to a defective trait or a deficiency that resides within the nonlearner; but in truth the nonlearning can be traced to a deficiency in task presentation. Suppose a teacher seeks to teach a property of an object to many individuals. She points to a picture of a shiny-looking yellow shoe presented in profile and calls it "getchum." (A nonsense word is used to disguise the intended meaning of the concept from the verbally facile reader, and to illustrate some programming principles. In truth, a label is only an arbitrary but consistent name for an object, some feature of it, or its relationship to other objects in space and time. For the instructionally naive, the labels for many objects and their features are functionally foreign to them; so the use of a nonsense word does not distort reality.)

What is the feature called getchum? It could be an example of shininess or yellowness, a nonliving thing, an article of clothing, something heavier than a toothpick, an object capable of being held in one hand, something usually kept in a closet, something that could be laced, a solid object, something made of leather (or plastic), something to put on after socks, something longer than an inch, an object presented horizontally, or a myriad of other features. The teacher had in mind only one of these attributes, say yellowness, and a few naive learners might identify getchum as that same attribute from the single illustration presented. Many will not be "correct," focusing instead on one of the hundreds of other stimulus properties, as Wilhelm and Lovaas (1976) report many mentally retarded learners will do when exposed to a compound stimulus. Large individual differences in classifications and incorrect interpretations are to be expected when only a single example of a positive instance of a stimulus concept, hereafter designated as S+, is used to show the essential characteristic of the concept.

The number of erroneous interpretations produced by just one S+ instance would be reduced by providing additional and diverse exemplars of the concept. Three-dimensional or pictorial presentations of a yellow sled, a miniature yellow car, a profile of a yellow chicken, and a piece of yellow shoelace, all presented in the horizontal plane, would result in a greater number of individuals identifying getchum as yellow. However, simply increasing the S+ range is insufficient to teach a concept (Tennyson, 1973). Individuals shown this expanded set of examples might not identify an upright glass filled with yellow water as getchum if the previous S+ examples resulted in the learner conceptualizing "solidness" as the correct concept. Similarly, if objects displayed in the horizontal plane are classified as getchum, then a blue crayon held sideways would be incorrectly labeled by some individuals as a positive instance of the concept. To still others, the next object in the sequence, regardless of its properties, might be identified as a concept instance simply because all previous examples were so labeled. Thus, considerable individual differences in concept acquisition would remain despite added S+ instances.

To teach what a concept is, instances of what a concept is not must also be presented. (Merrill & Tennyson, 1977). Those instances that demonstrate the absence of the essential stimulus feature of a target concept (e.g. nonyellowness) would be referred to as negative instances of nonexemplars (S−). As Tennyson (1973) and Granzin and Carnine (1977) have shown with college students and normal third-grade children, an enormous number of incorrect notions are eliminated by appropriate S− examples. If the relevant attribute is yellow, consider the kinds of misconceptions or misrules no longer viable when a red shoe, identical in all other stimulus features to a yellow shoe, is held vertically while the teacher presents an S−instance by saying, "not-getchum." Many more misinterpretations are alleviated when not-getchum examples include a glass of orange water, a blue shoelace, and a brown chicken.

Teaching Concepts Involves Multiple Discriminations

It is clear that there are always going to be stimulus properties inherent in objects (or in the relationship one object has to another) that will be irrelevant or nonessential to the status of a concept as either a relevant instance or noninstance. In the case of getchum and not-getchum, a few irrelevant stimuli (Si) mentioned dealt with the object's parts and its size, weight, use, usual location, orientation in space, texture, and composition. Infinitely more are possible if the Si includes a set or combination of characteristics. Because it is impossible to present a positive or a negative instance of a concept that is free of irrelevant stimuli, the learner may attach some significance to any of a number of Si's. When the learner falsely attends to or is controlled by some irrelevant stimulus or nonintended characteristic rather than the essential stimulus feature that is common to all concept instances (or generally what the teacher had intended to impart, e.g., getchum as yellowness), the unfortunate result is the formation of a misrule (Engelmann, 1975) or a misconception (Merrill & Tennyson, 1977). According to Engelmann (1975), once imparted, misrules may be difficult to unlearn, and they will most certainly impede further progress in the application and extension of the target concept.

According to Becker, Engelmann & Thomas (1975), concept learning involves a double discrimination, the nature or which is represented in Figure 1.

The learner must: (1) discriminate the relevant characteristics of a set of positive instances from a corresponding set of negative instances, for example, yellowness as S+ versus nonyellowness (any color except yellow) as S− and (2) discriminate relevant from irrelevant stimulus characteristics *within* successive positive instances and negative instances of the concept. Concerning within discriminations, if one example consisted of a yellow circle made of cloth and held in the teacher's hand, yellowness as an S+ would need to be sorted from such extraneous cues as shape, composition of material, and mode of presentation. Additionally presented examples of the concept would always involve positive instances of yellowness, but the added examples could introduce new irrelevancies and require some more within S+/S− discriminations. In the same manner, an example showing a negative instance of the concept, say a picture of a green square made of

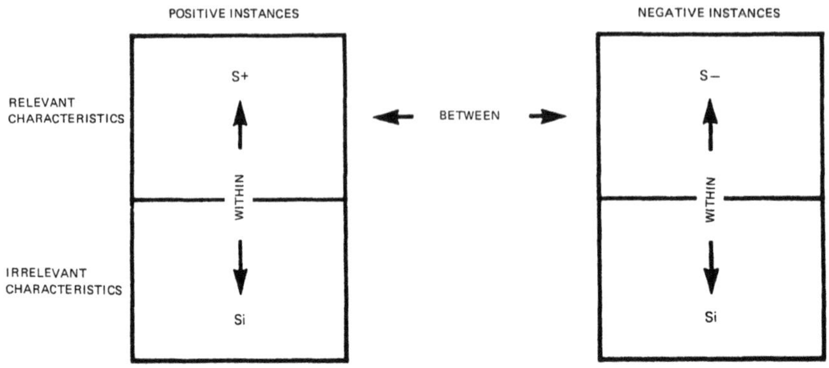

FIGURE 1. Types of *between* and *within* discriminations necessary for teaching a concept. Note that S+, S−, and Si can be a single characteristic or a set of characteristics. (From Becker, Engelmann, & Thomas, 1975.)

leather, would entail distinguishing a characteristic of nonyellowness from the myriad Si's that are part of that particular presentation. Similarly, further examples might bring into play other Si's that need to be distinguished from S−.

Between-Discriminations and the Importance of Negative Instances

Between S+/S− discriminations not only teach what is the essential feature among a set of positive instances, but they may also show what is essential among a set of negative instances. By being provided with negative instances, something is learned about the features of nonyellowness. This information is crucial for generalization purposes. In a generalization series, newly encountered positive and negative instances of the concept are provided, and the learner's job for correct classification is to accept the new S+ as a member of the concept as well as to reject the new S− as a member. If negative instances are not provided or S+/S− discriminations are not properly taught, this latter rejection process will be imprecise. New positive examples will be correctly classified, but some new negative instances, especially those examples high in difficulty level because they are somehow similar to the previously trained S+ instances, will be incorrectly treated as positive instances. Tennyson and Merrill (1977) have labeled this improper classification of novel negative instances as overgeneralization, indicating that the learner's range of acceptance is too great. A method to teach S+/S−

discriminations will be elaborated later but some mention needs to be made about the composition of S− instances.

Suppose squareness is the relevant feature of S+ instances, and the relevant feature of S− instances consists of only a *single attribute*, say circularity. (Assume further that a number of different Si are associated with S+ and S− instances, that is, the geometric forms used are varied in size, shading, pattern, position, etc.) The learner may master the square-circle problem, but what happens when other shapes—equilateral triangles, rectangles, parallelograms—plus versions of the original training objects, are presented as generalization or probe stimuli in transfer tests? Based on Carnine's (1976a) research with preschool children, the learner might respond to the negative instance's relevant characteristic before learning to respond to the desired relevant characteristic of positive instances, that is, newly encountered circles will be correctly classified as S− examples in transfer tests, but rectangles presented for the first time will be treated as S+ instances, in the same manner as squares. As a remedy, Carnine suggests that when negative instances in training that contain *several* relevant characteristics are presented, the likelihood of attending to the positive instances' essential characteristics is increased. Thus, by presenting circles as well as a *range* of other shapes as the set of S− instances, it would focus greater attention to squareness or to whatever is the relevant characteristic among the S+ instances. Obviously, for practical reasons, only a limited number of shapes can be used as S− examples—three to four are enough in the beginning stages—and as training progresses, the set may be enlarged to include others. Carnine's work also suggests that several S− attributes can be contained in a mixed shape, such as an object having two sides of an equilateral triangle joined by a circular third side; by these anomalous shapes, the disjunctive rule (an "or" statement) "squares cannot have circular or slanted sides" is implicitly taught and is thus helpful in showing what is the essential characteristic among S+ instances. Presenting objects containing several S− attributes is worthy of further research because of this practice's ramifications for facilitating generalization and reducing teaching time.

The programming of multiattributes among sets of S− instances rather than a single attribute has major implications for instructional practice. If the goal is to teach what is unique about the relevant characteristics of positive instances of typical classroom materials, such as identification of symbols (letters, numerals, and mathematical signs), common object characteristics (color, shape, orientation, etc.), or object groupings (singularity or oneness) then the negative instances should contain a range of other symbols, characteristics, and number groupings. Too often, however, discriminations are taught by using a single and constant attribute among a set of S− instances. For example, if singularity is the desired relevant S+ attribute, different groupings of two objects may be unfortunately presented as the only contrasting S− feature. If "twoness turns out to be a highly salient feature among naive learners, they will learn about the relevant S− feature rather than S+ feature of "oneness." The result may be that subsequently presented sets of three, four, or five objects will not always be treated as noninstances of singularity. Incidently, teaching separate discriminations involving paired members of the S−set (4 vs. 6; 2 vs. 5) will not necessarily show what is relevant about the target S+ attribute; to teach singularity, examples involving this concept need to be directly presented and responded to.

Presenting a range of new and different S− attributes for low-performing learners to label usually results in delays in acquisition and in naming errors. What should be labeled or verbally identified is the S+ attribute. If the target concept is yellow, objects of that color would be called, "yellow," and the diverse set of colors serving as S− called simply "not-yellow." Once yellowness is firm, a new color becomes the target concept, with yellow and the other nontarget colors functioning as S− instances. This process is repeated cumulatively until each remaining color serves as a target color and, at each step, the newly introduced color can then be identified by name. Periodically, the learner would be required to identify all previously taught colors by name. Working on the assumption that stimulus or sensory features of basic concepts be discriminated before embarking on the simultaneous instruction of concept names, Kincaid and Weisberg (1978); and Kincaid, Weisberg, and Sims (1980) were able to teach low performing preschool children such concepts as color, alphabet letters, and letter sounds to high and sustained levels of performance.

Within-Discrimination Considerations

As mentioned earlier, a range of within discriminations that differentiate S+ from Si's is necessary to avoid misrules. These discriminations, coupled with a number of S− versus Si distinctions, teach the learner about properties of the object other than the target concept. From a series of within discriminations, the learner is implicitly shown that other surface concepts of objects, namely their texture and pattern, have nothing to do with yellow or any other color. Also, the mass properties of objects, such as material, shape, size, parts, and weight, are similarly independent of the target color concept, and so are other properties, such as use, location, orientation, and space. An instructional implication of between and within discriminations is that to teach the relatively simple basic concept of yellowness, a host of other concepts must be taken into account.

A word of caution. Because one needs to program a host of irrelevant stimuli at various points in the instructional sequence in order to show that the essential concept feature holds despite the periodic intrusion of Si's, many overzealous teachers attempt to short-circuit the careful scheduling of Si's by flooding the learner with all types of nonessential details very early in the learning sequence. As will be argued later, this early bombardment by extraneous stimuli can have disastrous consequences for concept asquisition.

Selecting Minimally Different Examples

A question of immediate concern is how disparate should the pair of examples that constitute the S+ and S− instances be from each other. More specifically, should one neutralize the adverse effects of irrelevant stimuli by making the Si's highly similar within pairs of S+ and S− instances, and thus minimize their differences? If that is done, the relevant concept feature would become the major (and hopefully only) discrepancy. Or should one make the Si's within each S+ and S− pair highly dissimilar, and thus maximize their differences? If this were done, and the learner could somehow ignore the nonessential features imbedded in S+ and S−, it would facilitate the appropriate generalization of the target concept at the time when novel stimuli containing these nonessentials would be presented.

The first or minimal differences approach stresses training for a precise discrimination. However, if only a selected number of irrelevant stimuli are presented across pairs of stimuli, there is the danger that the concept will be mastered only in this limited training context; when novel Si's are suddenly introduced without further training before the transfer situation, generalization will probably be incomplete. The second or maximal-differences approach programs a number of different Si's within pairs of stimuli and stresses training for broad generalization of the concept. But, by being confronted with the mass of nonessential concept details, there is the danger that the target concept will not be learned at all. Adults and sophisticated learners usually have little problem dealing with varied Si's and can quickly learn to ignore them because of their vast experience with all kinds of stimulus dimensions. On the other hand, naive learners and those already exhibiting difficulty in learning concepts are likely to be trapped by the barrage of irrelevant details and unfortunately choose a highly salient Si as a basis for the formation of a misrule.

Based on the outcome of Carnine's (1978a) research on the effects of both approaches with regard to the achievement of appropriate generalization of the trained concept, making the differences minimal rather than maximal is better, at least in the case of the young child. Preschoolers were taught the concept *on*, which was called *flot* to reduce effects of previous knowledge, according to one of the five presentation precedures exemplified in Figure 2.

For condition I, the number of Si differences was small, the only difference between the S+ and S− pairs used being that the objects for S− instances were raised one inch above the horizontal line. For conditions II,

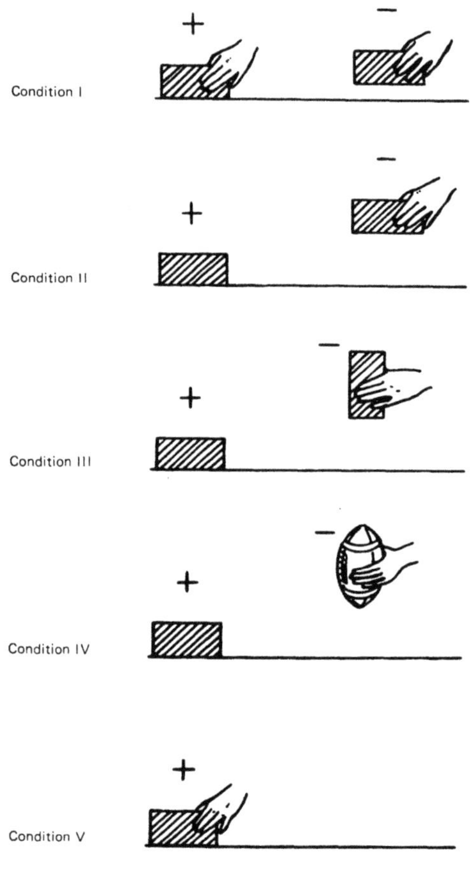

FIGURE 2. Number and kind of irrelevant stimuli used in the Carnine (1978a) study.

III, and IV, S− instances were always five inches above the line. In III, a second difference in Si was added by rotating each S− 90 degrees, and in IV, a third discrepancy appeared by making S− objects unlike S+ objects. Condition V did not employ an S− instance. Following training, novel S+ and S− instances were introduced: Condition I yielded significantly more correct transfer responses than any other condition, and II and III were better than IV and V. Carnine assumed that the children in conditions II to IV had learned one or more misrules, any of which was directly related to the number of Si differences separating S+ and S− instance pairs. As a result, these unchecked misrules were carried over into the transfer test. Carnine's findings support the contention that providing easy discriminations (maximal differences) throughout discrimination training is not necessarily helpful to the learner in the long run.

When positive and negative instances are sequenced so that only a single feature distinguishes them, the saliency of that relevant feature should be enhanced, and thus help focus the learner's attention to it. However, when many different features serve to differentiate S+ and S− instances, control by these other (irrelevant) features is greater than in the single (relevant) feature case. With only a single varient feature, not only is there increased stimulus saliency, but the memory load is reduced, since there is less information to recall from minimally different than from maximally different S+/S− pairs. (Note that the previous discussion which advocated the presentation of a range of S− values *across* a series of paired presentations in order to highlight the uniqueness of S+ is not contradictory to the present recommendation to keep the differences *within* selected pairs small.)

Dynamic Presentations

The problem in using minimally different instance pairs is that the differences may not be noted by the learner despite the opportunity for simple inspection of the pairs. Some more direct teacher action may be necessary. The preschoolers in the Carnine study were taught *flot* by having the teacher point to and name three successive pairs of S+ instances ("this is flot") and S− instances ("this is not flot"), with each instance followed by yes/no questions ("Is this flot?") and appropriate corrections. Judging from the high transfer scores of condition I, this six-trial concept demonstration of instances/noninstances-questioning procedure apparently sufficed to each the essential property of *flot*. There is no guarantee, however, that the same training procedure attempted with more difficult tasks would succeed with low-performing individuals in need of a more precise and powerful means to detect S+/S− differences.

In another study, Carnine (1978b) found that teaching the more difficult and unfamiliar task of diagonality to preschoolers by presenting minimally different pairs of the concept was not very efficient when the same type of concept instance identification-questioning procedure was used. Of the 12 children, 11 did not reach the learning criterion of 10 consecutive correct responses, and, of the one who did succeed, it took an average of 46 trials. Another method, in which S+ instances were dynamically and immediately converted into S− instances and vice versa, produced criterion performance for 11 children in 11 trials, with only one child failing to learn. Significantly higher transfer scores were also found for this dynamic conversion method.

In another study, the concept of convexity was taught to preschoolers, which Carnine admits was an easier task than diagonality. Criterion performance was attained quickly, in about four trials, when the child was told and questioned about minimally different instance pairs. Maximally different pairs were not employed, but a dynamic conversion procedure in which the curvature of a single pliable border was quickly transformed either into convex or nonconvex figures engendered even faster learning. It took only one trial to reach criterion following a six-trial demonstration of dynamic conversions in the object's border. Because of the ease of learning associated with both methods, significant group-training differences in a transfer test for convexity were not found.

The superiority of the dynamic method was again verified by Carnine (1978c) when kindergarten children quickly learned to discriminate drawings of a flower having leaves elevated upward at angles more than 90 degrees ("fleep") versus leaves angled exactly at 90 degrees or downward at less than 90 degrees ("not fleep"). In the dynamic method, a single movable leaf attached to a stem was rotated to create various angles conforming to either S+ or S− instances. For each rotation, the teacher named each of the changed instances ("it's fleep" or "not fleep"). The dynamically trained children met a six-consecutive-correct-response criterion in less than two trials, whereas another group receiving minimally different pairs took three times that number to learn the concept.

In summary, Carnine's research indicates that teaching procedures which immediately show the relevant feature of a basic concept will greatly improve and hasten discrimination and transfer performance in young learners. For many tasks, all that may be necessary is to present minimally different pairs coupled with teacher identification of each pair member as an instance or noninstance, followed by simple classification questions ("is this ______?"). If more rapid progress is desired, then one can use a single object and directly transform its concept feature into instances at one moment and noninstances at the next. Concept instance identification and questioning are also part of this dynamic approach. For more difficult tasks, the only training procedure expected to produce efficient and sustained learning is the dynamic approach. The instructional implications for the educable mentally retarded should be clear. Since discrimination of the relevant feature of many concepts may not be as obvious to this population, and otherwise easy tasks turn out to be difficult for them, it is recommended that, whenever possible, *all* basic discriminations be taught to them through a transformation or dynamic procedure. Before considering how this procedure may be engineered with one such concept, some traditional procedures for training concept discriminations in research settings will be briefly examined, and note will be made of their relevance to classroom settings.

TEACHING DISCRIMINATIONS

Discrimination by Trial and Error and Classroom Implications

Although the teacher seeks (or should seek) to impart a basic concept in the most immediate and simple manner to the largest number of learners possible, this same sense of urgency and efficiency is not necessarily the trademark of the researcher studying basic discriminations. Take the concept of *between*, defined as the spatial location of a relational object anywhere within two designated referent objects. How might someone schooled in traditional discrimination research train *between*? Pairs of stimuli, one member of which would exhibit the *between* relationship and the other *not-between*, might be presented, and the learner required to identify the correct stimulus by making a simple manipulatory response. The first six trials of such a possible two-choice, simultaneous discrimination task are given in Figure 3.

To widen the range of S+ instances, subsequent trials beyond the sixth one would feature the relational object (the block) in a variety of locations equidistant from the referent lines and, at other times, it would fall close to one of the end lines. Also systematically varied would be the range of S− instances: on a few trials the block would be located far away from one of the end lines, either to the left or right, and at other times at a distal space clearly

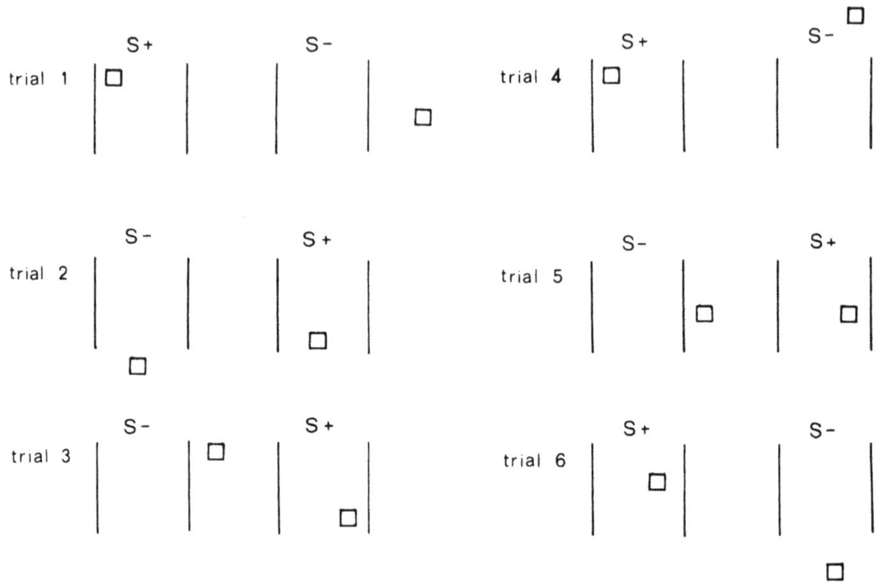

FIGURE 3. Hypothetical arrangement of stimuli for training *between* in a two-choice discrimination task. Only the first six trials are provided.

above or below one or both lines. On some trials it would occupy a space just outside the *between* vicinity, as is illustrated in trials 2 and 5. However, in the majority of S− instances, the block would fall at intermediate distances. Finally, to avoid a position habit, the side where the correct choice appears would be randomized.

With these conditions guaranteed (together with the proper motivation), the researcher waits for the learner "to discover," by trial and error, the relevant feature of *between*. Unfortunately, many instructionally naive and mentally retarded individuals required to discriminate *between* from *not-between* by this arrangement (Weisberg, 1980) never do correctly discover, but insted make errors which could easily number in the hundreds if training were allowed to continue. Nonlearning by self-discovery has been shown to occur for line orientation (Touchette, 1968), visual discriminations (Doran & Holland, 1979), geometric forms (Sidman & Stoddard, 1967), and prepositions (Dixon, Spradlin, Girardeau, & Etzel, 1974). Failure to learn, incidentally, is not limited to a dual response–choice setup; when six choices are provided but training is still by trial and error, high error rates prevail (Sidman & Stoddard, 1967).

It is important to understand that trial-and-error discrimination procedures were never intended or promoted to have ecological validity for the rapid teaching of unfamiliar concepts in large-group settings, as is the case in the classroom. Rather, their original purpose was largely evaluative in nature: to devise and test theories about the parameters that influence trial-and-error learning (Harlow, 1959; Spence, 1956); to serve as a standardized discrimination task in order to compare the rates of learning of members of different species (Schier, 1965) as well as the learning rates of the mentally retarded against normal controls (Zeaman & House, 1963); or to provide psychometric information for statistical prediction and classification purposes, that is to say, individual differences in performance based on trial-and-error learning are covaried with a wide assortment of other dependent variables to form the raw data for factor analysis and related correlational techniques (Latham, 1977). Although it is perhaps unfair to single out traditional discrimination methods as being unfit for classroom practice, the truth is that for a large number of behavioral psychologists their major and sometimes only experience with learning procedures is founded in trial-and-error, self-discovery methods.

This myopic view of learning, grounded on discrimination research methodology, is apt to invite certain preconceptions about the teaching process. Consider the role of errors. In presenting the concept of *between* according to a trial-and-error framework, errors would be a natural and acceptable outcome. Indeed, some theories of learning (Harlow, 1959; Spence, 1956) are predicated on the production of errors, and if only a few occur during training the training task is redesigned to permit a greater number, so that aspects of the theory can reasonably account for their presence or subsequent reduction. In contrast, in the classroom high error rates, especially for the low performer, should be highly unacceptable, unless the teacher wishes to prove that the instruction is unfitting. Errors for a theory or a research methodology that encourages and predicts their occurrence are not harmful, and are even welcomed. For the low-performing individual, their continual presence can cause much initial anguish until a noncaring attitude about academic achievement develops. For an ineffectual teacher, student errors can also be initially frustrating until the teacher begins to accept them as an attribute of the learner, rather than her teaching presentation.

In the hundreds of discrimination-learning studies done with young children and mentally retarded persons, the experimenter or examiner typically refrains from taking an active role in the training process, lest the solution to the target discrimination be given away. To prevent such contamination, the examiner understandably interacts minimally and in a perfunctory manner with the learner. When the examiner is the source of reinforcement and must interact, that process is carried out in a prescribed sequence, with the examiner cautioned not to provide any help in the identification of critical features that distinguish the training stimuli. In the best controlled situation, the human element is removed altogether by the substitution of automatic programming equipment. However, the impact of the teacher, charged with the deliberate instruction of groups of individuals, is not so easily ignored, nor should it be. The teacher should be motivated to "give the problem away" by taking the most direct and practical actions possible—by actively identifying stimulus features as instances and noninstances, by asking many relevant and well-placed questions, by precorrecting possible errors, and, generally, by setting the pace of the instructional sequence.

Because of the necessity to deemphasize human participation during trial-and-error training, it could be that research into the human factors that make for an efficient training strategy has not been as prominent as it should be, at least not from behavioral psychologists who study and posit theories about discrimination learning. As pointed out earlier, there have been major undertakings to examine characteristics of "good" teachers by behavior analysts, but these studies (e.g., Hall, Panyan, Rabon, & Broden, 1968) have been conducted within the framework of motivational, not instructional, variables. Teachers are usually judged on how well they can control the student's attentional and compliance behaviors through manipulation of teacher-imposed or experimentally specified reinforcement contingencies which we know can contribute significantly to the instructional process. Nevertheless, the target student behaviors in these studies are usually well-practiced routines.

What is needed is behavioral research in the effectiveness of teacher presentation variables on student learning of unfamiliar concepts or operations. Different teachers could be provided with special scripts that vary in certain instructional variables, such as specificity of directions, use of key instructional words, use of negative instances, frequency of questions asked, pacing rate, and so on. Functional relationships would then be established between these variables and the parameters of learner acquisition, maintenance, and transfer. There is some indirect research on this aspect (Hess & Shipman, 1965), albeit the role and degree of teacher presentation variables are determined *post hoc,* that is, the teachers are left to devise their own "styles" of instruction and, from televised recordings, the dimensions that underscore a particular style are summarized. Typically, no mention is made about whether the learner actually mastered the concept in these studies.

Finally, in traditional discrimination research, the arrangement of sets of discriminative stimuli are often not programmed according to a special plan to make it easy for everyone to learn. If anything, any programming bias that might favor a certain pattern of stimulus presentation for effective learning is carefully prevented by randomizing the order in which certain types of stimuli appear. For example, to "train" *between*, trials of the kind where S+ and S− instances reflect small differences (trials 2 and 5) would not predominate in the early trials, any more than those that show very large differences (trials 1 and 6). The experimenter may seek to create a favorable balance of hard, moderate, and easy discriminations across the aggregate of trials, but, in a trial-and-error procedure, these types are not usually placed in a circumscribed order. Because of this nonsystematic programming of stimuli, when a few individuals do discover the critical attribute of the concept, not much can be said about the programming features that led to the learning. When the vast majority do not learn, even though they were exposed to the same haphazard presentation of stimuli, these nonlearners most certainly cannot be turned into learners by offering them the same stimulus sequence as that which the few learners got.

The teacher who gives little or inadequate attention to the careful programming of stimuli in order to encourage a self-discovery strategy for student learning is in no better shape. Very few of the low performers will learn from a sloppy, illogical presentation, and the teacher will not be able to discern which variables contributed to concept mastery by the small minority of those who did learn. The teacher may admire star pupils and credit them with unusual powers, positing inner, nonspecifiable causal agents for the acumen. As Skinner (1971) points out, "the amount of credit a person receives [for learning] is related in a curious way to the visibility of the causes of his behavior. We withhold credit when the causes are conspicuous" (p. 45). To this may be added that, when a training setup is advocated, the very structure and function of which denies one from discovering the controlling variables for learning, we are in effect setting up roadblocks to developing a technology of instruction based on real and possibly powerful programming principles. The net effect of this impasse is to support a magical teaching methodology that works with only a few individuals.

It should be clear that the structure of traditional discrimination training within a research context does not translate well into practical teaching settings. (The same point has been made by Clark, 1971, with respect to the noncorrespondence in goals and procedures of laboratory research to determine whether adults can discover various kinds of conjunctive and disjunctive rules imbedded in concept-sorting tasks; cf. Bruner, Goodnow, and Austin, 1967; and how these projects differ from the practicalities of an academic milieu where concepts and rules must be explicitly taught to naive learners.) Yet, not to be forgotten are the strong parallels between traditional research and classroom practice, as is indicated by the similar kinds of unfortunate outcomes and dilemmas in interpretation that result when stimulus programming in both contexts turns out to be haphazard.

Training Concepts by Changing Stimulus Dimensions Across Time: Stimulus Fading

Between can be taught to a greater segment of instructionally naive individuals with minimum errors and less hardship by arranging a series of easier prior discriminations that gradually lead up to the target discrimination. Initial discriminative stimuli are selected that belong to markedly different and easily distinguishable stimulus dimensions, in order to keep S− responding at a low or errorless rate. In the case of *between*, an early discrimination task could present S+ instances as they would appear in the final discrimination task, that is, the relational block would be located anywhere between the end lines. Early S− instances, however, would differ from those in the final task. The beginning S− instances would show a larger-sized block located anywhere outside a square whose lines are the same length as the end lines in the S+ instances.

Success with this discrimination is likely to be high, since stimulus values on more than one stimulus dimension—block size and stimulus form—could control correct responding. (In traditional discrimination terminology, size is irrelevant and redundant or confounded with form.) Over time, stimulus aspects that are part of the S− stimulus dimensions are progressively changed in the direction of those dimensions desired in the final discrimination. Assuming success with the early training stimuli, the thickness and continuity of the top and bottom lines of the square could be gradually reduced or faded until only the side vertical lines remain. Subsequently and/or simultaneously with the programmed disappearance of the horizontal lines, the larger S− block would progressively get smaller to approximate the size of the S+ block. What would remain is the exact kind of discrimination displayed in Figure 3, except that now substantially fewer individuals taught by this method would fail to learn, compared to those trained by a trial-and-error procedure. And a technology for facilitating discrimination would be an important by-product.

There are undoubtably other fading procedures to train *between* versus *not-between*; however, Weisberg (1980a) followed the procedure just described to teach the concept to a group of four-year-old children from poverty level backgrounds. A series of 40 pairs of stimulus cards was presented: the first 10 discriminations emphasized the location of the S− block as outside the square, the next 20 faded out the square's top and bottom lines, and in the last 10 the size of the larger S− block was reduced until it equalled S+. When errors were made (choosing the S− card as *between*), the child was notified, and the pair of cards used just prior to the missed trial were represented; this backup correct procedure is common in fading experiments (Sidman & Stoddard, 1967; Touchette, 1968). There was little occasion to utilize these corrections, since the children made fewer than three errors, on the average, during the 40-trial series. Then, a series of target discriminative stimuli of the type shown in Figure 3 were given, and performance was almost perfect, resulting in less than two trials to reach a criterion of eight consecutive correct responses. No one in another group of 10 children begun immediately on the target discrimination mastered it, despite being given over 80 trials to learn via a trial-and-error fashion.

The fading procedure for teaching *between* followed the techniques employed by earlier investigators (Sidman & Stoddard, 1967; Terrace, 1963a); in that the S+ stimulus dimensions employed in initial training were identical or highly similar to those in the criterion task, whereas the S− dimensions between initial and later training were not so similar. Fading operations were thus largely employed with the S− dimensions. To train moderately mentally retarded adults to learn the spatial concept, *in front*, Dixon *et al.* (1974) also faded in distractor (S−) stimuli (under, in back, above) and produced a low error rate. Keeping the early and later S+ dimensions similar more nearly guarantees that attention to and responding to the relevant S+ dimension will be established. The opposite plan of maintaining high similarity between early and later S− dimensions may cause the learner to attend primarily to the relevant features of S− instances. When fading operations are employed with changing S− dimensions, it is possible that attention to the details of the relevant S+ dimensions will not be firm; the learner instead treating anything different from S− instances as an S+ instance. These assumptions about whether to act initially on the S+, S−, or both dimensions at once are currently without empirical support, and deserve investigation.

There is also the issue that those factors being attended to as aspects of the training dimensions are the ones being faded, and the learner left without the target discrimination. Investigators (Doran & Holland, 1979; Schilmoeller, Schilmoeller, Etzel, & LeBland, 1979; Wilhelm & Lovaas, 1976) have reported that performance may be errorless during the fading process; but selected probes conducted during or at the end of training show that the learner may not be picking up on the critical stimulus dimensions desired in the terminal performance. Schriebman (1975) has distinguished between two kinds of training or prompting procedures, which may help determine whether criterion discrimination performance will be high. With the within-stimulus prompt, the prompted (early) stimulus dimension is similar in part or in whole to the criterion stimulus dimension. With the extra-stimulus prompt, the early and final stimulus dimensions have little in common. Thus, if discrimination of line orientation is the criterion task, an extra-stimulus prompting procedure might teach an easier color discrimination first and fade-in by superimposing differently oriented lines. A within-stimulus prompting procedure starts with an already existing aspect of the lines (e.g., thickness, continuity) and emphasizes that aspect to make the initial discrimination easy before fading out the emphasizer. Schreibman (1975) showed that within-stimulus prompting was markedly superior to extra-stimulus prompting in teaching detailed visual and auditory discriminations to autistic children. Schilmoeller *et al.* (1979) also employed a within-stimulus fading procedure to teach difficult conditional discriminations to preschool children who failed to learn with traditional fading techniques. By using within-stimulus dimensional training, the learner is shown very early in training what is the relevant stimulus dimension. Once that is taught, redundant or irrelevant stimulus dimensions are either gradually introduced or removed.

The design of academic concepts via fading is often an arduous and time-consuming task for the designer. The actual product does not reflect these massive efforts. Moreover, experimental instructional programs have usually dealt with content that is limited in scope and rarely integrated with other concepts. For the most part, current fading procedures represent experimental illustrations of how particular discriminations can be acquired or remediated through innovative selection and planned modification of specific stimulus dimensions. As experimental demonstrations the target discriminations chosen for analysis are quite arbitrary, and, as such, they are often not the ones of immediate interest to the teacher. Guidelines for training and integrating other concepts related to the target one are not furnishmd, nor is there any consideration of the kinds of concepts that do not lend themselves to the same programming framework as that used to train the target concept.

Fading procedures, however, have been extensively used to teach reading to the moderately mentally retarded. The Edmark (1972) program is one such system. Whole words are introduced alone as S+ instances. In time, S− instances, which are at first grossly dissimilar from but eventually similar to the target S+ word, are introduced. To teach *horse*, the S− distractor items might include *ros*, *sho*, and *osr*. Apparently a horse–house discrimination is not programmed.) Compared to a picture-prompting and fading procedure, Walsh and Lamberts (1979) found that TMRs (CA = 12 years; IQ = 43) trained by the Edmark system showed significantly better performance on sight word recognition and labeling. However, as will be mentioned later as limitations of whole-word sight learning, though the Edmark system apparently teaches attention to the details in a word, it is questionable whether a general case decoding strategy is an outcome of this system.

Teaching by Transforming Stimuli

Static versus Dynamic Conversion Procedures

Engelmann and Carnine (1980) have outlined a new procedure that focuses one's attention on the critical differences between S+ and S− very dramatically and quickly. This procedure was previously discussed in connection with the dynamic transformation of stimuli, and, because of its promise for teaching basic concepts, it will now receive a more elaborate description and analysis.

Suppose the target discrimination is *longer than*. Various pairs of lines, matched for irrelevant features and different only in that one line is always longer, could be presented. Assume further that one, among many minimally different stimulus pairs, consists of a six-inch and a four-inch line. These stimuli along with other pairs always appear as *static* presentations, in that during their exposure none of the features of either line changes. The features of the shorter S− line, for example, are not suddenly transformed into a longer S+ line. Consider that on the next trial these stimuli are replaced by another static pair, say six-inch and seven-inch lines. How the previous six-inch line was converted into a seven-inch line during the intertrial interval is not demonstrated. That conversion process, if used at all by the learner as a means to spot changes in length, is left to the learner's own devices. (Although the classroom teacher might name the S+ instance to help the learner, whereas the researcher would probably not engage in concept label-

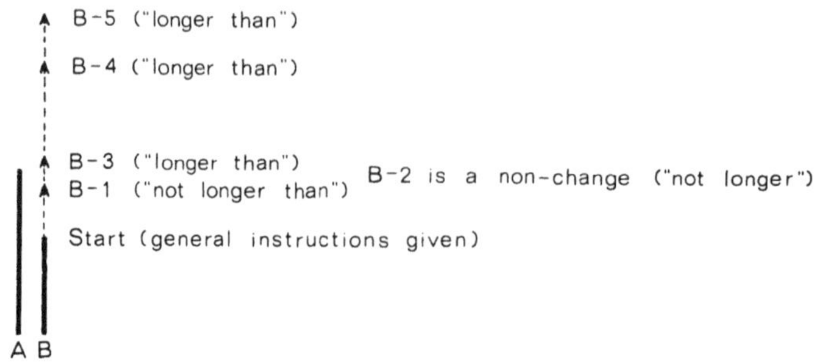

FIGURE 4. A stimulus conversion illustration for modeling *longer than*. See text for description.

ing, nonetheless in both situations the stimuli are compared on the basis of a static presentation procedure.) But think how much easier the discrimination would be if direct demonstration of the stimulus-conversion process became an integral part of the training process.

Figure 4 indicates one means for such a conversion.

The size of the left line (A) remains constant. The right one (B) changes, increasing in length by unequal but measured amounts, as indicated by the cumulative size attained by the series of dashed lines. Before any changes are made, line B, at the starting place, is about half the size of A. The trainer says, "Watch this line. I'll tell you if it gets longer than this one." Then two S− instances are created: (1) line B-1 is created by extending B upward until it is just a little shorter than A, and (2) B-2 is "created" by leaving B-1 unchanged. (To teach comparatives or relative amounts, it is important to show that nonquantitative changes in a previous example results in an S− instance.) On both S− occasions, the learner is told, "not longer than." An S− instance is then transformed into and verbally described as an S+ instance, by extending B-2 upward a little until its new length, B-3, is noticeably longer than A. Next, two more S+ instances are provided. B-3 is lengthened by relatively sizable and then moderate amounts to yield B-4 and B-5 respectively. The purpose of these changes is to vary the range of S+ instances: positive variation shows that the concept label, "longer than," applies despite small, large, and moderate increases in line length. Displaying an unpredictable variation in S+ instances during training also prepares the learner for future generalization tests, where successive sets of different sized objects will be unlikely to reflect a predictable and proportional increase in the size of one or more objects.

Line B-5 could next be shortened to show that the concept "longer than" holds under a descending series. What can be modeled is another no-change S− instance, and how an S+ instance is directly converted into an S− instance by making a small reduction in length. Additional information about the range of S+ and S− instances would also be conveyed by deliberately making nonproportional and unpredictable changes in line size. (Following the ascending and descending modeled instances, the learner would participate in a series of concept probe questions, details of which will be covered in a later section.)

Controlling for Irrelevant Stimuli

Not only can these instructional formats reveal relevant concept transformations; they can further reveal irrelevant concept attributes. If a manipulation acted on S− instances without a resultant change in concept classification, that operation obviously cannot serve as the relevant or essential concept feature distinguishing instances from noninstances. It must instead be an irrelevant feature. The fact that line B is always positioned to the right of A cannot be the basis for the concept, because *both* S+ and S− instances appeared on the right side. Upward extension of the line is also shown to be an irrelevant characteristic of *long than,* since, on some occasions, upward conversions resulted in "not longer than" (S−) and on others in "longer than" (S+) instances. (If relevant and irrelevant characteristics are learned with an ascending series, then a descending series may not be necessary for original concept instruction, although this series along with other length manipulations—changing the length of line A, using horizontal lines—can be used to illustrate application of the concept to other contexts.) If a descending series is used, downward movements (or line erasure) also cannot be a relevant concept feature, since these changes are similarly associated with S+ and S− conversions. For the same reason, certain overlooked or uncontrolled stimulus irrelevancies embedded in either line—differential width, shading, etc.—or those that are part of the stimulus situation—a smudge mark next to one line or the fact that the trainer always uses the left hand to make conversions—cannot serve as consistent cues for concept identification. Moreover, stimulus change or movement *per se* is also not the key; it is only certain movements associated with certain changes in the length of line B that indicate whether B is converted into a positive or negative instance of *longer than.* And, only when these particular stimulus changes are created, are the different verbal designations, "not longer than" and "longer than," given.

A single line can also be used to teach the concept. The general instruc-

Sequence of Examples	Teacher Talk	Line Size	Type of Instance
0	General instructions given	——	Stimulus displayed
1	"It got longer."	———	+
2	"It got longer."	————	+
3	"It got longer."	——————	+
4	"It didn't get longer."	——————	−
5	"It didn't get longer."	——————	−

FIGURE 5. Illustrative continuous-conversion series for teaching *longer*. Probe (test) trials are not shown.

tions are, "Watch this line. I'll tell you if it gets longer." This sequence is shown in Figure 5. The order of instance presentation is different from the dual-line order and is used here just to illustrate another workable procedure. The functional differences between S− starting and S+ starting instances for a conversion series will be discussed later in connection with teaching the concept of *between*.

After the initial display (example 0), the series starts with three S+ modeled instances, the first showing a slight but observable extension of the line, and the last two, where the lines again increase by different amounts, illustrating application of the concept to a range of line lengths. In example 4, an S− instance is created from a prior S+ instance by shortening its length a little. Example 5 presents a no-change S− instance. Further manipulations would involve varying line length in a scrambled order while the learner is probed. ("Did it get longer?"—or if verbal elaboration is desired, "Did the line get longer or not longer?" or "Tell what happened to the line.")

The series shows a continual change in only one end of the line. An acceptable series could modify both ends, so long as one end is not consistently associated with an S+ or S− instance. However, Engelmann and Carnine (1980) strongly recommend that as many elements of the teaching setup be kept the same for the initial illustration of positive and negative examples. Maintaining instructional constancy during the teaching of discriminations by a continuous conversion series lessens the chances of misrules. Too often, teachers beguiled by the acclaim received by a "creative" presentation pattern look to impose stimulus variety on their learners; the result of this "noisy" setting is possibly heightened and temporary interest in the variety, without any real progress being made in concept acquisition.

Teaching Details by Minimum Differences

According to Engelmann and Carnine (1980), the transformation of instances of S− into S+ (or S+ into S−) should be accomplished by making small changes in the relevant concept feature. And these changes should occur early in training. In the single- and dual-line situations, the line was lengthened by a slight but observable amount to create a "longer" example from the preceding "not longer" example. Small differences are likely to be detected because there is no interfering distraction or interruption that is in competition when one instance is instantly converted into another; the juxtaposition of examples must be done quickly, smoothly, and with conviction. When S+ and S− instances are instantaneously sequenced without interruption, they are referred to as a *continuous conversion* series. When a teaching sequence contains stimulus instances that disappear or are interrupted before the next instance, the sequence is a *noncontinuous conversion* series. The traditional discrimination tasks that present S+ and S− together (simultaneous discrimination) or one at a time (successive discrimination) and then remove them or cause some interruption before presentation of the next set of stimuli are tasks that conform to the noncontinuous-conversion (or static) arrangement. With a continuous-conversion series, prior examples do not completely disappear before the next example; rather they are *changed* to *produce* the next example. Continuous conversions reflect dynamic transformations of stimuli, whereas noncontinuous conversions represent static comparisons of stimuli.

To illustrate the point that small differences in the critical concept attribute are likely to be detected during continuous conversions, imagine a metronome adjusted to a specified beat. For subjects trained by continuous conversions, increase the speed by a few beats without any stoppage in the metronome's operation. For noncontinuously trained subjects, stop the metronome for a second or two before restarting it at the same increased beat provided for the former subjects. Chances are that the continuously trained subjects will detect the small differences in beats better than those noncontinuously trained. Noncontinuously trained subjects will require larger beat discrepancies before reporting the just noticeable difference. The psychophysical literature (Kling & Riggs, 1971) supports these contentions, showing that the difference threshold is lower for stimulus presentation procedures predicated on continuous-conversion methods (e.g., the method of limits) than on noncontinuous-conversion methods (e.g., the method of constant stimuli).

The same rationale pertains to visually presented stimuli. To teach the comparative, *wider than*, the teacher might hold her hands about six inches apart saying, "Watch my hands. I'll tell you if the space got wider." To create an S+ instance, by a continuous conversion, one hand is quickly moved slightly outward, by about half an inch, and "It got wider," is said. To create an S+ instance by a noncontinuous conversion, after the initial watch-my-hands instructions, the teacher removes her hands, places them at her side for about two seconds and then holds them apart again at about 6½-inches, which is the S+ distance used in the previous continuous-conversion case. Weisberg (1980b) showed the continuous-conversion demonstration of *wider than* on television to a class of 50 college students, all of whom reported with absolute confidence, in written comments, that the space got wider. In another class of 72 students shown the noncontinuous conversion, 48% reported a "got wider" answer, and of these, only 5% were absolutely certain of this response. The noncontinuous-conversion students reported that the interruption, even though not a serious one, prevented their recalling what the previous example looked like and that they were often distracted during the interruption by looking at the teacher's hands held at his side. Again, much larger increases in distance were necessary before all continuous-conversion subjects were certain of a "wider than" response.

The notion of using minimally observable differences to teach essential concept features may seem contrary to well-known discrimination principles that recommend large differences between S+ and S− for optimal discriminative performance. This apparent discrepancy is reconciled by reiterating that discrimination paradigms, including fading procedures, utilize noncontinuous-conversion procedures where transformations are not employed and the stimuli disappear from view between trials. To overcome the limitations of statically presented stimuli and the interfering effects occurring during the intertrial break, the S+/S− differences must be kept large.

Since, in continuous conversions, competing or interfering effects are not an obstacle, the learner can detect small stimulus changes. If the relevant concept feature is included in these changes, there is a good chance that the learner will note that feature. And, the earlier its detection, the better. If small but critical S+/S− differences are initially distinguished, so will more exaggerated differences given later in training. Training by reversing the sequence does not always hold: subjects initially able to distinguish large stimulus differences do not always succeed with finer discriminations later on (Honig, 1966). There is also the possibility that by trying to show the essential concept feature through the early use of pronounced S+/S− differences in a continuous-conversion series, some stimulus ambiguity may be introduced. Carnine (1978a) inferred that more misrules were introduced when the S − object in the *flot* experiment (see Figure 2) was held five inches off a table's surface compared to the smaller two-inch elevation. Taking this inference a step further, consider the ambiguity in concept interpretation, if to convert a not-*flot* (not on) example from a prior S + instance, the trainer removed the S − object from the table and carried it to the other side of the room while holding it in midair, or, to create the initial S + instance for longer, drew a gigantic line the entire length of the blackboard.

Although stimulus distractibility, such as being allowed to manipulate concrete reinforcers, has been shown to impair discrimination performance (Spence, 1970), the removal of obvious distractors *per se* does not necessarily bring about superior performance. As is proposed herein, the critical determinant is whether the learner is shown what kinds of stimulus events control the cross over from positive- to negative-concept instances, and the return to a positive instance. It just so happens that continuous-conversion procedures also have the distinct advantage of teaching concepts in a context of minimal distractibility.

Teaching Noncomparatives by Continuous Conversion

The structure of basic concepts involving comparatives (wider, heavier, darker, faster than, warmer) and concepts related to number (more blocks, fewer pencils) that are taught by continuous conversions have two major characteristics. First, the classification of each example as a positive or a negative instance depends on or is relative to the status of the prior example with which it is compared. The exception is the initial display example, which cannot be labeled as a S + or S −, and is used as a reference point for the first S + or S − instance. Second, when the preceding example is not altered, the next "converted" example is always a negative-concept instance.

There is a host of concepts that do not have the same features as comparatives. In teaching *between*, whether an instance is an S + or S − is independent of the object's prior location, and the first example displayed will be labeled as between or not-between. Additionally, the feature of a non-change negative example doesn't apply to between and concepts having similar structures. A prior example of between or not-between, if left unaltered, continues to be classified in the same way as its preceding instance. Concepts having the same properties as between, called by Engelmann and Carnine (1980) noncomparatives, include prepositions involving relative location

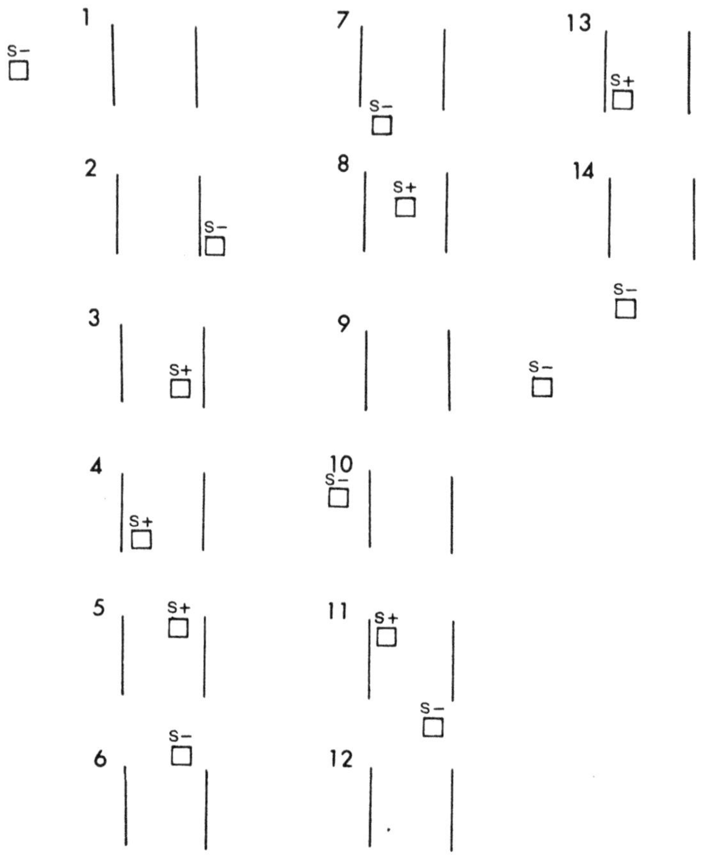

FIGURE 6. Sample continuous-conversion series for teaching the concept of *between*. The first six examples are modeled; the learner is probed on the remaining eight examples.

(under, in front of, near), polars (narrow-wide, near-far, old-young, hot-cold), some action verbs, (running, pointing), simple and complex adjectives (first, vertical, deep, convex, gradual), and some nouns (North, sadness). It is Engelmann and Carnine's general contention that basic concepts having the same properties as noncomparatives can be taught very efficiently if a continuous-conversion strategy is adopted. Moreover, the same instructional sequence appropriate to one noncomparative is also appropriate to all others.

A format that can be used to teach the noncomparative, between, appears in Figure 6.

Two referent lines are drawn on the chalkboard. Using a small block as a relational object, the teacher says, "Watch the block. I'll tell you if it's between or not-between." The first six examples are modeled with the appropriate concept description ("between" or "not-between") given for each example. Evaluation of training occurs for examples 7 to 14. Here, the learner is asked, "Is the block (it) between?"

The Role of Negative Instances

The first two S− instances show something about the range of negative examples. The sequence could have begun with three positive examples, as was done with the single line-longer format. According to Engelmann and Carnine, the formation of misrules is less for negative-first than for positive-first examples. Although without empirical verification, this assumption seems logical. By providing S+ instances first, one of several highly salient but irrelevant features can very quickly come to control discriminative performance. With S− examples first, however, there is no possibility for irrelevant stimuli correlated with the relevant (S+) concept feature to dominate, since the relevant feature has not yet been shown. Then, too, with S− instances the learner is essentially told, "This is not it yet—keep watching!" Thus, S− first instances may facilitate attentional behaviors. The limitation of S+ first instances is not serious in a well-planned continuous-conversion series, since the sequence specifies the early presentation of S− instances that will probably contain the irrelevant stimulus as well as S+ instances that do not contain it. Both kinds of instances, if presented within the first 14 examples, should mitigate against misrules. Moreover, probes are required rather early in training, so that misrules can be spotted and corrective measures taken. All these considerations suggest the use of S− first examples for teaching most basic concepts, but well-engineered sequences that start with S+ examples will not be deleterious and should be employed to avoid memorization of a particular order.

Despite the logical necessity for S− instances in a continuous-conversion sequence and supportive research based on nontransformational-discrimination approaches (see Clark's, 1971, review) that recommend the inclusion of S− instances at least somewhere in the sequence of discrete trials, many teachers and psychologists are probably not sensitive to these suggestions. Weisberg (1980c) asked 48 experienced special-education teachers and 19 third-year psychology graduate students to design a format to teach *between* to a young child. Only five and seven individuals in the respective groups directly specified the inclusion of S− instances, and in no format was an S− first example used. The reluctance to use S− instances can be traced to at least three research sources.

First, results from operant work using fading procedures seemingly cast doubt on the utility of presenting the negative stimulus at its full value early in discrimination training, and investigators (Sidman & Stoddard, 1967; Terrace, 1963b) warned of the many developing and persisting error patterns likely to occur if repeated and early responding to S− was allowed. To avoid impending incorrect S− responding, teachers using continuous-conversion sequences are required to point out directly by modeling and identifying negative instances of the concept. The learner is not allowed, so to speak, to strike the manipulandum and discover nonreinforcement. Rather, modeled S− pretraining with a range of S− values is provided. The direct-modeling aspect is not possible in animal research, of course, and fading research with mentally retarded individuals has never or rarely included that aspect, leaving instead acquisition of nonresponding to S− to a slow and carefully arranged program. Second, traditional concept acquisition studies (Clark, 1971) have consistently shown that provision of *only* S− trials is the least useful means of imparting a basic concept. Could it be that a false reading of this finding has led to the total rejection of S− instances (mixed with S+ instances) in a series? Third, there was some early evidence for the superiority of presenting S+ instances over S− instances (Bruner *et al.*, 1967), but these studies dealt with complex (multidimensional) conjunctive-type concepts presented to sophisticated adult subjects. Recent adult research has repeatedly shown that, even with conjunctive concepts, the provision of negative instances is critical for concept attainment (Markle & Tiemann, 1974, Tennyson, 1973). And, almostr all investigators, including Bruner *et al* (1967, agree that, for complex disjunctive concepts, negative instances are indispensable. It would, therefore, be good practice to provide exemplars containing both S− and S+ instances at every level of concept complexity.

Minimal Differences

Returning to Figure 6, the two transformations where S− is converted to S+ on examples 2 and 3 and from S+ to S− on examples 5 and 6 reflect small stimulus differences. As with the comparative concept of *longer*, the critical detail that distinguishes S+ from S− features of a noncomparative concept are detectable by making small changes, because continuous conversions do not submit to interference effects. By showing these critical details as soon as possible, the programmer is betting on the more or less immediate selection of the relevant concept feature. The rest of the examples are to confirm that the selected concept feature is valid, and to show that it still applies despite irrelevant stimulus variation in the remaining S+ and S− instances. Quite clearly, such programming logic is different from stimulus-fading paradigms, where early S+/S− features contrast markedly, and where it is not until the end of the program that, finally confronted with the target discrimination, the learner must attend to the small but critical differences between S+ and S−.

By recommending minimum overt changes during early conversions, the stimulus differences should be well above the detection threshold of all sensory-intact individuals. If this is done, individual differences in recognition will be less of an obstacle. The object is not to run a detection contest by producing a hardly noticeable difference, acknowledging those few observers who spot the change while leaving everyone else unaware that a concept instance was converted into a noninstance or vice versa. By a minimum difference is meant the smallest practical and *observable* stimulus manipulation. Minimally observable S+/S− differences in continuous-conversion series enable one to attend to the relevant concept details in the most economical way, but these benefits will be demolished in the hands of a teacher mistaking minimum with trickery and stimulus ambiguity.

Evaluation and the Sampling of the Range

Evaluation of training occurs for examples 7 to 12. Here the learner is asked, "Is the block between?" Probes should be instituted as early as possible, both to have overt learner participation and to check for misrules. Resorting to a lengthy preprobe modeling sequence could make for attentional drifts and lessens academic engagement time.

The present probe series, in keeping with Engelmann and Carnine's (1980) suggestions, contains new instances of S+ and S− presented in an order different from that used in training. Also, the probe examples do not admit of a predictable pattern. In the present probe series, earlier examples are not repeated, albeit if the S+ or S− range for the concept is extremely narrow, repeats are inevitable. A third minimum-observable-difference conversion occurs during examples 10 and 11, but this conversion is optional, useful largely as a check by which low performers may see whether they are still attending to the details that separate *between* from *not-between*.

The S+ and S− values presented during the 14-example series obviously cannot be exhaustive. Rather, the range of values constitutes a sample from which other values, never included in the training set, can be correctly discerned by the learner. There are two programming procedures to facilitate the generalization process (Becker *et al.*, 1975). In *interpolation*, if the boundary conditions representing S+ or S− are adequately shown, then the learner is likely to make similar responses to intermediate values. Examples 1 and 10 in Figure 6 establish the boundary conditions for *not-between* when the block is outside one of the (left) end lines, and examples 2 and 9 define the S− range for the other end line. Examples 6 and 12 and 7 and 14 sample the ranges for intermediate positions above and below the lines. Thus, any S− values within these coordinates should be identified as *not-between* by interpolation. Interpolation also applies to how later presented novel S+ instances will be classified by the learner. If the early S+ block locations in examples 3, 4, 5, and 8 are sufficiently scattered, then intermediate S+ values given later will be similarly classified. Because of the greater restriction of the S+ range in teaching *between*, the interpolation process is not so obvious. In the second procedure, called *extrapolation*, the learner is likely to treat any S− more deviant than that presented in the training set as an S−. Thus, more distal S− locations farther away from the block locations in examples 1, 9, 12, and 14 would also be called *not-between*.

Rapid Pacing

The execution of the modeled conversions is critical. The block needs to be held stationary for about two or three seconds, and its movement to the next position done quickly and with certainty. If there is any interpretation in the sequence, caused perhaps by vacillation in the placement and repositioning of the block or by nonessential teacher talk, then these and other kinds of distractions, however momentary and nonintentional, will compete for attentional control and serve to increase the learner's memory load, making concept comparisons difficult. Execution of the probe examples should also be rapidly paced. Detection of the stimulus changes, if observable, should be immediate, and recall of what happened should be tested at once. The learner therefore should be required to answer the teacher's (yes/no or other) binary-type questions very soon after the block is placed in its new location. If perception is immediate, giving extra thinking time or engaging in extraneous tasks, such as do-you-remember-what-happened-last guessing games, is wasteful and may, in fact, induce attentional drifts away from the task demands.

The recommendation for brisk and rapid pacing holds for all basic discriminations and concepts taught by continuous conversions. Even the teacher presenting forms of stimuli that appear statically on the printed page, but have the feature of being immediately processed because of highly distinctive differences, should subscribe to this recommendation. Thus, quickly paced tasks could include teaching and review of the identification of common objects, dissimilar looking letters and numerals, groupings of objects that are opposite in some obvious feature (e.g., recognition of a fat vs. a skinny man) or different in some distinct manner (color, size, number), and literally hundreds of discriminations that are now being taught in a painfully slow manner.

So important is the pacing rate for effective teaching that it is well to elaborate on this variable. Engelmann and his collaborators have documented successful academic programs (ABT Associates, 1977) for teaching low performers and the mentally retarded (Becker, Engelmann, Carnine and Maggs, 1979) language, reading, and arithmetic by a direct-instruction method known as DISTAR. Each program calls for the rapid presentation of material wherever possible. With faster paced tasks, a greater number of opportunities for learner-participation practice and on-task behavior is possible. Carnine (1976b) compared a fast rate of presentation (12 questions per min) with a slow rate (5 questions per min) for teaching decoding skills to two very low-achieving first graders. The percentage of correct answering was substantially greater for the faster than the slower rate (80 vs. 30), and the percentage of off-task behavior was lower (10 vs. 70).

Obviously, the pace for some tasks will be slower than that for others, particularly those calling for the application of a recently trained strategy involving a sequence of activities, as in the teaching of subtraction problems by counting backward or those invoking recall of remote material. Sometimes the pace must be intentionally varied; for example, when following a few fast-moving tasks, the pace for the next one should be slowed a little (Engelmann, 1969b). This latter tactic suggests that when a long series of different tasks is presented, the pace should be deliberately varied in the sequence. In all of the DISTAR programs, the opening task is usually one that is rapidly paced, evoking a great deal of active and frequent participation. Slower paced tasks featuring, for example, the application of rules associated with longer learner thinking times and somewhat concentrated teacher talk are usually bounded by tasks accomplishable in a shorter period of time.

Suggesting that the teaching pace be picked up whereever possible appears illogical when applied to the retarded learner. The individual is slow in thinking; so the pacing, it is claimed, should match that slowness. However, part of the problem resides in the inhibiting variables commonly correlated with a slowly paced task. There is generally less opportunity for frequent questioning, participation, and review and corrections (Bereiter & Engelmann, 1966). Moreover, when the teacher encourages open-ended, divergent-type discussion among low-performing individuals, these slower paced routines are correlated negatively with academic achievement (Rosenshine, 1976).

Given a continuous-conversion series that is rapidly paced, a basic concept can be taught incredibly fast. Subscribing to the 14-example format in Figure 6, Weisberg (1980a) was able to present it for 4-year-old disadvantaged children in less than a minute, general instructions included. Following such training, the children were then evaluated by the two-choice static examples of the *between* concept like those in Figure 3. All children responded correctly in eight consecutive trials without error on the criterion task. Those trained with the 40-trial fading procedure took about 8 min, averaging three errors per child. Criterion performance was achieved in two trials. Relative to the fading procedure and a trial-and-error group begun immediately on the criterion discrimination where learning was not evident after 80 trials, altogether taking about 15 min, the faster paced conversion training was thus beneficial both in terms of accuracy and in speed of initial learning.

Stimulus Change and Attention

Aside from what rapidity of presentation has for maintaining attention and what the transformation of stimuli has for showing critical concept details, consideration must be given to the role of stimulus change as the fundamental operation for all conversion-training procedures. Sokolov (1963) has proposed that stimulus change will consistently elicit orientational responses in all sense modalities from all organisms, and there is a large body of supportive literature based on conditioning and dishabituation studies (Reese & Lipsitt, 1970). For the concepts of *between, longer than,* and *wider than,* the stimulus change operation involved movement, which could be of service to teach a large number of other kinds of visually presented concepts. The kind of stimulus-change operation employed depends on the concept taught and the modality addressed: for felt experiences (heavy, heavier, hot, hotter, etc.), immediate changes in pressure, temperature, or surface texture will be necessary; for auditory discriminations, it will be intensity and frequency; and for certain kinds of visual discriminations, changes in area, distance, curvature, denseness, density (fatter, deeper, convex, transparent, fewer than, etc.), in intensity (brighter), or in color may be necessary. Concerning movement cues, Trabassco & Bower (1968) note that they are highly salient and easily discriminated by naive learners. However, if movement stimuli have the status of being irrelevant concept features associated with a not-so-obvious relevant concept feature, the natural "eye-catching" characteristics of movement can greatly hamper concept learning, as Gelman (1969) and Watson (1968) have argued. In other words, misrules founded on movement acting as a strong stimulus feature can be easily and inadvertently taught. The continuous-conversion series for teaching *between* and similar concepts takes advantage of the fact that movement is an attention-getter (as are other stimulus change operations), but attempts to avoid the possibility of misrules by associating movement with both S+ and S− instances. An inspection of the conversion sequence in Figure 6 also reveals that the directionality of movement (left, right, up, down) is not consistently identified with a set of S+ or S− instances.

Keeping the Teaching Setup Constant: Restricted-Phase Teaching

In every example of the series, scores of irrelevant features remained the same. The same relational object was used throughout and was always oriented in the horizontal plane. The end lines were of a fixed length, and oriented vertically, with the distance between them constant, the block always held in the same hand, and so on. The advantages of programming early S+ and S− instances so that they share the greatest number of irrelevant features has already been mentioned in connection with the simultaneous presentation of minimally different pairs of stimuli. In continuous conversions, the successive juxtaposition of a single stimulus that produces the fewest number of changes will make it easier to compare and remember important details.

This simple principle is not always appreciated. The programmer may be tempted to vary one or more irrelevant stimuli while at the same time trying to show what is the relevant positive feature as well as the range of instances to which it applies. Take block orientation. To rule out this irrelevant feature, it seems perfectly adequate as a control procedure to vary orientation systematically among all positive instances or, as an alternative, to vary it in some of the positives and some of the negatives. One programming consequence of this tactic is the necessity of adding more examples to illustrate the permissibility of block orientation as an irrelevant feature. Another outcome is the possibility that such intermittent variation will make inter-example comparisons harder, because each variation requires another new feature for the learner to process. The difficulty of the task is infinitely increased the greater the number of irrelevant features added. Although sophisticated college student learners confronted with a fairly difficult concept can handle such variation, even if several irrelevancies are introduced at once (Tennyson *et al.*, 1972), there is evidence that less sophisticated learners, namely first graders, cannot do so well (Granzin & Carnine, 1977). The literature on selective responding by animals (Reynolds, 1961), young children, and low-IQ individuals (Wilhelm & Lovass, 1976) to a compound stimulus, where one or more features are equally relevant, is worth mentioning. If special training is not provided, these subjects will often choose only one among the set of available relevant features. Also, intersubject consistency in the one overselected is not high. The programming implication for present purposes is that to inundate the naive learner with a large number of irrelevant stimuli very early in concept learning is effectively to create a compound stimulus. Although there may be a single relevant feature—in the case of *between*, it is relative spatial location of a relational object—the rather sudden imposition of the irrelevancies can cast too many other interpretations, causing selective responding to any of them rather than to the one intended.

It is thus far safer for original concept training of low performers to keep the teaching setup—the materials used, the questions asked, the mode of presentation—as restrictive as possible. Once criterion concept performance is achieved in the limited setting, new irrelevancies should be immediately introduced in ever expanding settings. Not only is this expansion of activities desirable, it is necessary. Should the blocks-line task be unnecessarily overpracticed in the restricted setting, the learner may act as if *between* applies only to that setting. When presented with new relational and reference objects and different task demands, the learner may fail to generalize appropriately. As a result, one or both kinds of the generalization errors previously discussed may occur—undergeneralization (overrejection of newly encountered positives by classifying them as negatives) and overgeneralization (overacceptance of negatives by classifying them as positives). Whatever the case, these errors are likely to occur in low performers who have been overtrained in a fixed routine and the newly encountered examples are unlike and entail more difficult discriminations than those in the original training

Discrimination Tasks not Permissible by Continuous Conversions

Discriminations tasks where a positive instance of a concept differs from a negative instance on a single relevant characteristic lend themselves to continuous-conversion training sequences. It is a relatively simple matter quickly to relocate, reorient, or reshape objects that have absolute values in order to create instances and noninstances of: on and not on, next to and not next to, suspended and not suspended, diagonal and not diagonal, pointing North and not North, convex and not convex, flat and not flat, and so on. Continuous conversions are further possible with the relative or comparative aspects of objects by making a single quantitative change in an object or object configuration to transform it from: thicker to not thicker, higher to not higher, deeper to not deeper, louder to not louder, warmer to not warmer, and more to not more. Although the nature of the materials used to teach the different concepts will vary, the principles adhering to continuous conversions will not (e.g., modeling, rapid pacing, providing a range of examples, keeping early S+/S− differences minimal, using the S+ first or S− first order of presentation, probing early). Thus, although the concepts vary, the same instructional structure is used for all.

Concepts that differ from each other on more than one relevant feature do not easily permit discrimination training by continuous conversions. Concepts, such as shapes, letters, numerals, common objects (or nouns), and items presented on the printed page do not avail themselves to transformations. It is difficult to convert a triangle into a square, an *S* into *J*, a 3 into a 5, a penny into a dime, or a cow into a shoe by using a single step, stimulus change. Since these concepts differ on more than one relevant dimension, making a minimal observable change with respect to a single stimulus change is impossible.

Multidimensional discriminations should be taught by modeling a few instances of the new item, and presenting it in an evaluation set with other items. The number of positive instances of the concept presented depends on the concept's range: noun concepts like shoe or bottle have a wide S+ range, whereas symbols have a very narrow range, and demand fewer positive instances. The other concepts in the set, or negative-concept instances, should be limited to members that have been previously taught and are extremely familiar. Since the names of the objects have probably been taught, the response used in the noun sequence is usually a labeling response to the question, "What is this?" The format is thus an object identification task.

Given that noncontinuous (static) rather continuous conversion formats will be used, the differences between positive and negative instances for nouns, symbols, and other multi-dimensional stimuli will need to be large. Thus, in the initial teaching of the sound for *f*, the other (S−) stimuli, all of which should have been previously taught, might be *m*, *s*, and *a*. Sounds similar in appearance (*t*) and in name (*v*) should be delayed in time. If it is necessary to teach similar items immediately, the physical appearance between the relevant characteristics of similar concepts may be exaggerated (e.g., making the normally circular component of the *d* oval and/or changing the length of its line segment to make it discriminable from *b*). An extrastimulus prompt might be added to emphasize the relevant differences (e.g., employing diacritical marks with all short vowel sounds). However, the programmer should have a readily available procedure to maintain whatever discriminable performance has been established with the added prompt after it is removed.

Expanding the Concept Set

Teaching in the Expanded Phase

Since the original teaching samples the range of S+ and S− instances only with respect to a narrow set of examples under restricted task demands, it does not imply the range to other examples and other demand characteristics. For this reason, the meaning of the concept must be expanded to a wider context very soon after performance in the restricted setting is firm. Moreover, continued teaching in a limited context must not go on forever; and therefore, at some point, programmed generalization must begin. The implementation of expansion activities is thus a practical measure to speed up the generalization process.

As a rule of thumb, the selection of initial expansion activities should not differ too greatly from original learning, and the slower the learner's performance mastery, the smaller the difference. For a very low performer, if new relational objects for *between* are used, it is wise to utilize the same reference objects for the first several trials and to probe by continuous conversion using the same response form. More advanced learners can tolerate greater initial changes in objects, questions, and mode of presentation. For them, immediately presenting a picture of five different objects on a printed page and asking where various objects are located might cause little difficulty, whereas the lower performer might initially struggle with the new format.

Generally speaking, teaching in the expanded phase for generalization purposes, according to Engelmann and Carnine (1980), should not require extensive modeling or telling the learner about the various examples. Teaching is done largely through testing or probing. After the original series in Figure 6, new relational and/or reference objects would be presented and the learner evaluated briefly for each combination. Few or no minimal-difference conversions are necessary if the learner recognized the relevant variable controlling the original concept. Acknowledgment for correct answers is given and mistakes are corrected by providing the proper information, including limited modeling. As a greater diversity of new objects is successively incorporated into the teaching set, the necessity for modeling and minimum conversions will rapidly disappear.

Selection of Expansion Activities

The relational and reference objects selected for expansion activities should all be familiar to the learner. Over the entire set of activities, the objects should be as dissimilar as possible from each other and from those used in the original, restricted setting. Tasks that constitute both a continuous conversion and a static mode of presentation are also necessary. The instructions and questions should embody different forms, from yes/no questions to identification of the concept through verbal description (who, what, where, which, etc. questions) to manipulation requests where the learner points or constructs a response ("Move the pencil so it's between"). One possible set of tasks for evaluating *between* in the expanded phase is as follows:

1. Teacher asks:
   a. "Hold your finger between your eyes."
   b. "Where is your finger?"
2. Off to one side are two small boxes with a red toy car between them; to the other side are two boxes with a blue car under one of the boxes,
   a. "Is one of the cars between the boxes?"
   b. "What color is the car that's not-between?"
   c. "Move the car so it is between the boxes."
3. The words shown represent objects that appear on a printed page:

   owl truck rabbit wagon cow

   a. "What kind of animal is between the truck and the wagon?"
   b. "Touch the object that's between the owl and the rabbit."
   c. Teacher touches cow and asks, "Is this between the rabbit and the wagon?"
4. A spoon and knife are made parallel to each other on the horizontal plane. The spoon is about four inches higher than the knife. The teacher holds up a penny and says, "Tell me if the penny is between or not-between."
   a. Teacher places penny above the spoon.
   b. Teacher places penny between the objects.
5. Teacher positions self between a chair and wastebasket:
   a. "Where am I standing?"
   b. "Show me where to stand so I'm not between the chair and wastebasket."

The tasks reflect diversity in number and kind of objects, response forms, and mode of presentation. Three- and two-dimensional representations of *between* are shown using inanimate and animate objects, including an action format (Task 1). Two yes/no questions (2a, 3c), six verbal-identification questions (1a, 2b, 3a, 4a, 4b, 5a), and four manipulation requests (1a, 2c, 3b, 5b) are intermittently dispersed for evaluation. Greater emphasis is given to verbal-identification and manipulation requests, partly because original learning probes featured only yes/no questions, also for expediency and because of the present goal of expanding the learner's response repertoire. Manipulation responses are usually good indicators of concept understanding if they require the learner to create the relevant S+ and S− instance, as they do in 1a, 2c, and 5b. Those examples where the teacher or learner is required to transform an S+ to S− or S− to S+ represent continuous conversions, and they appear in 1a, 2b, 4a, 4b, and 5b. The remaining examples start with S+ or S− instances fixed in space, and the task does not require a stimulus to be changed. These thus conform to a static or noncontinuous presentation mode.

The learner must be thoroughly trained to deal with the different response forms and to reco nize the objects in the expansion activity. Mistakes made because of a failure to understand "where" questions or unfamiliarity with an owl rather than a misconception about the target concept, will cause the unknowing teacher to reach the wrong conclusion about concept knowledge. The expanded phase is not the time or place to teach object identification of the necessary question forms; if answers to "where" and other question forms have not been pretaught, it is better to substitute a yes/no question or a manipulation request. Individuals with expressive language problems could be required to answer by making head nods or some standardized gesture or manipulatory response. (Procedures for the questioning at the receptive level can be found in Chapter 9.)

Choice Situations

The choice situations in 2b and 3a require familiarity with two concepts: the target one (of between) and some other concept, color in 2b and animals in 3a. An answer describing some characteristic of the other concept is necessary, and to arrive at it the learner must first utilize some implied information about the target concept. Such evaluation procedures are called implied-conclusion tasks. Because two (or more) concepts can be tested at once, considerable economy in teaching is attained. Their use is recommended as long as the features about the other concept are well understood; if not, the teacher should switch to some already trained concept and, if necessary, reword the question. Someone weak on color, but familiar with big and little, could be given different-sized cars for 2b and asked a multiple-choice question: "Tell me which car is not between—the big car or the little car?" If animal names are not firm, the critical items in 3a can be replaced with familiar people (boy, girl, man), and the implied concept probed by a "who" question: "Who is between the truck and the wagon?" The alternative choices in implied conclusions must contain one or more negative instances of the other concept; that is, if the red (long)________ is to be identified, then other-colored (sized) distractors must be displayed.

An unrecognized danger of choice situations is that correct identification of the target concept may be reached because of spurious prompting about characteristics of the other concept. Here are some questions to avoid: "The object that's not-between the boxes is like the color of the sky. Tell me what's not between." "The animal between the rock and the tree has long ears. What's between?" Another task to eschew is the no-choice, can't-miss situation. For example, the learner is directed to sit between two individuals where there is only one empty seat, or to place a peg in the only unfilled hole of one side of the pegboard that occupies the in-between position separating two pegs.

Concept examples can be portrayed on worksheets. Whenever possible, step-by-step directions and close monitoring of the initial tasks should be given before the rest are done independently. If the learners are in a group, the teacher could give a clear auditory signal to control some distinct form of responding: "When I clap, everybody touch (or "make a mark like this on") the object between the ________and the ________. Get ready," and then clap. Unison-responding to a signal also enables one to check several individuals at a time and to correct immediately those off target. By requiring an obvious marking response (circling, crossing out, drawing lines, coloring), this same form can be used as a vehicle for completing the remaining tasks independently. Simple worksheet items could present pictures illustrating positive or negative instances of *between*, and a single or a dichotomous marking system used, depending on the learner's skill. Incomplete pictures showing only two reference objects could also be presented, and learners, through previous instruction, asked to "make an X between them." To gauge understanding of *not-between* relationships, sets of four distinct pictures, only one of which reveals the negative instance, could be given, and the correct choice indexed by some easy marking system.

Fooler Games

Fooler games provide an enjoyable means of instilling interest in academic detail. The teacher enticingly announces that she is going to trick or fool the group. They are warned to stop her when she makes a mistake. About 10 examples are then run off. For seven of them, S+ and S− instances are correctly identified, and the group is to remain silent. For the others, scattered throughout the series, the teacher commits an obvious error, making sure not to provide facial and intonation cues. Anyone catching the mistake stops her from going on. The teacher, in mock disbelief, insists that she is correct but soon challenges someone to "tell me what I should do" or "show me the right way." If possible, the correction should involve the teacher or learner making a transformation. For example, in task 4, the penny is placed between the spoon and knife, and the teacher says, "not-between." After being caught and defending herself, the teacher says, "so, where should it go to be not-between? Here. . . (No!) . . .Here. . . (Yes!) . . ." or "Show where the penny should go." The teacher belittles herself for being so silly, announcing something like, "I'd better be thinking next time!" If the mistake is not picked up, the teacher gleefully announces that, "I fooled you. . .this penny is not-between." Training naive learners to be conscious of teacher error can be done in another context by deliberately misidentifying the students' names, or confusing some obvious facts about them or classroom materials—for example, calling a chair a dog. Bereiter and Engelmann (1968) have detailed a set of fooler-game activities.

The Fooler Game enables one to apply academic information in an educationally and socially significant way. Learners come to understand that accident or luck had nothing to do with catching the errors of an authoritative figure, such as the teacher. Rather it was mastery of the concept that made them "smarter than the teacher," and they were the ones to furnish the proof. Spivack and Shure (1974) have proposed that these kinds of activities elevate confidence in academic achievement. If done properly, the game will have the students on the edges of their seats carefully attending to task details, even though they recognize that the situation is a sham. Occasionally, without any advance notice, a mistake is made in order to perk up an otherwise disinterested group. The teacher fouls up some easy step in a chain of events to draw interest to the more difficult events to come. Vigilance and related research (Charlesworth, 1964; Holland, 1958) has shown that attentional behavior to an otherwise habituating task can be increased and maintained if unpredictable and novel events are occasionally programmed.

Fooler Games require some playacting, but it should not be overdone, since the group can get carried away and academic engagement time will suffer. Running off 10 items should take less than two minutes, histrionics included. The game should also not be overplayed, perhaps scheduled once after every five expansion activities. One hard and fast rule: Never utilize it for information of concepts where performance is weak or unstable. To trick the student on material that is already difficult could promote escape-and-avoidance behaviors from academic-learning situations.

SEQUENCING CONCEPTS

Criterion Performance

Before consideration can be given to the introduction of new material, the programmer must be positive that performance for the recently trained concept is solid. There are two general approaches for determining when to move on to the next concept in a sequence. In the *fixed-trials* method, a concept is presented for some predetermined number of occasions. For instance, a new word is presented 10 times on a flash card, along with six familiar words. Often, calendar events establish how long a concept will be taught; the teacher prepares a weekly lesson plan or follows the order of lesson specified in some commercial program and teaches one lesson per day, more or less, independent of the learner's performance level.

In the *mastery learning* approach (Bloom, 1976), some performance standard, based on speed of task completion or on some minimum number or percent of errors, is adopted beforehand, and new material is withheld pending satisfaction of these criteria. Almost all educational practitioners (Cronbach & Snow 1977) favor mastery learning; yet the majority of commercial programs do not specify behavioral criteria for learning, leaving that decision completely to the teacher. Some programs (e.g., DISTAR) have built-in mastery- or criterion-referenced tests. Given periodically, each learner is tested on the highlights of recently instructed material. Explicit performance criteria determine whether the learner is to be remediated or advanced to the next level.

It is probably the case that high performers can survive academically with correct performance at 75% or 80%, whereas low performers should be maintained at levels close to 95% to 100% throughout training. Part of the reason for the double standard is that when making errors, high achievers more than low achievers are likely to ask questions in the classroom or seek the answers elsewhere (Cronbach & Snow 1977). It has been experimentally demonstrated with the severely and profoundly retarded that high error rates tend to promote persistent guessing patterns (Sidman & Stoddard, 1967), and that difficult word discriminations, taught by matching to sample designs (Sidman, Cresson, & Willson-Morris, 1974), can temporarily suppress the performance of formerly mastered material.

Selection and Order of Introduction of New Members

Four major sequencing guidelines can be discerned from the programming suggestions of Becker and Carnine (1978), Carnine (1980), and Engelmann and Carnine (1980).

1. *Introduce higher utility material before lower utility material.* Concepts that have greater potential application to the learner should be introduced early. If the prepositions *on* and *over* are used more often in daily interaction than *between*, they should be taught before it. If primary reading material reveals a greater use of *m* than *j*, the higher-utility item should be taught earlier. Carnine (1980) notes that if students are to learn a phonics strategy for decoding words, teaching highly functional sounds (*m, a, s, r, d,* etc.) will facilitate the decoding of more words than less functional ones (*x, y, v, w,* etc.). Carnine and Silbert (1979) have provided a list of the differential incidence of letter sounds appearing in the English language, as well a list of the 400 most common words, derived from the familiar Thorndike-Lorge and Dolch lists. In addition, basal readers (e.g., Houghton Mifflin, 1971, 1976) typically create their own lists of some highly frequent and useful words for beginning readers. Concerning language concepts, Palmer (1971) has ordered descriptive adjectives dealing with size, position, tactile, motion, color, and other concepts, according to three levels of usefulness. Carnine and Silbert (1979) provide a list of the basic vocabulary words that the beginning reader will need. The items are classified according to colors, prepositions, common objects and locations, pronouns, parts of objects, opposites, and important occupations.

2. *Introduce easier examples before difficult examples.* Empirical data may disclose that some members are harder to discriminate and should perhaps be scheduled later in the sequence. For example, the unvoiced *f, s,* and *p* are more difficult to learn than their voiced counterparts, *v, z,* and *b*. Also, stop sounds (*p, k, t,* etc.) are more difficult than sounds that can be held or are said to be continuous (*m, r, l,* and long vowel sounds). Therefore, an

unvoiced stop sound (*p, j*) should be quite hard for the beginning reader to produce. However, they may be easier to learn following a great deal of prior phonics instruction with more easily enunciated sounds. Introducing easier examples earlier not only enhances teaching efficiency but can also contribute to greater learner success, which, in turn, can lead to a better learner attitude and to better performance when more difficult material is introduced later on in the sequence.

Research on example difficulty exists for letter sounds and words. Carnine (1975) considered the relative difficulty of sound-symbol correspondences for three short vowel sounds (*e, i, u*) and three consonants (*c, s, m*). In one experiment, preschool children of normal IQ were taught each of these sounds in the context of five previously introduced letters. In terms of number of criterion trials, the *u* was the most difficult (92 trials), followed by *e* (83), *i* (76), *c* (48), *m* (24), and *s* (12). A second experiment also showed that the vowels were significantly more difficult than the consonants, and *e* was harder than *i*. In a study comparing the relative difficulty of decoding three classes of regular words by first and second graders taught by a phonics-based program, Carnine and Carnine (1978) found the order to be in increasing difficulty: CVC words with an initial stop sound (*tan, gum*), CVCC words with an initial continuous sound (*mast, rock*) and CCVC words (*slip, them*). Mean correct performance for each word class was 71%, 40%, and 22%, respectively. Research on the relative decoding difficulty of possibly easier word types, such as two-letter words (*an*) and CVC words with an initial continuous sound (*sit*), remains to be done.

When empirical validation of concept difficulty does not exist, a logical analysis of potential difficulty becomes necessary. Becker *et al.* (1975) performed a component analysis of five closed geometric forms (circle, equilateral triangle, square, rectangle, parallelogram) based on the number of identical components. Overlapping components considered were the number of equal sides, 90° angles, non-90° angles, straight sides, and points equidistant from the form's center. Although no experimental data were provided, it was expected that the greater the number of common components, the more difficult the discrimination. Thus, three common components were predicted to be the most difficult when presented as pairs (e.g., square-rectangle, rectangle-parallogram), followed by two overlapping components (square-parallelogram, rectangle-equilateral triangle), and the easiest had one identical component (circle-square, circle-parallelogram). A similar analysis was done with the five lower-case letters *c, a, d, l,* and *t*. Assigning differential weights based on the number of common components, for example, *l* and *t* have one element in common, whereas *c* and *t* have none and should therefore be easier, a hierarchy of discrimination difficulty in terms of letter configuration was calculated for all possible 10-letter pairs. One note of significance is that the pair *a-d* was expected to be the most difficult of the set, with the *e-a* pair the third most difficult; yet, these two pairs are usually among the first to be presented in teaching lower-case alphabet letters.

Becker *et al.* (1975) have suggested that, when concepts differ in many ways, only a sampling of ways in which they differ needs to be taught. If two concepts differ in many ways (*horse* from *dog*), it is only necessary to respond to one of the differences to be right. When there are fewer differences (*dog* from *wolf*), each of the essential differences must be taught, and more practice must be given to this discrimination than in the multistimulus case.

Allowing the learner early in learning to focus on only one among many potentially relevant characteristics as a basis for distinguishing one item from another can have its drawbacks, depending on the nature of the new members added to the set of discriminations. If the newly added member contains the same relevant component as the one controlling the early discriminations, the learner will encounter trouble. For example, assume that in the initial *s* versus *b* discrimination, the basis for the distinction was that *s* is shorter and has no straight parts. When *r* is introduced, one of the rules for identifying *s* must be modified. "Shortness" will not permit the learner to discriminate *s* from *r*, because both are shorter than *b*. Through the addition of members that show similar features with earlier introduced members, discriminable performance is continually shaped. When *c* is presented, further modification is necessary for identifying *s*, because it is no longer the only member without straight parts.

Several possible solutions exist. One is to model different instances of non-*s* examples (*c*, *r*, and *o*) and to contrast them against *s* when it is shown as a positive instance. The learner does not label the S− instances, but merely answers yes or no to "is this *s*?" questions. Another is to call attention to the specific features of *s* in expansion activities, for example, requiring the learner to copy *s* or to engage in cross-out games where only *s*'s are to be marked off on a page containing three or four other letters.

There is also the problem of the learner's selecting as a basis for discrimination a stimulus component that is salient, but is not the major or relevant characteristic. If, in teaching the concept about vehicles, the initial S+ instances contained a truck, a plane, and a car, a perfectly salient cue is that vehicles have wheels. Possible confusion with the subsequent presentation of a canoe, a sailboat, and a rocket can be prevented if some nonwheel vehicles were included in the modeling of objects in the class of vehicles.

All these points should caution the programmer to prepare well in advance a complete list of the items expected to be taught and to search the list for highly similar material appearing close in time. It is not just the appearance characteristics of items that might be screened but their auditory components as well. For example, if the learner said "*de*" for *the*, the prepositions *on* and *under* might sound alike, as in "The ball was on the (de) table." Less auditory similar stimuli would thus need to be interspersed between the two items.

3. *Separate materials that are similar in sound and/or appearance.* Stimuli may be confused because they look alike (*m* and *n*), sound alike (the sounds *f* and *v*), or share both characteristics (*b* and *d*, *m* and *n*). To arrive at a practical order of introduction, the members should be arranged so that highly similar members are separated by two or more nonsimilar members. In the acceptable sequence, *b m* s e k *n* j v *d*, seven members separate *b* and *d* and three members are interspersed between *m* and *n*. A potentially difficult order would be *b* s *d m* k *n* v e. Another rule is to avoid two or more successive introductions that involve minimally different discriminations. Accordingly, this sequence would be inappropriate: *m b* s e k *n d* because when *n* is introduced the troublesome *m–n* discrimination is invoked, and introducing *d* as the next item causes a second (*b–d*) difficult discrimination. By altering the sequence to *m b* s e *n* o k *d*, the two relatively easy items, *o* & *k*, prevent the learner from dealing with two difficult pairs in a row.

Carnine (1976c) investigated the procedure of separating the auditorily similar sounds of short e and i by contrasting a similar-separated order (*e* c m u s *i*) and a similar-together order (*e i* u c m s). The *e–i* order was counterbalanced. The learners had to achieve criterion performance on all the preceding sounds when presented together before the next one was introduced. First graders made significantly more correct training responses when trained by the similar-separated condition (52%) than by the similar-together condition (33%). Using a trials-to-criterion measure to assess performance in another experiment with preschoolers, a mean of 178 trials versus 293 trials was necessary for the similar-separated and similar-together groups, respectively.

To lessen the deleterious effects associated with high stimulus similarity, the response requirements in the presence of several similar stimuli should be simplified. The form of the response to the newest member of a set that includes one or more similar members can initially consist of yes/no answers while the previously trained members can continue to be verbally identified. If the newest member is hard to enunciate, but must be verbally identified, then it should first be trained within a set of easy-to-label stimuli, and more opportunities given to the newest member. The general recommendation is therefore to provide simpler forms of discrimination training if response labeling will impede further learning.

4. *Teaching regularities before exceptions.* The programmer must comb the academic material to determine where irregularities exist and to insert them intermittently after the learner is shown that regularity exists with some content. In teaching decoding skills, the strategy for sounding out regular words, where each letter in the word is represented by its most common sound, should be taught before irregular-sounding words are introduced. Carnine and Silbert (1979) suggest introducing irregular words after students are proficient at reading regular CVC words (e.g., *mad, fin, not*) The first irregular words selected should be "moderately irregular" in that, when the letters are blended and then said quickly to form the word, the word should not greatly distort its normal spoken pronunciation. Initial irregular words creating less distortion (e.g., *was, is, put, look*) should appear earlier than more complex irregular words (*does, said, walk, boat*). Since learning to decode irregular words involves somewhat of a new strategy, all things being equal, the first several irregular words should be interspaced by a greater number of lessons than the next set of irregular words. However, as the third guideline suggests, the newest irregular word should not be similar to the words the student is having difficulty with.

Although several forms of information are traditionally arranged in a fixed order, for example, alphabet letters, they should not necessarily be taught in that order for all concepts. An analysis of the order may reveal exceptions with respect to a rule that the teacher is trying to establish. If the rule is to teach the correspondence between upper- and lower-case letters, those pairs which are similar in configuration (*Oo, Tt, Ss*) should be introduced before less generalizable pairs (*Aa, Gg, Dd*). Ironically, among the first five alphabet pairs (*Aa* through *Ee*), there is only one similar pair (*Cc*). As another illustration, students frequently have trouble recognizing and labeling the lower-teen numerals (*10, 11, 12, 13*) but do better at recognizing other teens (*14, 16, 17, 18, 19*). Because the second digit is a reliable cue for correct performance, these "regular" teens should be introduced in numeral-identification tasks before the exceptions, which should be added into the set one at a time. Note that the suggestion to modify heretofore fixed orders to produce regularity for symbol identification tasks does not mean that other activities, such as reciting the alphabet and counting, should be altered.

Sometimes a classification rule which is only partially correct is taught because it adequately describes a sufficient number of cases for the novice.

The full dictionary definition of the rule may not be taught because to do so would imply knowledge of unfamiliar concepts. Consider the rule for vehicles: "If it takes you places, it is a vehicle." The rule is only partly correct, because the man-made aspect is not mentioned and, strictly speaking, beasts of burden would incorrectly fit the rule. The manufacturing component to the rule, which is a difficult concept for naive learners, can be taught much later with the rule modified: "If it's made to take you places, it's a vehicle." Meanwhile the rule in its initial form is fine to use, because it benefits the learner by ordering so many different environmental objects. The exceptions to the rule can be dealt with later on, after the establishment of valuable classification behavior.

Whenever feasible, the irregular features of a concept should be modified to fit a normal and familiar basis for responding. Orthographic changes in size and shape can create such regularity. If a macron is used over all long vowels and unheard letters are written smaller in size than normal, irregular words such as *boat, fate,* and *tail* (bōat, fāte, tāil) are no longer irregular. The same is true for digraphs. By joining *s* and *h* to look like sh, *c* and *h* to look like ch, and *w* and *h* to look like wh, the reader is prompted to say the correct sound. The outcome of these functional prompts is that the learner is able to treat the modified form in the same way as regular words.

To modify irrelevant features so that single or selected cases are more efficiently dealt with is a waste of instructional efficiency and often leads to a dead-end skill. It is not infrequent to find suggestions to alter specific words in commercial programs and teacher journals. For instance, the irregular words, *feet* and *see,* are prompted by making *legs* and *eyes* out of the "ee" sounds in these words. (Note that by adding diacritical marks to the double letters, the beginning reader will have an effective decoding strategy for dealing not only with these words but with words not easily and conveniently pictorialized (*between, indeed, sixteen*). Another technique to avoid is to teach beginning readers complex phonic rules that apply to only a few words, for example, spending considerable time dealing with the silent *t* in *listen.*

Sometimes a concept which is considered irregular in the early part of the instructional program may not be treated as irregular at a later point of the program. For example, *soil* and *eat* would be considered irregular if a single sound is taught for each vowel. However, if later in the program the sounds *oi* and *ea* were taught as letter clusters, these and words in the same class would be decoded in the regular manner. (The reason that letter combinations should not be taught initially is that sounding out words is easier for beginning and low-performing readers if they decode letters one at a time, without having to attend to letter clusters.) The chief criterion for attempting to create regularity from exceptions to the rule is whether the revised form will apply to a large number of cases. Silent *e* and letter cluster training, and the prompts for long vowels, are necessary because they greatly expand the number of words correctly read.

Programming Trade-Offs

In actual practice, it is difficult to specify an order of introduction that satisfies all four guidelines. What is often necessary is a reasonable compromise that engenders the most highly generalizable and practical behaviors in the long run. Teaching the decoding of irregular words, such as *to* and *said*, may be scheduled for early introduction into a reading program because of their high utility in creating sentences. This means that the guidelines of easiness and regularity (and possibly, similarity, if *do* and *sad* were formerly taught) will need to be sacrificed for functional reasons.

Providing initial instruction in letter sounds will not result in word reading as quickly as introducing highly discriminable sight words. However, by teaching identification of sounds and how to blend them together, this difficult strategy will eventually result in a greater number of correctly read words.

Teaching how to count from a number located anywhere in a series to a higher number, for example, from 5 to 9 or from 19 to 22, may seemingly be difficult to do in early arithmetic training. Yet, once this component skill is mastered, it will prove to be extremely useful for doing subsequently presented adding problems of the type $5 + 4 = \square$ or $19 + 3 = \square$. The learner identifies the number in the first group (5 or 19), then draws in the appropriate number of lines under the second group (4 or 3), and, using the counting-from-a-number skill, starts with the first number and successively counts the lines to achieve the answer. It may be functionally easier in the beginning to do the $5 + 4 = \square$ problem by having concrete objects stand for 5 and another set for 4 and, to solve the problem, counting all objects beginning with one up to nine. However, the problem of $19 + 3 = \square$ can be formidable if 19 concrete objects are to be represented for the first group and all objects in the first and second groups counted beginning with one. Teaching the counting-from-a-number strategy permits one to do normal addition problems plus algebraic problems, such as $5 + \square = 9$, and, if a counting-backward-from-a-number skill is taught, normal and algebraic subtraction problems can be accomplished as well. These illustrations show that task simplicity was compromised in favor of training in a highly useful, regular mode of doing problems. The similarity issue appears when counting-forward tasks are intermixed with counting-backward tasks.

Concept Integration and Cumulative Review

After original teaching and expansion, a particular concept is integrated and reviewed in a context containing previously trained concepts. Those concepts sharing common stimulus characteristics with the one trained should be selected for integration. Since *between* belongs to the stimulus class of relative spatial location, it should be integrated with other members of that concept class, namely, *on, over, in, under, in front of,* and similar prepositional terms.

The general procedure for sequencing concepts is to teach concept A in isolation and in expansion activities, repeat the process for B, then integrate and review B with A, teach C, integrate C with A and B, and so on. The nature of the integration-and review-process would consist of expansion tasks where questions about five or six of the previous related concepts would be probed. Table I reflects this procedure by showing the nature and sequencing of the teaching activities both preceding and following *between,* and its eventual consolidation with the prior concepts in the same class.

Assume that *on, over,* and *in* were the first three concepts taught, which altogether took nine lessons before they were integrated. Table I duplicates the process for the next three concepts: *in front of, in back of,* and *between.* One new concept is introduced every four lessons. Two lessons are provided for the restricted-phase teaching to enable some manipulation of the reference and relational objects: for example, during the 16th lesson, the new reference objects for *between* might be horizontally and vertically positioned, whereas, possibly, in the 15th lesson only vertical alignments may have been used. The second lesson also enables training for absentees, and provides extra practice for some learners, but not enough for the phenomena of undergeneralization and overgeneralization to occur because of overpractice in the restricted setting.

Fink and Brice-Gray (1979) compared a method of presenting new concepts in isolation before each was cumulatively reviewed in conjunction with all previously taught concepts (as is done in Table I) with a method where concepts were also taught in isolation, but were reviewed by all possible pairs. In the pairwise method, each pair was brought to criterion before the next pair was introduced. The concepts were five functional words (*entrance,*

TABLE I
Hypothetical Sequencing of Activities for Introduction, Expansion, and Integration of Concepts

Activity	Lessons 1-9	10	11	12	13	14	15	16	17	18
Concept(s) introduced in restricted setting	(on, over, in)	in front of	in front of		in back of	in back of		between	between	
Expansion activities	The last concept trained (in)	(in)	in front of	in front of		in back of	in back of		between	between
Integration and Review	Related concepts (RC) (on, over, in)	RC	RC	in front of plus RC	in front of plus RC	in front of plus RC	in back of plus RC	in back of plus RC	between plus RC	between plus RC

women, exit, danger, poison) taught to moderately and severely handicapped preschool children. Touching the word on cue was required for a correct response. The rate of acquisition and that of recall were both substantially better for the cumulative-review group than the pairwise-review group. The median number of trials to master all words both in isolation and in review was 173 for the cumulative-review group and 244 for the pairwise group. When the five words were presented together and evaluated at the end of training, 90% of the words were correctly recalled by the cumulative-review group, as against 48% for the pairwise group.

Carnine (1976c) demonstrated the superiority of cumulative programming for teaching a set of six letter-sound correspondences (*e,s,m,u,c,i*) to intellectually normal children. A cumulative-review-trained group required 178 trials to reach terminal criterion, whereas a control group presented with the letter–sounds one after another without opportunity for integrated review took 261 trials. Letter–sound retention scores were also better: 84% for the cumulative review group, compared to 66% for the control group.

The cumulative-review sequence has been urged and is being employed in an increasing number of experimental settings dealing with academic material, from geometric forms (Becker *et al*, 1975) to colors, alphabet letters, and letter sounds (Kincaid & Weisberg, 1978; Staats, Brewer, & Gross, 1970), to number–object equivalencies (Ferster & Hammer, 1966) and addition facts (Carnine, 1978d). However, the advantages of this method have not been fully realized. In many curricula material and commercial programs the learner reads short *a* words one day, short *i* words the next, and short *e* words the next. However, the learner is not required to read short *e* words that are interspersed with words having different vowel sounds in them. As long as the learner receives words of a particular type during a given period (e.g., only short *e* words), performance may be adequate. This performance does not prove that the learner can discriminate between short *e* and short *i* words.

Cumulative programming is easy to follow when about six to eight members have been taught, but after that point requiring criterion performance on all old members before the introduction of the next one is time-consuming. Moreover, presenting a large number of different elements simultaneously for cumulative review poses logistic problems. As a consequence, criteria for review selection must be adopted. Becker and Carnine (1978) offer four guidelines. Select six to eight members that include: (1) the member(s) most recently taught; (2) troublesome members as defined by high-error rates; (3) members not recently reviewed; and (4) members that are similar either in stimulus configuration (*m* & *n*, *9* & *6*) or auditorily (*v* & *f*, *7* & *17*).

Kincaid and Weisberg (1978) have suggested giving more opportunities to relatively unpracticed material in the review set so that the extra practice can facilitate the acquisition process.

The criteria for the selection of formerly trained items in the review set are different from those governing selection of items to contrast against a newly introduced item. A new item should be presented in a context with previously trained items that are maximally dissimilar to it, but, once adequately taught, the newest item should be reviewed among some items that are similar to it. There should thus be two formats in an instructional program: introductory tasks where item discrimination is relatively easy, and review tasks where discrimination can be expected to be harder.

READING

Historical Perspective

Reading instruction for the mentally retarded has historically been considered a tool subject. Blodgett and Warfield (1959), Ingram (1953), Perry (1960), and Wallin (1924) represent the thinking of the first half of the century advocating teaching functional reading skills, such as traffic sign recognition, the names for common objects, and completion of a job application. It was widely believed that EMR children could sometimes learn to read up to a second- or third-grade level by the time they left school (Blodgett & Warfield, 1959; Ingram, 1953; Perry, 1960), and that a trainable mentally retarded child would not advance far enough to make reading a very useful tool. Reading instruction was generally delayed for several years, until the mentally retarded child was deemed "ready" to begin reading. In the case of normal children, the prevailing opinion was that a mental age of 6.0 to 6.5 was required in order to start the process of reading (Morphett & Washburne, 1931). This required delay implied that mentally retarded youngsters would not receive actual reading instruction until they were around 10 or 11 years old.

Three Components of the Reading Process

Reading can be considered the translation of symbolic material (written words) into either communication that is oral (spoken) or covert (silent reading). Oral language communicates directly through sounds, whereas written language communicates through a visual code of letters which represent these sounds. The selection and organization of materials designed to teach reading is based on the theoretical and speculative emphasis that curricula programmers place on the reading process. In other words, the definition of reading one subscribes to specifies the selection and sequencing of reading material in an instructional program.

McCracken and Walcutt (1969) offer three meanings of reading which can coexist in time but have unique features. Reading I is decoding or turning the written word into its spoken equivalence. This means that the word may be correctly deciphered but not understood. A difficult poem, for example, or nonsense words, can be "correctly" pronounced but carry no meaning. Reading II emphasizes the comprehension components that words convey. If a Shakespearean sonnet is correctly decoded and not understood, it is no different from reciting that sonnet or hearing it recited and not understanding it. One would not go to a remedial-reading teacher for help here, but to an expert on Shakespeare. Reading III takes us into "the world of art and intellect that is accessible only through the printed word" (p.9). It involves literary forms and styles, and eventuates in higher qualities of spoken discourse which do not usually occur in spontaneous spoken language.

There are several approaches to the teaching of reading, but they generally fall into phonic-linguistic approaches, which emphasize explicit teaching of decoding strategies (Reading I and then Reading II and III), and whole-word reading, which immediately stresses the attachment of meaning to the printed symbol (Reading II and III), with minimal consideration of the grapheme–phoneme (letter–sound) relationship. Most commercial programs are whole-word reading programs containing basal readers and phonic components. Those programs which claim to be phonic-oriented incorporate meaningful reading along with decoding.

BASAL READERS AND THE WHOLE-WORD APPROACH

Background

Basal reader instruction constitutes what has come to be known as the traditional method of teaching reading with all populations (Williams, 1979). Flesch (1979) estimates that this approach is used in about 75% of the classrooms in the United States. Carnine and Silbert (1979) report that three basal-reading programs (Houghton Mifflin, Ginn, and Scott Foresman) account for approximately 45% of the reading programs used from kindergarten to eighth grade.

Briefly, authors of basal readers assume that words should be taught as meaningful wholes. Accordingly, high-frequency and discriminable words are initially presented in the context of colorful pictures, and the students are urged to predict what the word might be, based on an assortment of cues—pictures, word length and letter shape, beginning and ending letters, sentence or story context, and group discussion about word meaning. Phonics, or the relationship between the sounds that single letters or letter clusters make, is not usually taught directly; the learner is expected to deduce phonetic structure indirectly after much reading has occurred.

Historic Rationale for Whole-Word Approaches

Several basic discoveries between 1879 and 1910 had a significant effect on the adoption of whole-word reading approaches. Cattell in 1885 and 1886 (see Gibson & Levin, 1975) found that, with tachistoscopic exposures of 10 msec, "connected materials" could be recognized better than "unconnected materials," that is, only three to four connected letters could be read in the same time frame as four connected short words. Moreover, when single words were briefly exposed they were recognized as quickly as single letters, and, in fact, it took longer to name letters than to name words. Cattell concluded from this tachistoscopic reading research with adults that words are perceived and read as wholes, not letter by letter.

Other pertinent findings revealed that the eye makes quick jumps (saccades) from one fixation to the next and that the information is extracted almost, if not entirely, during the fixation. Within a single scan, about an inch and a half of a line of print held at the ordinary reading distance is possible. Still further, one need not see distinctly all the letters, or even all the words, to recognize the group of words. These investigators concluded that the span of fixation of a sophisticated adult reader's eye movements reflect a whole-word reading pattern. According to Gates, Jersild, McConnell, and Challman (1950), these discoveries led to the development of whole-word reading approaches emphasizing learning to: (1) recognize words as total configurations instead of letter by letter; (2) read by getting meaning directly from perception of the symbols without the intervention of oral reading or complete articulation of the words; and (3) utilize rapid and rhythmic eye-movement progressions along the line.

Given Gestalt theory (Hilgard & Bower, 1966), which advocates learning from wholes to parts and that initial recognition of an object or person is immediate and holistic, followed only later by part–whole discriminations, it is easy to appreciate how this approach was applied to reading. The new reader should be presented with a whole story (on an experience chart) and led to pick first certain sentences out of this whole and finally individual words. According to this system, it is absolutely wrong to teach the letters (parts) first, because doing so would reverse the fundamental learning process. The naive reader seeing letters instead of whole words would have his attention captured by these small shapes and fail to look at the whole words out of which meaning is made.

Limits of Tachistoscopic Research and Gestalt Applications

The early influential research efforts of Cattell and of Erdman and Dodge (see Gibson & Levin, 1975) on the adoption of whole-word approaches is open to criticism partly because prose reading for adults is similar to spoken language, whereas letter reading is a novel response (Brewer, 1976). Second, an analysis of the final polished reading performances of the adult reader does not necessarily indicate the same forms of behaviors that are to be expected from the beginning reader. For example, an adult reads silently, takes in large units, does not point, and reads rapidly (about 400 words per minute). Although whole-word reading approaches usually try to promote these behaviors very early in the reading process, some proponents of phonic-based programs (Engelmann, 1975) have suggested that the very opposite reading behaviors be instilled in the beginning reader, before adultlike reading takes over. The DISTAR reading program (Engelmann & Bruner, 1974) emphasizes oral reading, blending individual letter sounds to make words, encourages pointing, and initially stresses accuracy rather than speed.

Deductions from Gestalt theory applied to reading and similar phenomena are highly suspect. It has been suggested that the whole-word-recognition method of teaching reading is not a valid application of the Gestalt theory (Terman & Walcutt, 1958). For example, in learning to "read" the Morse code, whole-word approaches were not successful (Keller, 1943). A greater number of telegraphic receivers taught the letters of the code learned it much better than those taught whole-word patterns, from which it was expected they would deduce the letter symbols. Terman and Walcutt (1958) point out that, as in the case of Morse code receivers, the budding musician must first learn to read notes and practice playing scales for hours, before being able to play several pieces of music spontaneously. Finally, when encountering unfamiliar words, sophisticated readers look at letters or letter patterns, rather than at the whole words (Terry, Samuels, & LaBerge, 1976).

CHARACTERISTICS AND LIMITATIONS OF THE WHOLE-WORD APPROACH

Picture Prompting

Whole-word programs usually make extensive use of pictures in teaching beginning readers. These pictures appear with the text of the story. Pictorial presentations have frequently been justified in terms of providing interest to the reading material and helping to focus attention on the story meaning (Singer, Samuels, & Spiroff, 1973–1974). Since an unfamiliar printed word cannot be correctly read at first, a picture is used to prompt verbal identification. The problem then becomes one of shifting stimulus control, from the picture to the relevant stimulus of the printed word.

Corey and Shamow (1972) demonstrated that nonreading preschoolers could read words orally after the picture in each of six picture-printed word pairs was gradually blackened out over five trials, with the word appearing alone on the sixth trial. This fading condition produced better performance (5.7 words correctly read) than a superimposed condition (.33 words) where picture-printed word combinations appeared together for five trials before the word suddenly appeared by itself on the sixth trial. Dorry and Zeaman (1973) compared the effects of picture-fading and non-picture-fading (or stimulus superimposition) procedures for four training trials on the ability of severe and moderately retarded children (IQs of 23 to 55) to read eight words presented alone one at a time in a cumulative test. The fading procedure engendered higher reading scores (3.6 words) than the superimposition group (1.2 words).

Taken together, these findings seemingly suggest the adoption of picture-fading procedures for whole-word reading in the classroom. However, the educator is cautioned against such adoption. In the Corey and Shamow (1972) study, the mean of 5.7 correct words or 95% accuracy was based on the critical sixth trial, which was really a test for short-term memory of the recently presented picture–word pair. A delayed and more adequate test for sight word reading where the six words were individually presented without prior picture prompts lowered reading accuracy for the fading trained group to 50%. Reading performance for the mentally retarded children in the Dorry and Zeaman study approached the same level (3.6 of eight words, or 45% accuracy). Duell (1968) reported recall accuracy scores for eight sight words of 40% for kindergarteners trained by a two-trial picture–prompt procedure. In trial one, a single picture–word pair was exposed. In trial two, that same pair plus another picture–word pair appeared in a choice situation. Given the need for reading procedures that promote strong performance, the accuracy scores of 50% or lower fall greatly short of this ideal. Moreover, in none of the studies were control conditions conducted, that is, just presenting printed words alone in traditional flash card style to see whether picture prompting and fading actually facilitated reading accuracy over what is normal classroom practice.

The composition of the words must also be considered: all were highly discriminable nouns (e.g., *apple, ball, horse, dog, elephant,* and *book*) that began and generally ended with different letters and varied in length and in configuration patterns. Parenthetically, it would seem that, given any or all of these distinguishing features, accuracy scores much higher than 50% should have been found. Even if picture fading does result in superior performance for nouns, there is the double problem of reliably representing other syntactical structures by pictures and also making sure that *all* the words chosen will continue to be distinctive. Grammatical forms failing on these two accounts include articles (e.g., *the, a, an*), pronouns, (*they, their, those, that, these, this*), direct and indirect objects (*them, it*), conjunctions (*and, or*), certain prepositions (*at, in, on, about*), adverbs (*there, then*), and dozens of other "little" words that appear in reading material but are frequently confused with each other by readers taught to attend to the whole word.

Taber and Glaser (1962) earlier advocated the teaching of words signifying colors by first surrounding the words with appropriate colored lines radiating outward. The lines were gradually removed and replaced by color prompts that appeared on the letters within each word. The color–letter prompt was also faded, until all eight training words were printed in black on a white background. The results were mixed. Of five kindergarten children, all above average in IQ, two had learned all eight words while three failed to read any word. Duell and Anderson (in Duell, 1968) extended the color-fading procedure to a larger number of nonreading primary-grade children and failed to demonstrate a shift in control from the actual color to the word. "Reading" was perfect with the color prompts intact, but, after their complete removal, none of the 14 children read any word correctly. Not surprisingly, nine of the 14 called every word "black," since each word at the end of the training was now in black print. The remaining five children guessed freely.

In light of what was said earlier about selecting reading material that emphasizes word regularity, the use of color words seems to emphasize the exception rather than the rule: of the eight color words used in color-fading experiments, three could be construed as sounding out regular (*black, green,* and *red*); the rest are irregular (*brown, purple, blue, orange, yellow*). It thus appears that beginning readers cannot easily extract letter-sound regularities. Lacking this skill, they would be forced to adopt a whole-word strategy and learn words prompted by colors, pictures, word configuration, and other cues.

Samuels (1970) notes that using picture–word pairings produces a dependence on picture cues, and the new reader operates according to the principle of least effort: when a picture–word compound stimulus is presented, that aspect of the compound is selected which most easily evokes the correct response. Instead of looking at the printed word, the reader selectively responds to the picture, as long as it is presented with the word. Duell's (1968) data support these claims. Kindergarteners were required to point to either the picture or the word of a picture–word pair in a choice oral-reading test. Of 40 subjects, 29 or 72% chose the picture as the "reading" response. Many low-performing students will spend months, unbeknownst to the teacher, "reading pictures." As long as word presentation and syntax are controlled, picture reading will be identical to word reading. When more text and less syntactic control occurs and when rhebuses are removed, there is the discovery that picture reading and not word reading was taught.

In a review of picture-prompting methods to facilitate whole-word sight recognition, Samuels (1967) concluded that pictures can hamper performance. When pictures accompanied four printed nouns, kindergarten children required a longer time to read the words and made more errors than when pictures were not present during acquisition training. Harzem, Lee, & Miles (1976) varied the nature of picture prompts accompanying 16 noun words taught to normal-IQ first-graders. The order of increasing reading scores was: (1) no pictures, (2) nonsense pictures (3) inappropriate pictures (noncorrespondence between picture and word), and (4) appropriate pictures. These results suggest that appropriate-picture prompts can distract the reader's attention from the printed word, the result of which is less focused attention to the word itself. Gibson and Levin (1975) state that the sooner one learns that what is read is determined by the letters that make up the word, the better.

Pictures can be even more distracting for poor readers. Samuels (1967) found that pictures had no deleterious effect on the better readers, but among poorer readers, the presence of pictures interfered with learning a sight vocabulary. Baker and Madell (1965) noted that when distracting stimuli were presented, such as pictures, the performance of underachievers suffered greater disruption than did the performance of more capable students.

Other Cues

Besides pictorial support, semantic information is used to narrow down the choices to guess the meaning of the word. (When he passed the test he felt *terrific*. . . the word terrified makes no sense). Sentence syntax is also useful to determine the form of the word (He is feeling sick. . . The sickly look on his face.). The beginning or ending sound, word length, or a combination of cues is helpful in making correct word guesses. However, as reading becomes more complex, it is more likely that incorrect guessing will increase, given the phonetic irregularity and the visual similarity of words appearing in basal readers (Groff, 1976).

The appropriate selection and utilization of these complex strategies may be impossible for the low performer. Yet, the use of contextual cues as an appropriate reading strategy has been advocated by such authorities as Goodman (1965). Although beginning readers probably do not have adequate reading experience to depend completely on semantic and syntactical cues, these same strategies may indeed be very useful to more advanced readers. Samuels (1970) argued that context cue strategies are actually detrimental in the beginning reading acquisition. Instead, decoding should be emphasized as the most efficient way to attack early word reading. Samuels suggests that Goodman's endorsement of context-cue effectiveness results from studying the reading process of fluent readers, not beginning readers.

Prompting Comprehension

Basal-reading programs advocate the use of pictures in stories because they lead to greater comprehension. The research on the comprehension issue is not so clear as it is on the acquisition issue. Studies (Guttman, Levin, & Pressley, 1977; Miller, 1938) of comprehension through picture inclusion have usually not separated effects according to reading ability. Picture reading may facilitate comprehension for poor readers, who lack decoding skills, but the inclusion of pictures does not improve comprehension for good readers. If the poor readers cannot decode, then logically including pictures will improve their comprehension scores. Samuels (1970) suggests that pictures may indeed improve interest in the reading material, but including them on the same page as the story will result in the least-effort phenomenon—attending to pictures rather than to words. Because of the strong control exerted by interesting and colorful pictures, inducing less sustained attention to words, it is suggested that pictures be shown after the story has been read, to encourage comprehension questions and discussion.

Word Selection

Basal-reading programs select highly occurring words from word lists generated from children's library literature. The actual words selected vary somewhat across programs, but, once chosen, the goal is to present them with sufficient repetition for instant recognition. The term, *basal words,* means those high-frequency words found within a particular basal-reading series. Other words of low frequency are chosen from word lists when they are considered essential for telling specific stories. For instance, the word *zoo,* although frequently found in literature for children, was not considered a high-frequency word by Houghton Mifflin (1971), and is thus not considered a basal word. Houghton Mifflin makes "no serious attempt . . . to provide enough repetition of these [low-frequency words] to insure their becoming a part of each pupil's recognition vocabulary" (*Teacher's Guide,* pp. 21–22), although this may occur.

Teaching New Words and Rate of Introduction

The method of introducing new words is left to the discretion of the teacher. Those preferring to introduce words in advance by listing them are strongly urged by Houghton Mifflin (1976) to do so with the help of context cues. That is, specific sentences containing the new word are provided as samples. However, the series also recommends not listing and giving pretraining of new words prior to story reading. If too much help is offered, independent word-attack strategies are assumed not to develop so rapidly. Indeed, context cues, picture prompts, and beginning and ending grapheme–phoneme identification appear to be the most favored early word recognition strategies employed. The Houghton Mifflin manual suggests that an accelerated introduction of new words will improve reading; and so there is presently a more accelerated rate of new sight words introduced than in earlier basal editions. Analyzing words found in eight popular basal-reading series, Bernard and DeGracie (1976) found the rate of introduction of new words and the vocabulary load to differ significantly between those basal series and, in addition, current basals have 56% more words than those analyzed ten years ago.

Decoding Strategies and the Basal Reader

Since basal readers are the most popular means of reading instruction, the fact that, at a specific series level, only one-third of the words studied by Barnard and DeGracie (1976) were common to two of the eight programs is an alarming finding. In addition, when all words in these series were analyzed, only 47% of the words were common to two or more programs. In the case of low performers, the relative nonoverlap of words strongly suggests that one stay with a specific series or run the risk of increasing the sight word memory load and creating reading failure. Stated differently, the publishers of a particular basal series may introduce and review words consistently, but the concern for a controlled vocabulary across series is not evident. Since children's literature purportedly provides the basal words, there is no stated consideration of the phonetic regularity of the words selected. For example, perusing the preprimer, *Tigers* (Houghton Mifflin, 1971), reveals that, of the first eight *a*-vowel words, only four of them have the short *a* sound (*and, can, cat,* and *have*), which is the most common sound the vowel makes. The other words, *a, are, real,* and *want,* do not contain the most common sound for *a,* and are considered irregular words. Engelmann (1975) examined the 1966 Harper and Row basal series and similarly discovered great phonetic irregularity in the introduction of new words for beginning readers.

Carnine and Silbert (1979) found that, of the first 50 words introduced by three major basal-reader series, the incidence of irregularity was 32 (Scott Foresman), 33 (Ginn), and 28 (Houghton Mifflin). With this high incidence of irregularity, it is understandable why attending to letter–sound regularity is not intensely used for early decoding. Mason (1977) points out that most basals avoid major pattern regularity in vocabulary and opt instead for a reading vocabulary that contains the most frequently occurring words.

What is frequently used in the name of phonics—or, as Flesch (1979) calls it, "phonics window dressing"—is the encouragement of attention to the beginning and/or ending sounds in words. These grapheme–phoneme relationships are almost always consonants and consonant blends which are highly regular and consequently easy to teach.

To select correct words by using consonant sounds and context cues, students are urged to adopt a fill-in-the-blank strategy, which is programmed to be guaranteed correct guessing! According to Houghton Mifflin (1976), "Suppose a pupil knows all of the words. . .except the last one: I went to the zoo with my ______" (p. 19). Context cues would rule out inappropriate words, and "just a few letter–sound associations together with contextual clues will yield a certain identification of an unknown word." Thus, if a reader knows the sound of *m* "he should have no real doubts about the unknown word's being mother." The fact that many appropriate-context *m* words would fit (such as *mom, mama, monkey mittens*) is totally overlooked by Houghton Mifflin (1976). Carnine and Silbert (1979) report that Scott Foresman introduces the new word, *duck,* in part by drawing attention to the *d* and *k* in the word and distinguishing it from the alternative possibility, *bird,* because *d* and *k* are not the beginning and ending sounds in *bird.* That *duck* cannot be *deck, dick,* or *dock* is not even presented for word analysis.

Vowels get less attention than consonants, even though they should probably get more because of the various sounds they make. Accordingly:

> The task of learning a large number of sound associations for vowels in addition to. . . consonants would be a heavy burden. . . they are not essential and. . . would tend to lead pupils to "puzzle out" unknown words as if they were in isolation rather than in meaningful context. (Houghton Mifflin, 1976, p.8)

In trying to further their advocacy of the use of context cues for decoding, they present the following example of two sentences with words that have letters missing. Although it may be "easy" to read some material without knowing all the letter sounds, the missing letter example is not easy even if one *tries* to use context cues! Consider this:

> L--rn-ng t- r--d c-n b- l-ts -f f-n. I- -oe- -o- -a-e -o -e -a-- -o--. (Learning to read can be lots of fun. It does not have to be hard work.) (Houghton Mifflin, 1976, p. 10)

Semantics and Teacher Talk

Purportedly, basal readers develop enthusiastic readers through selecting or writing highly interesting stories. However, if one were to peruse the literary nature of the stories, the amount of presumed knowledge by the low-performing reader is great. Complex semantics, even in third-grade basals, such as "cleaning out the ants. . . dawn crept into the tent. . . tried everything under the sun" (Holt, Rinehart, & Winston Series, 1977), are common. The concepts within the first-grade reader can presume considerable sophistication. "A man named Mr. Groan groans a lot. . . . Someone saw something in the paper. . . . It's spooky out here in the country," are common examples (Laidlaw Reading Program, 1976).

In the very first lesson of *Sundrops* (Economy Company Keytext Series Readiness Books, 1978) is a section intended to develop rhyming skills for individuals having reading difficulties. There are eight words in the *ake* family (*cake, wake,* etc.) which are initially read to the group. The teacher is told to "elicit the response that the words end with the same sound." Then a formal definition of what such words are called becomes the focus of group discussion, presumably in an open-ended manner. If all else fails, the teacher finally volunteers the answer, "They are called rhyming words." Next, without even stopping to offer a single example of a not-*ake* word to determine whether the concept of rhyming was ever learned, or what is meant by "sound," "word," or "end with," another rhyming family is immediately introduced, "Say words that rhyme with *cat*." Following this, pictures of various objects (*hoe, boat, goat, fan, can, fly, car*) are displayed, and the children urged to find the pictures whose names rhyme (*boat–goat* and *fan–can*). Note that there is no assurance that the names of pictures not rhyming with *oat* and *an* (e.g., *hoe, fly*) are familiar to the low performers.

By this time, four diverse word families have been presented, but at no time are any explicitly reviewed. In the same lesson, four more rhyming-word families are then introduced, in the form of short poems. A picture card, "whose name rhymes with a word in the poem and completes the poem," is to be chosen. Consider just one poem: "He stubbed his toe on the garden ______." Even if *hoe* is chosen, its selection could be based merely on contextual rather than on rhyming appropriateness. If an error occurs, the teacher is not prepared to remediate, because the factors causing it are unknown: it could be vocabulary unfamiliarity with the words (*hoe* and *stubbed*), lack of a rhyming strategy, or failure to understand certain directional words (*poem, completes, whose name rhymes with*).

The jumble of activities just cited moves so quickly, and the sheer load of assumed vocabulary knowledge embedded in the teacher talk so great, that it is highly unlikely that a naive learner, much less one with reading difficulties, could learn what rhyming words entail.

The Stanwix Beginning Functional Reading Series (1968) is expressly designed for use with mentally retarded children. It introduces vocabulary words at a very slow pace and emphasizes sight word recognition strategies. Early reading is primarily a discussion of pictures to teach comprehension, matching to sample configuration (word shape) and context—picture cues for decoding purposes. The first reader, *About King*, has seven vocabulary words, all auditorily and visually dissimilar: *King, Bill, and, Mary, run, to, jump*. None of these words begins or ends alike, and three are proper nouns, which guarantees that, wherever they are positioned in a sentence, they will begin with a capital letter, which considerably lessens the occurrence of visual-discrimination difficulties. The first reader has over 60 pages, enabling a good deal of review of the seven words taught.

Ironically, it is this very slowly paced introduction of new words, coupled with the absence of effective word analysis or phonome-grapheme training as well as the great emphasis paid to picture reading, that probably undermines the program's effectiveness with low performers. Of the 81 words in the first four readers, about one-quarter are regular. Here too the irregularities are principly owing to vowels; yet, no attention is given to vowels and their sounds in early reading training. Discriminations of words which may look alike (*house, here*) are taught by purely visual matching tasks. When attention is drawn to sounds in words, they are usually beginning sounds, making the *house-here* distinction when it appears much later in the series a difficult one.

Since most words in Stanwix are not simple to decode through phonetic analysis, it is easy to see why other strategies are employed. However, it is also clear that when the sight word load becomes too great, the reading mastery of students can plummet. Typically, the first two readers (totalling 19 words) are easily mastered within a year. The next two readers often take two years (62 additional words) to complete.

An analysis of the programming of the word, *run*, will reveal the problems mentally retarded children will encounter in this series because there is such minimal attention given to phonics.

1. In the first reader, *About King, run* is initially taught midway through the book, introduced as *Run* and *run*, and the teacher's guide indicates that the teacher should point this out to the children. Indeed, the sound of *r* is also discussed. However, this occurs only once. All the remaining story pages have *run* on them, but rarely are *Run* and *run* together, to review that capital and lower-case letters are functionally the same. Most of the time *Run* is the first word in the sentence (in the 24 of the 30 pages containing *run*, it is so). There is a strong possibility that a slow learner will be learning that all words which begin with *R* say *run*.

2. In the second reader, *About Bill and Mary* (94 pages, 12 new words), there is no other *r* word taught, and, most of the time, *run* is capitalized at the beginning of a sentence. There is a continuing possibility that a slow learner discriminates *Run* more easily than *run*, and the increasing likelihood that words beginning with *r* are to be called *run*, since, out of a total of 156 pages, the only *r* word is *run*.

3. In the third reader, *About Friends* (109 pages, 26 new words) there is no other *R* or *r* word taught; which perpetuates further a possible misconception about *r* words all being *run*.

4. In the fourth reader, *About Fun and Play*, the pupil is introduced to *rope*. This is followed by *ran, ride,* and *rest*. It is in this reader that phenome-grapheme characteristics of *initial letters* is introduced, first through auditory- and then through visual-discrimination training.

Because no effort is made to teach phoneme-grapheme relationships beyond the initial sound, even an average pupil may have difficulty in discriminating among *r* words, especially if they appear in word lists without the familiar picture prompts or sentence context cues. Indeed, *ran* and *run* are so similar, that without actual discrimination training they are probably not easily distinguishable from each other by low performers.

Teachers who use the Stanwix Books are initially very enthusiastic because their students appear to be reading early. However, as the number of sight words increases, more and more failures occur, and the teacher is unable to remediate. A sufficient number of decoding skills (phoneme-grapheme relationships, discrimination training between similar words) have not been taught and, instead, there is reliance on imprecise stimulus cues (picture reading, word shape and length, story context) to create apparent rather than actual reading. The low performers, who primarily learn through sight word strategies, have not learned any generalizable rules to apply with certainty to determine what new words are.

Mason (1978) analyzed the strategies used by educable mentally-retarded teenagers (mean IQ = 63) to identify different classes of words. Concrete words (names for real objects) were better read and remembered than both nonconcrete words (verbs, adjectives, and nonconcrete nouns) and uncommon words, compared to control groups of normal second- and fifth-graders. The EMRs turned unfamiliar words into familiar words (*ship* for *skimp*, *coat* for *coax*), read only a common shorter word embedded in the uncommon word (*ear* for *earl*, *yes* for *yeast*, *bus* for *bush*), made more errors on the end than the beginning of a word (*seem* for *seep*), and frequently misread consonant clusters (*class* for *clash*, *much* for *mush*). Also, they guessed at words and discounted letter-sound relationships, choosing instead short and common word patterns. In contrast, the normal grade school children made more errors on common words because they were applying letter-sound strategies which did not work with irregular vowel sounds. Although the type of prior reading instruction given to the EMR group was not explicitly stated, it was most likely whole-word training, since the nature of their errors is exactly the kind exhibited by subjects not trained in individual sounds or letter clusters.

Even though English is quite regular at the letter cluster level of analysis (Venezky, 1967, Mason's findings indicate that the EMR child may, unfortunately, never notice this regularity. The outcome may be overuse of context cues, guessing, whole-word memorization, and a disregard of letter information. The development of precise and reliable instructional strategies is obviously needed; and, if none are available, reading for the EMR child is bound to become a chance phenomenon.

PHONIC-LINGUISTIC READING PROGRAMS

Overview

Reading programs which emphasize decoding as a first step in the reading process (Merrill Linguistic Readers, SRA Linguistic Readers, Lippincott Readers, DISTAR) organize the introduction of new words around particular linguistic elements. Sound-grapheme relationships are taught and appear in word lists, and these words then appear in stories. Some programs incorporate a sight word vocabulary in order to facilitate story reading (Merrill, Lippincott); others do not (DISTAR). All programs introduce regularly decoded words (sound-symbol relationships which are most predictable) before irregular words. These programs use a synthetic phonics approach to reading; that is, the readers learn the relationship of letters to the sound they make, learn to read in a left-to-right direction, and learn to telescope these sound into words. Linguists claim (McCracken & Walcutt, 1969) that these methods of decoding ensure precision in reading, which is a necessary prerequisite for understanding what is read. If a reader says that a word is *father* instead of *uncle* because a picture was misinterpreted, then word reading has not occurred.

Since basal-reading series account for the most of the reading-instructional material, it is critical that what their interpretation of phonics is be addressed. Spache and Spache (1969) report that Clymer analyzed manuals, wordbooks, and readers of four basal series and calculated over 121 statements about phonic principles. Basal-reader proponents (Durkin, 1970) endorse the use of phonics, but, according to Flesch (1979), essentially they treat phonics as an incidental component to whole-word reading. Typically, a sight word reading vocabulary is first taught and then an analysis of these words is made to deduce the rules which govern their pronounciation (Durkin, 1970). Because this approach is so typically understood to be *the* phonics approach, it is understandable why reading-series and basal-reader advocates are cautious about its use.

The DISTAR model: General Description.

This model is singled out for description because it is one of the few phonics-oriented programs receiving wide use with the mentally retarded. The successful academic results attained by DISTAR with low-performing children in the Follow-Throught Project has been previously mentioned in this chapter's introduction, as has the encouraging progress made by Maggs (see Becker *et al.*, 1979) with the mentally retarded.

The DISTAR model attempts to teach the maximal amount in the shortest time. Pretested scripts specify how to deliver tasks, and thus allow some quality control over teacher instructional behavior which, in turn, permits the discovery of functional relationships between teacher presentation variables, instructional variables, and student performance. The scripts also provide explicit correction procedures to deal immediately with common errors. No incorrect response is left uncorrected. There are mastery tests given periodically to assess performance, and there are associated remedial tasks.

The size of the instructional group varies as a function of level of performance—4 to 6 for EMRs and 7 to 10 for normal and higher performers. Students answer on signal, so that no one student leads the group, and responding is mostly in unison. As many as 200 to 300 group responses can occur in 30 minutes, and, as a result, extensive practice is provided, and teacher pacing is brisk and rapid. New or difficult material is taught more slowly, with sufficient thinking time given when needed.

Teaching new discriminations is done by a three-step procedure—the teacher models what is to be done, then leads the group through the task, and finally tests the group and/or individual learner. With more complex material where a learning strategy was taught, the teacher prompts the learner to apply the strategy. The higher performers sit at the ends of a semi-circle, and the lower performers in or near the middle, receiving as much as three times the number of opportunities to respond individually as the high performers.

Major Characteristics of DISTAR Reading

Early reading instruction emphasizes correct decoding of regular words through the teaching of requisite skills and their integration (Carnine & Silbert, 1979). A critical strategy is to have learners "sound out" words. Starting at the beginning of the word, the most common sound represented by the first letter is said, then advancing in a left-right progression, the sounds for successive letters are blended without stopping between sounds. The word *man* is sounded out as "mmmmaaaannnn," after which it is immediately said at its normal spoken rate, "man"!

Reading is not begun with the sounding-out-of-words strategy, however. The prior subskills are:

1. *Sound identification.* The letter-sound correspondences for the first few words to be decoded are taught.
2. *Telescoping* (or, "Say it fast"). The teacher says the sounds in a word slowly, "mmmmaaaannnn," and the student creates the word by saying it fast, "man"!
3. *Segmenting of words into component sounds* (or, "Say the sounds"). The teacher says, "man," at a normal rate and the student says the sounds in the word slowly, "mmmmaaaannnn"!
4. *Directionality.* Moving from left to right across the page is done by imitation games and by following arrow prompts.

Telescoping and segmenting are auditory skills in that printed letters or words are not presented. The students respond to orally presented examples.

Once a student can sound out regular words, then phrase reading, sentence reading, and finally passage reading are introduced. By this time, the students are able to read whole words at sight, without the deliberate use of the oral-blending or sounding-out strategy. Concurrently, high-frequency phonetically irregular words (*is, was, said*) are introduced. The introduction of these irregular words is carefully controlled, so that students do not become confused regarding when a sounding-out strategy will and when it will not work.

This method of teaching reading is assumed to result in students becoming fluent, capable readers. Comprehension is taught concurrently with phrase, sentence, and passage reading. Comprehension moves from literal responding and recall of facts to literary and interpretive responding. As the process of decoding becomes more automatic, the sophistication of the stories read increases, and the nature of the comprehension expected shifts from simple to more elaborate forms of responding.

Also the following instructional suggestions distinguish DISTAR from meaning-emphasis programs:

1. Letter sounds are taught before letter names. Although knowledge of letter names is necessary for later spelling and dictionary tasks, it is not needed for sounding out words in beginning reading instruction. Since early emphasis should be directed toward decoding, letter sounds should be taught first.
2. Decoding of words are taught through sounding out rather than by sight. Whole-word sight reading increases the likelihood of error in early reading. For example, *truck* and *trunk* are so similar that, without attending to the sounds within each word, a naive reader

may not differentiate them. The sounding-out operation is a general case strategy, such that by training the operation with several words, the decoding of new words is possible. Conversely, the whole-word sight learning is not likely to have these same generalizable features. When presented with new words, the whole-word sight reader must memorize each word or guess at new words using various extra-stimulus prompts.

3. New words are taught in isolation during the beginning reading stage; later, words can be introduced in context. By presenting the word in isolation initially, DISTAR prevents errors in later context reading. This practice also focuses the beginning reader on the letters in the word, rather than allowing context or other cues to dominate the beginning reader's attention.
4. Reading is taught for accuracy initially, rather than fluency. As the sounding-out strategy becomes more automatic and words are recognized by sight, fluency can be improved.

Issues and Research in Phonic Programs

Several significant research reviews indicate that code emphasis programs are more effective than meaning emphasis programs in teaching reading. Chall (1967) analyzed 25 acceptable studies and reported that programs emphasizing decoding tended to surpass meaning-emphasis programs in the areas of word recognition, oral reading, and spelling. Phonics-based programs were generally more effective for both below- and above-average-ability children. Gurren and Hughes (1965) reviewed 22 comparative studies on slow learners and found significant differences favoring the code-emphasis programs in comprehension as well as in decoding. More recent research reviews (Diederich, 1973) are consistent with earlier comparisons.

Despite the overwhelming evidence in favor of a code-emphasis approach, many still doubt its effectiveness with the low performer. Spache and Spache (1969) encourage the teaching of phonic rules in an orderly fashion and teaching only those rules which apply to the greatest number of words, but they warn:

> Our outline is quite feasible for average and bright children, while slow learners and those lacking in auditory skills or in aptitude for using phonics will need delayed or prolonged presentation of skills. We do not assume that all children will profit from this training. . .and phonics training will be approached cautiously, if at all, with these pupils, (pp. 395, 396)

Even if the application of phonic-based programs is able to impart effective decoding strategies, there is still the additional problem of teaching word meaning or vocabulary development. DISTAR-trained low-performing children learn to decode words extremely well. Becker (1977) reported their performance on this skill reached the 70th percentile, as assessed by the Wide Range Achievement Test. Their performance on third grade reading comprehension, however, reached the 40th percentile, which although significantly higher than other educational models, is still not within normative levels. And, there are indications that reading comprehension scores will drop even lower as the children move on to higher grades unless they are given explicit training in vocabulary meaning. Becker (1977) points out that, in the first two or three grades, textbook writers tend to use the same vocabulary words but that, by about the fourth grade and thereafter, the vocabulary load swells and becomes highly variable as different content areas and literary styles are stressed. Currently, schools are not systematically teaching the language concepts that are necessary for disadvantaged performers to compete with advantaged children who may otherwise receive language training at home. Becker (1977) estimates that about 25 new basic words will need to be taught each week if students with vocabulary deficiencies are to attain the full adult vocabulary and to master material presented by upper-grade and high-school textbook writers.

The fact that an excellent technology now exists to produce accurate decoding skills is significant, since it allows for more attention to be paid to the more difficult tasks of vocabulary building and comprehension, or language understanding. For low-performing populations especially, the emphasis on selection of efficient programs is critical if they are to ever have the chance to "make significant gains."

Concluding Remarks

Changes in academic training for the mentally retarded in the 1980s will probably be more marked than in the previous decade. Training programs for the mentally retarded now in the community, or for those presently being deinstitutionalized, will need to consider the application of instructional training to real-life settings. There is presently an emphasis on teaching functional survival skills, such as money usage, shopping skills, traffic and pedestrian concepts, time-telling, telephone usage, and following printed material in menus and recipes. Teaching strategies that attempt to impart general knowledge merely on the basis of single purpose, rote-learning procedures, when more effective general-case, instructional strategies are available, should become the object of focus by behavior analysts and educational programmers. For instance, though it is possible to teach, by sight word training, a number of key functional words (*poison, exit, flammable, danger*), it is shortsighted and unrealistic to think that the natural environment will always feature these words invariably in their trained form. Instead, words, in modified form or changed altogether, are just as likely to occur. What is the mentally retarded person, who is unable to decode and read words, to do when confronted with, *nonpoisonous, not an entrance, nonflammable, not dangerous,* or, *watch out—man hole!* Teaching one to work the problem, 24 + 6, by drawing 24 lines, then six more lines, when a more effective strategy of learning how to count from a number to a higher (or lower) number produces fewer mistakes and is applicable to a greater number of similar problems, is another case in point.

The future of educational programming for the mentally retarded should no longer be based on training single-purpose, dead-end skills but must, instead, consider the development of instructional strategies based on logical and long-term programming objectives that consider the integration of related tasks. Behavior analysts, sophisticated and confident in designing reinforcement systems, must become more knowledgeable about instructional programming. They should begin to question certain commonly-held conceptions about the nature of prerequisite skills for more complex learning. Is learning the alphabet necessary for reading? Is learning to discriminate a square and triangle critical for teaching how to discriminate numerals and other symbols?

With the implementation of PL 94-142, greater concern in the 1980s for mentally retarded children will be manifested in two ways. Fewer of these children will be identified as mentally retarded, since the definition of this condition in educational circles is no longer only intellectual deficiency but includes deficiency in adaptive behavior. Because the American Association for Mental Deficiency has revised its criteria by stating that mental retardation exists if IQ scores are two or more standard deviations below the mean, the regular classroom can be expected to serve more youngsters who were formally labeled educably retarded and placed in special-education classes. Additionally, the concept of least restrictive environment from PL 94-142 (or "mainstreaming") will result in increased numbers of mentally retarded individuals being placed in regular classes. Special education and regular classrooms for the mentally retarded will thus house more seriously academically handicapped children than in the past, which raises more emphatically the need for appropriate instructional programs and methodology.

REFERENCES

ABT ASSOCIATES. *Education as experimentation: A planned variation model* (Vol. 3). Cambridge, Mass.: ABT Associates, 1976.

ABT ASSOCIATES. *Education as experimentation: A planned variation model* (Vol. 4). Cambridge, Mass.: ABT Associates, 1976.

BAKER, R., & MADELL, T. A continued investigation of susceptibility to distraction in academically underachieving and achieving male college students. *Journal of Educational Psychology*, 1965, *56*, 254–258.

BARNARD, D. P., & DEGRACIE, J. Vocabulary analysis of new primary reading series. *The Reading Teacher*, 1976, *30*(2), 177–180.

BECKER, W. C. Teaching reading and language to the disadvantaged: What we have learned from field research. *Harvard Education Review*, 1977, *47*, 518–543.

BECKER, W., & CARNINE, D. *Direct instruction: A behavior theory model for comprehensive educational intervention with the disadvantaged.* Paper presented at the VIII Symposium on Behavior Modification, Caracas, Venezuela, February 1978.

BECKER, W., & CARNINE, D. W. Direct instruction: An effective approach to educational intervention with the disadvantaged and low performers. In B. B. Lahey & A. E. Kazdin (Eds.) *Advances in CLinical Child Psychology* (Vol. 3). New York: Plenum Press, 1980.

BECKER, W., ENGELMANN, S., & THOMAS, D. *Teaching II: Cognitive learning and instruction.* Chicago: Science Research Associates, 1975.

BECKER, W., ENGELMANN, S., CARNINE, D., & MAGGS, A. Direct instruction technology—Making learning happen. In P. Karolz & J. Steffen (Eds.), *Advances in child behavior and therapy* (Vol. 2). New York: Garden Press, 1979.

BEREITER, C., & ENGELMANN, S. *Teaching disadvantaged children in the preschool.* Englewood Cliffs, N.J.: Prentice-Hall, 1966.

BEREITER, C., & ENGELMANN, S. *Language learning activities.* New York: Anti-Defamation League, 1968.

BLODGETT, H., & WARFIELD, G. *Understanding MR children.* New York: Appleton-Century-Crofts, 1959.

BLOOM, B. S. *Human characteristics and school learning.* New York: McGraw-Hill, 1976.

BRACEY, S., MAGGS, A., & MORATH, P. The effects of a direct phonic approach in teaching reading with six moderately retarded children: Acquisition and mastery learning stages. *The Slow Learning Child*, 1975, *22*, 83–90. (a)

BRACEY, S., MAGGS, A., & MORATH, P. Teaching arithmetic skills to moderately mentally retarded children using direct verbal instruction: Counting and symbol identification. *Australian Journal of Mental Retardation*, 1975, *3*, 200–204. (b)

BREWER, W. F. Is reading a letter-by-letter process? A discussion of Gaugh's paper. In H. Singer & R. Ruddell (Eds.), *Theoretical models and processes of reading.* Newark, Del.: International Reading Association, 1976.

BRUNER, J. S., GOODNOW, J. J., & AUSTIN, G. A. *A study of thinking.* New York: Krieger, 1967.

CARNINE, D. W. *Relative difficulty of three vowels and three consonants.* Unpublished manuscript, University of Oregon, 1975.

CARNINE, D. W. Establishing a discriminative stimulus by distributing attributes of compound stimuli between instances and non-instances. In W. C. Becker & S. E. Engelmann, (Eds.), *Formative research on direct instruction.* Eugene: University of Oregon, Project Follow Through, 1976. (a)

CARNINE, D. W. Effects of two teacher presentation rates on off-task behavior, answering correctly, and participation. *Journal of Applied Behavior Analysis*, 1976, *9*, 199–206. (b)

CARNINE, D. W. Similar sound separation and cumulative introduction in learning letter sound correspondences. *Journal of Educational Research*, 1976, *69*, 368–372. (c)

CARNINE, D. W. The effects of progressive increases in the number and/or magnitude of differences between positive and negative concept instances. In D. W. Carnine (Ed.), *Formative research studies on direct instruction*. Eugene: University of Oregon, Follow Through Project, 1978. (a)

CARNINE, D. W. Two procedures for sequencing instances in discrimination learning tasks: Simultaneously presenting minimally different instance pairs and changing a single stimulus to generate successive instances. In D. W. Carnine (Ed.), *Formative research studies on direct instruction*. Eugene: University of Oregon, Follow Through Project, 1978. (b)

CARNINE, D. W. Three procedures for presenting minimally different positive and negative instances. In D. W. Carnine (Ed.), *Formative research studies on direct instruction*. Eugene: University of Oregon, Follow Through Project, 1978. (c)

CARNINE, D. W. *Research on designing and implementing procedures for teaching sounds*. Unpublished manuscript, University of Oregon, 1980.

CARNINE, D. W., & SILBERT, J. *Direct instruction reading*. Columbus, Ohio: Charles E. Merrill, 1979.

CARNINE, L., & CARNINE, D. W. Determining the relative decoding difficulty of three types of simple regular words. *Journal of Reading Behavior*, 1978, *10*, 40–41.

CHALL, J. *Learning to read, the great debate*. New York, McGraw-Hill, 1967.

CHARLESWORTH, W. R. Instigation and maintenance of curiosity behavior as a function of surprise versus novel and familiar stimuli. *Child Development*, 1964, *35*, 1169–1186.

CLARK, C. Teaching concepts in the classroom: A set of teaching prescriptions derived from experimental research. *Journal of Educational Psychology Monograph*, 1971, *62*, 253–267.

COREY, J., & SHAMOW, J. The effects of fading on the acquisition and retention of oral reading. *Journal of Applied Behavior Analysis*, 1972, *5*, 311–315.

CRONBACH, L., & SNOW, R. *Aptitudes and instructional methods: A handbook for research on interactions*. New York: Irvington, 1977.

DIEDERICH, P. B. *Research 1960–70 on methods and materials in reading*. Princeton, N. J.: Educational Testing Service, January 1973. (TM Report 22, EPIC Clearinghouse on Tests, Measurement and Evaluation.)

DIXON, L., SPRADLIN, J., GIRARDEAU, F., & ETZEL, B. Facilitation of acquisition of an "in front" spatial discrimination. *Acta Symbolica*, 1974, *5*, 1–22.

DORAN, J., & HOLLAND, J. Control by stimulus features during fading. *Journal of the Experimental Analysis of Behavior*, 1979, *31*, 177–187.

DORRY, G., & ZEAMAN, D. The use of a fading technique in paired-associate teaching of a reading vocabulary with retardates. *Mental Retardation*, 1973, *11*, 3–6.

DUELL, O. K. An analysis of prompting procedures for teaching a sight vocabulary. *American Educational Research Journal*, 1968, *5*, 675–686.

DURKIN, D. *Teaching them to read*. Boston: Allyn & Bacon, 1970.

Economy Company keytext series readiness books. Oklahoma City, Okla.: The Economy Co., 1978.

Edmark reading program. Bellevue, Wash.: Edmark Associates, 1972.

ENGELMANN, S. *Conceptual learning*. San Rafael, Cal.: Dimensions Publishing, 1969. (a)

ENGELMANN, S. *Preventing failure in the primary grades*. Chicago: Science Research Associates, 1969. (b)

ENGELMANN, S. *Your child can succeed*. New York: Simon & Schuster, 1975.

ENGELMANN, S., & BRUNER, E. *DISTAR reading level 1*. Chicago: Science Research Associates, 1974.

ENGELMANN, S., & CARNINE, D. W. *Instructional design*. Unpublished manuscript, University of Oregon, 1980.

FERSTER, C., & HAMMER, C. Synthesizing the components of arithmetic behavior. In W. K. Honig (Ed.), *Operant behavior*. New York: Appleton-Century-Crofts, 1966.

FINK, W., & BRICE-GRAY, K. The effects of two teaching strategies on the acquisition and recall of an academic task by moderately and severely retarded preschool children. *Mental Retardation*, 1979, *17*, 8–12.

FLESCH, R. Why Johnny can't read. *Family Circle*, November, 1979, pp. 26, 43–45.

GATES, A., JERSILD, A., MCCONNELL, T., & CHALLMAN, R. *Educational psychology*. New York: Macmillan, 1950.

GELMAN, R. Conservation acquisition: A problem of learning to attend to relevant attributes. *Journal of Experimental Child Psychology*, 1969, *7*, 167–187.

GIBSON, E., & LEVIN, H. *The psychology of reading*. Cambridge: M.I.T. Press, 1975.

GOODMAN, K. S. A linguistic study of cues and miscues in reading. *Elementary English*, 1965, *42*, 639–643.

GRANZIN, A., & CARNINE, D. W. Child performance on discrimination tasks: Effects of amount of stimulus variation. *Journal of Experimental Child Psychology*, 1977, *24*, 332–342.

GROFF, P. Limitations of context cues for beginning readers. *Reading World*, 1976, *16*(2), 97–103.

GUESS, D., SAILOR, W., & BAER, D. M. *Functional speech and language training for the severely handicapped. Part I: Persons and things*. Lawrence, Kansas: H & H Enterprises, 1976.

GURREN, L., & HUGHES, A. Intensive phonics vs. gradual phonics in beginning reading: A review. *The Journal of Educational Research*, 1965, *58*, 339–347.

GUTTMAN, J., LEVIN, J., & PRESSLEY, M. Pictures, partial pictures, and young children's oral prose learning. *Journal of Educational Psychology*, 1977, *69*, 473–480.

HALL, R., PANYAN, M., RABON, D., & BRODEN, M. Instructing beginning teachers in reinforcement procedures which improve classroom control. *Journal of Applied Behavior Analysis*, 1968, *1*, 315–322.

HARLOW, H. F. Learning set and error factor theory. In S. Koch (Ed.), *Psychology: A study of a science* (Vol. 2). New York, McGraw-Hill, 1959.

HARZEM, P., LEE, I., & MILES, T. The effect of pictures on learning to read. *The British Journal of Educational Psychology*, 1976, *46*, 318–322.

HESS, R., & SHIPMAN, V. Early experiences and the socialization of cognitive modes in children. *Child Development*, 1965, *36*, 869–886.

HILGARD, E., & BOWER, G. *Theories of learning*. New York: Appleton-Century-Crofts, 1966.

HOLLAND, J. G. Human vigilance. *Science*, 1958, *128*, 61–67.

Holt, Rinehart, & Winston reading series. New York: Holt, Rinehart, & Winston, 1977.

HONIG, W. K. *Operant behavior: Areas of research and application*. New York: Appleton-Century-Crofts, 1966.

Houghton Mifflin reading series. Boston: Houghton Mifflin, 1971.

Houghton Mifflin reading series. Boston: Houghton Mifflin, 1976.

INGRAM, C. *Education of the slow learning child*. New York: World, 1953.

KELLER, F. S. Studies in International Morse Code: I. A new method of teaching code reception. *Journal of Applied Psychology*, 1943, *27*, 407–415.

KINCAID, M., & WEISBERG, P. Alphabet letters as tokens: Training preschool children in letter recognition and labeling during a token exchange period. *Journal of Applied Behavior Analysis*, 1978, *11*, 199.

KINCAID, M., WEISBERG, P., & SIMS, E. *Using tokens as instructional stimuli to teach skills to children during a token exchange period*. Unpublished manuscript, University of Alabama, 1980.

Kling, J. W., & Riggs, L. A. *Experimental psychology*. New York, Holt, Rinehart, & Winston, 1971.

Laidlaw reading program. Summit, N. J.: Laidlaw Brothers, 1976.

Latham, L. L. *Construct validity of short-term memory measures in retarded subjects*. Unpublished doctoral dissertation, University of Alabama, 1977.

Maggs, A., & Morath, P. Improving problem solving skills in 130 moderately and severely mentally retarded school aged children. *Rehabilitation in Australia*, 1975, *12*, 22–24.

Maggs, A., & Morath, P. The effects of direct verbal instruction on intellectual development of institutionalized moderately retarded children: A 2-year study. *Journal of Special Education*, 1976, *10*, 357–364.

Markle, S. M., & Tiemann, P. W. Some principles of instructional design at higher cognitive levels. In R. Ulrich, T. Stachnik, & J. Malory (Eds.), *Control of human behavior* (Vol. 3). Glenview, Ill.: Scott, Foresman, 1974.

Mason, J. Refining phonics for teaching beginning reading. *The Reading Teacher*, 1977, *31*, 179–184.

Mason, J. M. Role of strategy in reading by mentally retarded persons. *American Journal of Mental Deficiency*, 1978, *82*(5), 467–473.

McCracken, G., & Walcutt, C. C. *Lippincott's basic reading* (teacher's ed.). Philadelphia: Lippincott, 1969.

Merrill, M. D., & Tennyson, R. D. *Teaching concepts: An instructional design guide*. Englewood Cliffs, N. J.: Educational Technology Publications, 1977.

Miller, W. Reading with and without pictures. *Elementary School Journal*, 1938, *38*, 676–682.

Morphett, M., & Washburne, C. When should children begin to read?. *Elementary School Journal*, 1931, *31*, 496–503.

Palmer, F. H. *Concept training curriculum: For children ages two to five* (5 vols.). Unpublished manuscript, State University of New York at Stony Brook, 1971.

Perry, N. *Teaching the mentally retarded child*. New York: Columbia University Press, 1960.

Reese, H. W., & Lipsitt, L. P. *Experimental child psychology*. New York: Academic Press, 1970.

Reynolds, G. S. Attention in the pigeon. *Journal of Experimental Analysis of Behavior*, 1961, *2*, 203–208.

Rosenshine, B. Classroom instruction. In N. L. Gage (Ed.), *The psychology of teaching methods*, Seventy-fifth yearbook of the National Society for the Study of Education. Chicago: University of Chicago Press, 1976.

Samuels, J. S. Attentional process in reading: The effect of pictures on the acquisition of reading responses. *Journal of Educational Psychology*, 1967, *58*, 337–342.

Samuels, J. S. Effects of pictures on learning to read, comprehension and attitudes. *Review of Educational Research*, 1970, *40*, 397–407.

Schier, A. *Behavior of non-human primates* (Vol. 1). New York: Academic Press, 1965.

Schilmoeller, G., Schilmoeller, K., Etzel, B., & LeBlanc, J. Conditional discrimination after errorless and trial-and-error training. *Journal of the Experimental Analysis of Behavior*, 1979, *31*, 405–420.

Schreibman, L. Effects of within-stimulus and extra-stimulus prompting on discrimination learning in autistic children. *Journal of Applied Behavior Analysis*, 1975, *8*, 91–112.

Sidman, M., & Stoddard, L. The effectiveness of fading in programming a simultaneous form discrimination for retarded children. *Journal of the Experimental Analysis of Behavior*, 1967, *10*, 3–15.

Sidman, M., Cresson, O., & Willson-Morris, M. Acquisition of matching to sample via mediated transfer. *Journal of the Experimental Analysis of Behavior*, 1974, *22*, 261–273.

Singer, H., Samuels, J., & Spiroff, J. Effects of pictures and context in learning sight words. Reading Research Quarterly, 1973–74, *9*, 555–567.

SKINNER, B. F. *Beyond freedom and dignity.* New York: Knopf, 1971.

SOKOLOV, E. N. Higher nervous functioning: The orienting reflex. *Annual Review of Physiology,* 1963, *25,* 545–580.

SPACHE, G. D., & SPACHE, E. B. *Reading in the elementary school.* Boston: Allyn & Bacon, 1969.

SPENCE, J. T. The distracting effects of material reinforcers in the discrimination learning of lower- and middle-class children. *Child Development,* 1970, *41,* 103–111.

SPENCE, K. W. *Behavior theory and conditioning.* New Haven: Yale University Press, 1956.

SPIVACK, G., & SHURE, M. B. *Social adjustment of young children.* San Francisco: Jossey-Bass, 1974.

STAATS, A., BREWER, B., & GROSS, M. Learning and cognitive development: Representative samples, cumulative-hierarchial learning, and experimental-longitudinal methods. *Monographs of the Society for Research in Child Development,* 1970, *35,* 8 (Whole No. 141).

Stanwix beginning functional reading series. Pittsburgh: Stanwix House, 1968.

TABER, J., & GLASER, R. An exploratory evaluation of a discriminative transfer learning program using literal prompts. *The Journal of Educational Research,* 1962, *55,* 508–512.

TENNYSON, R. D. Effect of negative instances in concept acquisition using a verbal learning task. JOURNAL OF EDUCATIONAL PSYCHOLOGY, 1973, *64,* 247–260.

TENNYSON, R. D., & MERRILL, M. D. *Teaching concepts: An instructional design guide.* Englewood Cliffs, N. J.: Educational Technology Publications, 1977.

TENNYSON, R. D., WOOLLEY, F., & MERRILL, D. Examplar and nonexemplar variables which produce correct concept classification behavior and specified classification errors. *Journal of Educational Psychology,* 1972, *63,* 144–152.

TERMAN, S., & WALCUTT, C. C. *Reading: Chaos and cure.* New York: McGraw-Hill, 1958.

TERRACE, H. S. Errorless transfer of a discrimination across two continua. *Journal of Experimental Analysis of Behavior,* 1963, *6,* 223–232. (a)

TERRACE, H. S. Discrimination learning with and without errors. *Journal of Experimental Analysis of Behavior,* 1963, *6,* 1–27. (b)

TERRY, P., SAMUELS, S. J., & LA BERGE, D. The effects of letter degradation and letter spacing on word recognition. *Journal of Verbal Learning and Verbal Behavior,* 1976, *15,* 577–586.

TOUCHETTE, P. E. The effects of graduated stimulus change on the acquisition of a simple discrimination in severely retarded boys. *Journal of Experimental Analysis of Behavior,* 1968, *11,* 39–48.

TRABASSCO, T., & BOWER, G. H. *Attention in learning: Theory and research.* New York: Wiley, 1968.

VENEZKY, R. L. English orthography: Its graphical structure and its relation to sound. *Reading Research Quarterly,* 1967, *2,* 75–106.

WALLIN, W. *The education of handicapped children.* Boston: Houghton Mifflin, 1924.

WALSH, B. F. & LAMBERTS, F. Errorless discrimination and picture facing as techniques for teaching sight words to TMR students. *American Journal of Mental Deficiency,* 1979, *83,* 473–479.

WATSON J. Conservation: An S–R analysis. In I. Siegel & F. Hooper (Eds.), *Logical thinking in children,* New York: Holt, Rinehart, & Winston, 1968.

WEISBERG, P. *Teaching the prepositional concept of between by continuous conversion, fading, and trial and error procedures to preschool children.* Unpublished manuscript, University of Alabama, 1980. (a)

WEISBERG, P. *Adult judgments of differences between positive and negative instances for comparative concepts taught by continuous and noncontinuous conversions.* Unpublished manuscript, University of Alabama, 1980. (b)

WEISBERG, P. *Analysis of instructional strategies used by teachers to design programs to teach basic concepts.* Unpublished manuscript, University of Alabama, 1980. (c).

WILHELM, H., & LOVAAS, O. Stimulus overselectivity: A common feature in autism and mental retardation. *American Journal of Mental Deficiency*, 1976, *81*, 227–241.

WILLIAMS, T. Reading instruction today. *American Psychologist*, 1979, *34*, 917–922.

ZEAMAN, D., & HOUSE, B. The role of attention in retardate discrimination learning. In N. R. Ellis (Ed.), *Handbook of mental deficiency*. New York: McGraw-Hill, 1963.

Index

www.ingramcontent.com/pod-product-compliance
Ingram Content Group UK Ltd.
Pitfield, Milton Keynes, MK11 3LW, UK
UKHW051451290926
15471UKWH00008B/1140
9781461571315